THE NEW ILLUSTRATED

MEDICAL ENCYCLOPEDIA

FOR HOME USE

VOLUME 4

Edited b

WITH ILLUSTRATIONS BY SYLVIA AND LESTER V. BERGMAN

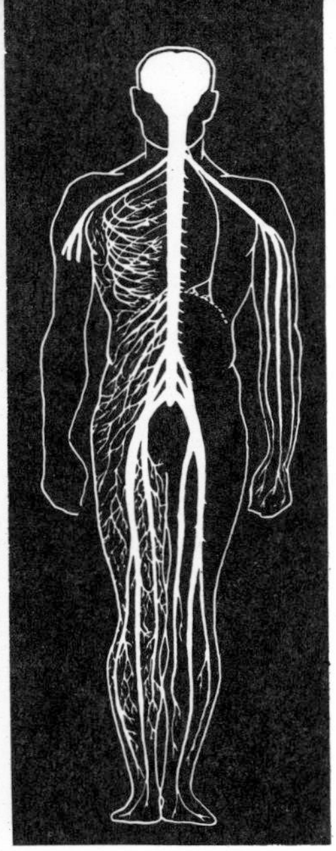

The NEW Illustrated MEDICAL ENCYCLOPEDIA *FOR HOME USE*

A PRACTICAL GUIDE TO GOOD HEALTH

COMPILED AND PREPARED BY MEDBOOK PUBLICATIONS, INC.

ROBERT E. ROTHENBERG, M.D., F.A.C.S.

ABRADALE PRESS *Publishers / New York*

NOTE TO THE READER

The reader is advised that for disorders requiring individual examination and treatment, a doctor must be consulted, for no prescription or course of treatment is intended to be recommended in these volumes.

ENLARGED AND REVISED EDITION

Library of Congress Catalog Card Number: 67-14553
Standard Book Number: 8109-0284-2

DESIGNED BY HOWARD MORRIS
PRINTED IN THE UNITED STATES OF AMERICA

Table of Contents

This Table of Contents lists all topics in this particular volume only. For a complete Table of Contents listing all topics in the entire four volumes of this *New Illustrated Medical Encyclopedia,* see Volume One. A special section of Definitions of Common Medical Terms will be found at the end of this volume.

THE NEW ILLUSTRATED

MEDICAL ENCYCLOPEDIA

FOR HOME USE

CHAPTER 55

Preoperative and Postoperative Routines

(See also Chapter 8 on Anesthesia; Chapter 25 on First Aid)

PREOPERATIVE MEASURES

Can the patient, by proper preoperative preparation, improve his chances for a smooth operative and postoperative course?

Yes. There are many things a patient can do to make the surgeon's task easier and his own discomfort less.

What can the patient do to help himself before entering the hospital?

a. Smoking. It is much better for the patient to smoke as little as possible for a few days before he is to be operated upon. This will lead to a smoother anesthesia, with less chance for postoperative complications such as coughing, inflammation of the trachea, lung congestion, etc.
b. Alcohol. It is wise not to drink heavily for a few days before contemplated surgery. Excessive drinking may have harmful effects upon the liver, and it is important that liver function not be impaired when major surgery is being performed.
c. Sleep. Patients should have at least eight hours' sleep for a few nights before major surgery. A rested body will respond better to the trauma of surgery.
d. If there are loose teeth, they should be pulled prior to hospital admission, and if the planned operation is an elective one, infected gums should be treated and decayed teeth should be taken care of.

What are some of the routine procedures which will be carried out in the hospital?

a. Bowel function. As the bowels may not move for several days after an operation, an enema is given the night before most surgical procedures. This is not carried out where there is an acute inflammation within the intestinal tract or abdomen.

b. Food intake. It is always best to operate upon a patient whose stomach is empty. Fasting for ten to twelve hours before surgery is a routine procedure.

c. Sedatives. In order to insure a good night's rest before surgery, adequate doses of sleeping pills are usually prescribed.

d. Narcotics. In order to have the patient in a calm semiconscious state, an injection of demerol, morphine, or a similar drug is given one or two hours before the patient goes to the operating room.

e. Preparation of the wound area. It is customary to shave a very wide area around an operative site. This is done in order to insure surgical sterility. Thus, the entire abdomen is shaved for an abdominal operation and an entire limb may be shaved for surgery upon an arm or leg.

f. Teeth. Before the patient goes to the operating room, all false teeth or dentures are removed, so that they are not dislodged during the giving of anesthesia. It is always wise to inform the anesthetist if you have a loose tooth in your mouth, so that this may be attended to before the operation.

g. Intravenous injections. If a patient is dehydrated or if he is in need of special medications, such as vitamins, proteins, sugars, or antibiotic drugs, these may be given prior to surgery.

h. Blood transfusions. Surgeons find that their patients react much better to major operative procedures when there is no anemia. Therefore, people who have lost marked amounts of blood, or who are exceptionally anemic, may be given blood by transfusion before surgery.

i. Stomach tubes. For certain kinds of abdominal operations, particularly those upon the gastro-intestinal tract, it is advisable to have the stomach completely empty. A rubber tube is therefore inserted through the nose into the stomach and attached to a suction apparatus. This may be done the night before surgery or early the morning of surgery. These tubes are often left in place throughout the operative procedure and for a few days thereafter.

j. Catheterization. Patients will be much more comfortable postoperatively if their bladder is empty. In order to insure this, a rubber tube (catheter) is sometimes inserted into the bladder before the patient goes to the operating room; the tube may be left in place during the operative procedure and for some time thereafter.

k. Wearing apparel. No matter how minor the operative procedure and no matter how limited the area to be subjected to surgery, it is general practice to remove all clothing before a patient goes to the operating room. He will then be dressed in a cap and a short gown, and will have something to cover his legs. This is done because the patient's clothes are not surgically clean and therefore should not be worn in an operating room.

POSTOPERATIVE MEASURES

What are the usual measures carried out immediately after an operation?

a. Recovery rooms. More and more hospitals have installed recovery rooms staffed by personnel specially trained in the care of the postoperative patient. In such rooms are all the various types of apparatus necessary to combat any possible postoperative complication. It is customary for patients not to return directly to the preoperative room but to remain in the recovery room anywhere from a few hours to as long as a few days.

b. Position in bed. Patients are usually placed flat in bed, on returning from the operating room. It is customary for children to be placed lying face-down on their abdomen and for adults to lie flat on their back. If the patient's blood pressure has dropped as a result of the surgery, it is sometimes customary to raise the foot of the bed above the level of the patient's head. This allows more blood to flow to the head and will help to raise blood pressure. In operations upon the neck or chest, the patient is often placed in a semi-sitting position immediately after operation.

Surgeon Scrubbing Prior to Donning Operating Gown and Gloves. Despite the fact that surgeons wear sterile rubber gloves, they scrub their hands thoroughly with antiseptic soaps or detergents before operating. This is done as a safeguard, so that if a glove should accidentally be pricked or ripped during surgery, bacteria will not contaminate the operative wound.

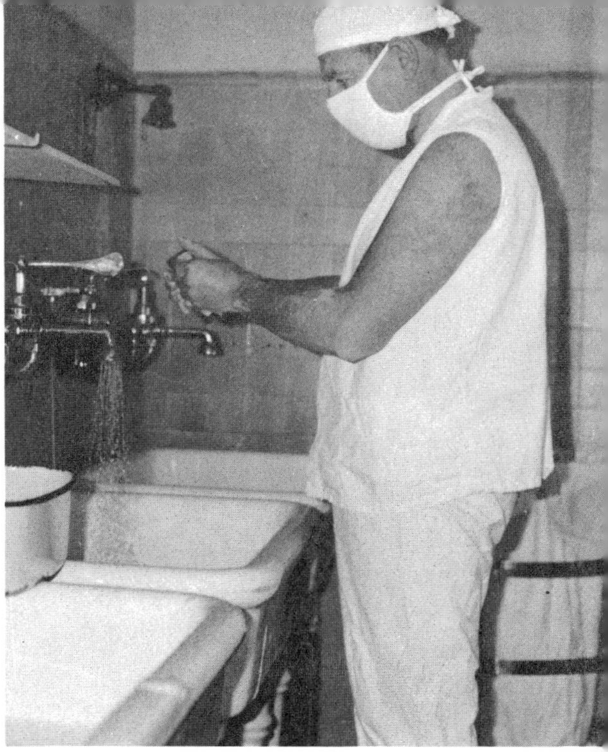

Below: Operating Room Scene. Each doctor and nurse in an operating team has a specific job to perform. No one can be operated upon by one person alone—it requires a team of six or seven to carry out all the duties which attend even the most routine surgical procedure.

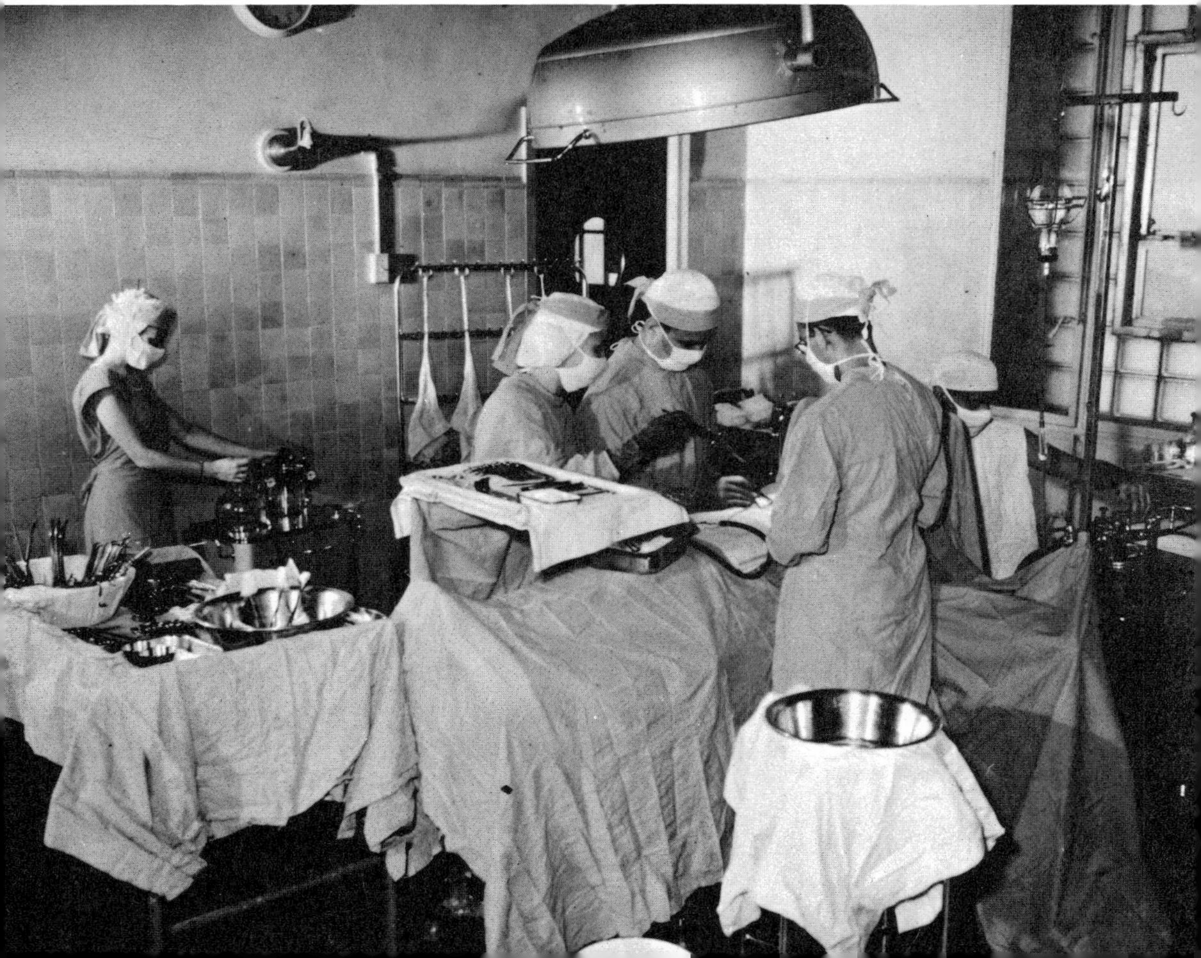

After full reaction and recovery from the anesthesia, the patient is urged to change his position frequently and to move his limbs about in bed. This stimulates circulation, thus reducing any tendency toward the development of blood clots in the veins of the extremities.

c. Airways. The anesthetist will often place in the mouth of the patient an airway which extends into the back of the throat. The airway will prevent the patient from swallowing his tongue or developing an obstruction to the free passage of air from the outside into his lungs. It will stay in place until he regains consciousness. As soon as he awakens, the patient will cough up the airway or remove it himself. Airways are small black plastic tubes shaped to conform to the curvature of the mouth and pharynx.

d. Ambulation. Modern surgery advocates that the patient get out of bed as soon as he possibly can after surgery. This practice, called early ambulation, has been found to minimize lung complications and circulatory disturbances. Many patients can get out of bed the day after major surgery; others can be gotten up and walking within two to three days after surgery. There are, however, a small number of patients who must remain in bed for a week or longer after an operation.

e. Stomach tubes. Distention of the stomach after an operation is a common occurrence which can cause great distress and discomfort. To avoid this, a rubber tube is passed through the nose into the stomach and allowed to remain there for a day or two. In order to make sure that the stomach remains deflated, this rubber tube is sometimes attached to a suction apparatus.

f. Food and fluid intake. Most patients are extremely thirsty after operation, particularly when fluids have been withheld preoperatively. Small amounts of water or tea may be taken within a few hours after surgery, if patients have not been operated upon for a condition within the stomach or intestinal tract. (Such patients are usually forbidden to drink or eat for two to three days and are fed by intravenous fluids.) When the latter situation is not applicable, patients may have small amounts of a soft bland diet the day following surgery and may return to a regular diet within three or four days.

Patient Receiving Intravenous Solution and Medications. When people are unable to take fluids, foods, and medications by mouth, they are given these ingredients by injection into their veins. They can be maintained in this manner for several days until their digestive tract can resume its normal function.

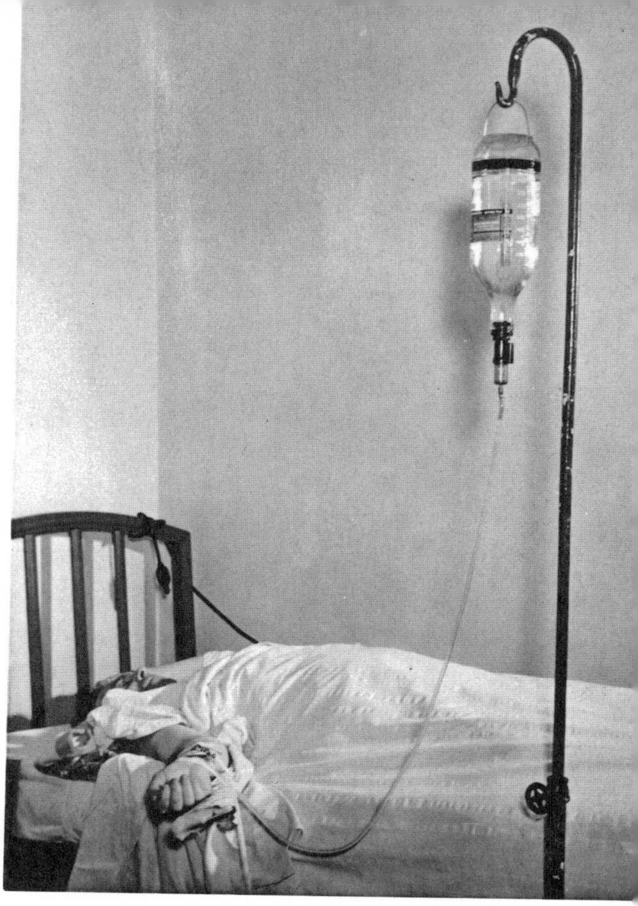

g. Catheterization. Difficulty in urinating for a day or two after surgery is a common occurrence. This is particularly true when spinal anesthesia has been used or after an operation involving the lower abdomen, the female organs, or the rectum. In order to avoid the uncomfortable feeling of a distended bladder which cannot be emptied, it is routine procedure to pass a rubber tube into the bladder at regular intervals. In certain cases, the catheter may be left in place for a few days.

   The ability to urinate always returns, but repeated catheterization may be necessary for several days.

h. Narcotics. Since all people will have varying degrees of pain following surgery, it is customary for narcotics to be prescribed. Pain-relieving narcotics or sedatives are given, if necessary, every few hours for the first day or two after surgery. The patient should be cautioned not to seek these medications unnecessarily, as they may retard the rate of recovery. However, there should be no fear of drug addiction, because this does not occur within the short space of time it takes a patient to convalesce.

i. Antibiotics. Whenever there is a chance that infection may retard operative recovery, the surgeon will order antibiotic drugs to be given either by injection or by mouth. It is very important for the patient to inform his surgeon if he is sensitive or allergic to any of the antibiotic drugs. Fortunately, the large number of antibiotic drugs available makes it possible to find one to which the patient is not sensitive or allergic.

j. Blood transfusions. Every major operation is associated with a certain amount of blood loss. If this amount is sizable, the surgeon will order a transfusion to replace the loss. It should not be concluded merely because blood is being given that the patient's condition is precarious.

k. Enemas. Bowels often do not function satisfactorily for the first four, five, or six days after abdominal surgery. Failure to have a bowel movement should be no cause for alarm. Enemas are often prescribed on the third, fourth, or fifth day to remedy this situation.

l. Wound dressings. Dressings of operative wounds vary according to the type of procedure that has been performed. Wounds with drains may be dressed every day or every other day after surgery. Clean, tightly closed wounds may not be dressed until the sixth, seventh, or eighth day, when the sutures or clips are to be removed. Most dressings are not painful, but if pain is to be associated with the dressing, the surgeon will often prescribe a sedative or narcotic.

m. Suture or clip removal. As mentioned above, sutures or clips may be removed on the sixth, seventh, or eighth day after surgery. There is very little pain and discomfort associated with the removal of clips or sutures.

CHAPTER 56

The Prostate Gland

(See also Chapter 34 on Kidneys and Ureters; Chapter 39 on Male Organs; Chapter 72 on Urinary Bladder and Urethra)

Where is the prostate gland, and what is its function?

The prostate is a part of the male genital apparatus, located near, and surrounding, the outlet of the urinary bladder. It is the size of a horse chestnut and its main function is to secrete a liquid which comprises the bulk of the seminal fluid.

What are the principle diseases affecting the prostate gland?

a. Infections (prostatitis).

b. Enlargement of the gland associated with the aging process (benign hypertrophy).

c. Cancer.

How is the prostate examined?

a. Because of its proximity to the rectum, the examining physician can obtain much information about the gland by inserting his finger into the patient's rectum.

b. Additional information can be obtained by examination through a cystoscope.

What is the usual route by which infection reaches the prostate gland?

a. By direct extension from the outside, up the urethra.

b. Less often, by bacteria being brought to the gland through the bloodstream.

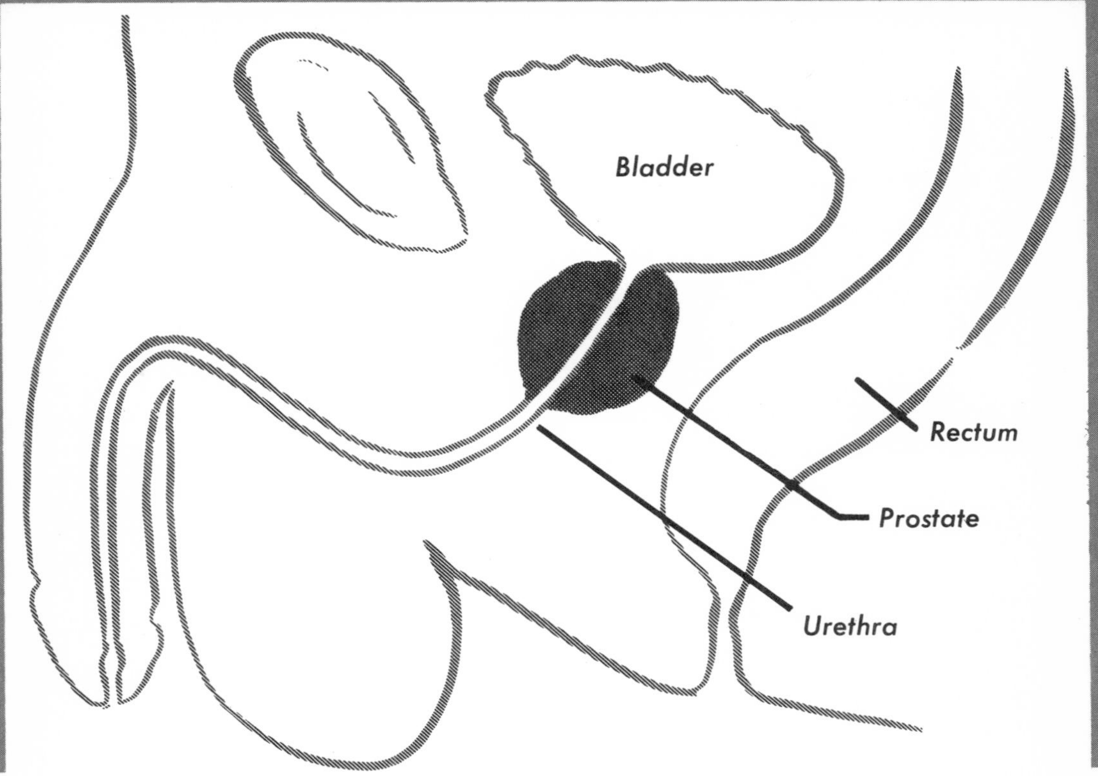

The Prostate Gland. This diagram shows the location of the gland as it surrounds the outlet of the urinary bladder. The prostate gland, for some unknown reason, tends to enlarge as a man ages. The function of the prostate is to secrete the fluid in which the sperm are carried.

What bacteria are most likely to infect the prostate?

The gonorrhea germ; also other bacteria, such as staphylococcus, streptococcus, or colon bacillus.

What are the symptoms of infection in the prostate?

Fever, pain in the lower part of the back, frequency of urination, pain upon voiding, infected and bloody urine.

What is the treatment for prostatic infections?

a. Bed rest.
b. Administration of the appropriate antibiotic drug.
c. Liberal intake of fluids.
d. Avoidance of alcoholic beverages and spicy foods.

e. Administration of sedatives to relieve tension and pain.
f. Avoidance of sexual intercourse.
g. In chronic cases, repeated gentle massage of the gland.
h. Hot sitz baths.

Is surgery often necessary in the treatment of prostate infections?

Usually not, except when an abscess has formed.

What is chronic prostatitis?

A low-grade, persistent inflammation which manifests itself by low back pain, urinary disturbance, sexual disturbance, and sometimes a morning discharge from the penis.

What is the treatment for chronic infections of the prostate?

a. The use of the antibiotics.
b. Periodic gentle massage of the prostate by insertion of the finger into the rectum.
c. Hot baths.
d. Rectal diathermy.

Are most infections of the prostate curable?

Yes, although there is a tendency for the more stubborn and chronic infections to recur from time to time.

BENIGN ENLARGEMENT OF THE PROSTATE
(*Prostatism*)

What is benign enlargement of the prostate?

A condition in which portions of the gland slowly enlarge over a period of years. Malignancy does not occur in this type of enlargement.

Is it natural for all men to have enlargement of the prostate when they grow older?

Yes. Beginning at forty to forty-five years of age, almost all men have a slowly enlarging prostate.

Will all men develop symptoms from prostatic enlargement?

No. Most men go through life without having difficulty. It must be remembered that enlargement of the prostate accompanies normal aging processes.

How can one tell if the enlargement of his prostate requires medical attention?

There will be interference with normal urination.

Why does enlargement of the prostate interfere with urination?

An enlarging prostate compresses the outlet of the bladder.

What may be the eventual outcome of prostatic enlargement?

It may cause a sudden inability to urinate. This condition is known as acute urinary retention.

Is there any relationship between the amount of sexual activity and enlargement of the prostate?

No.

Do all men with enlargement of the prostate have to undergo surgery?

No. Only one in four men will have any symptoms at all . Of those who do have symptoms, only one in four will require surgery.

Is there any satisfactory medical treatment for enlargement of the prostate?

Treatment with hormones, advocated by some physicians, does not help this condition! Massage of the gland may help at times to relieve symptoms partially but will not actually reduce the size of the gland. If there is an infection associated with the enlargement, its control may relieve symptoms.

What are the most common symptoms of enlargement of the prostate?

a. Frequency of urination during the day.
b. The need to void several times during the night (nocturia).
c. Hesitancy in starting the flow of urine.
d. Diminution in the size and force of the urinary stream.

e. Dribbling before and after urination.
f. Burning on urination.
g. Eventual inability to void (acute urinary retention).
h. Bleeding on urination.

The greater the enlargement of the gland, the more the obstruction and the more pronounced will be the symptoms.

What is the effect of enlargement of the prostate upon the bladder and kidneys?

Since the main function of the bladder is to expel urine, it is obvious that an obstruction such as enlargement of the prostate will force the bladder to work harder to discharge the urine. As a result, the wall of the bladder becomes thickened, more muscular, and heavier. Eventually, the bladder fails to empty itself completely with each voiding. This residual urine increases in amount, and will ultimately create abnormal back pressure up the ureters toward the kidney. Along with the dilatation of the ureters there is some impairment of kidney function and the general health of the patient suffers. Permitted to progress untreated, such a condition may lead to complete kidney failure, with resultant uremia and death.

What harm does incomplete emptying of the bladder do to the patient?

It results in stagnation of the urine, with consequent infection. The infection usually spreads up the ureter to the kidney as well. Ultimately, from stagnation of the urine over a period of years, stones may form in the bladder. The increased work and pressure on the bladder wall may cause local "blowouts," known as diverticula. These are sac-like protrusions from the wall of the bladder; they may contain stagnant urine, or stones may develop within them.

What operations are carried out for enlargement of the prostate?

a. Suprapubic prostatectomy. This is an operation in which an incision is made in the midline of the lower abdomen, and the bladder is opened. The prostate gland is removed through the open bladder, in either one or two stages. A rubber tube is then placed in the bladder for a period of days. When the tube is removed,

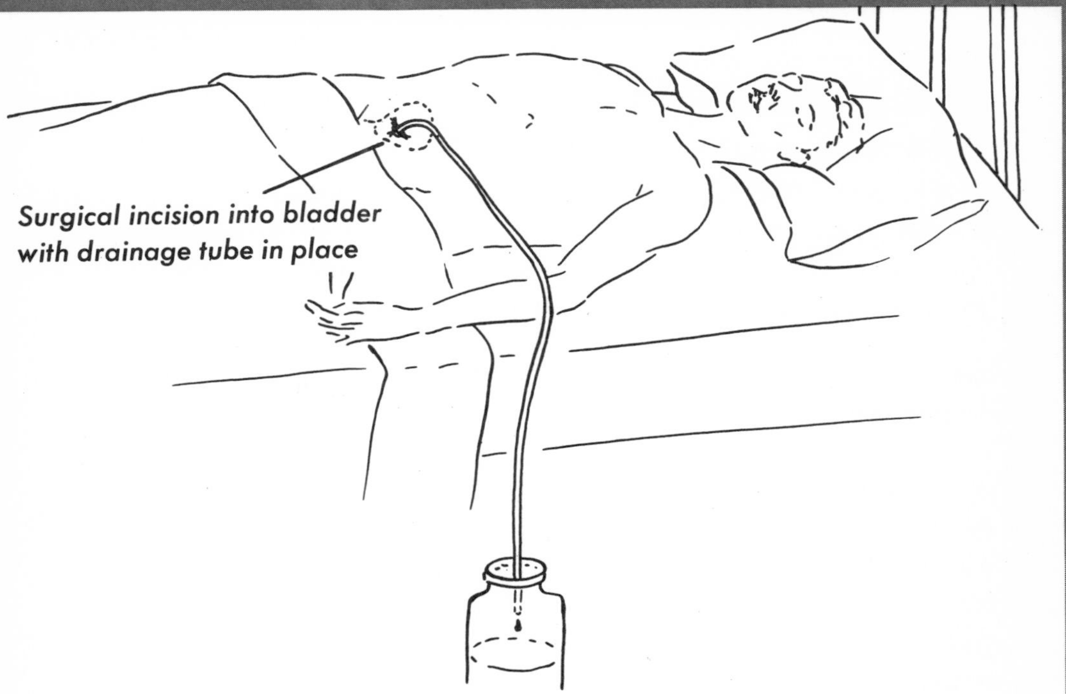

Suprapubic Cystotomy. This shows an operative procedure in which a surgical opening has been made into the bladder to relieve urinary obstruction caused by an enlarged prostate. Such an operation is often done as a preliminary procedure to the removal of the enlarged prostate.

the normal urinary stream flows through the urethra as it did preoperatively.

b. Retropubic prostatectomy. This is a surgical procedure in which the incision is made in the lower abdomen directly over the prostate, and the prostate is removed without opening the urinary bladder.

c. Perineal prostatectomy. This is an operation in which an incision is made in the perineum (the space below the testicles and in front of the rectum). The prostate is removed through this incision.

d. Transurethral resection of the prostate. This is a procedure in which part of the obstructing portion of the prostate is burned away with a cutting loop which is passed through a cystoscope. No incision is made for this procedure.

What will determine which procedure is chosen?

a. The size of the prostate gland.

b. The presence or absence of stones or infection in the bladder.
c. The presence or absence of bladder diverticula.
d. The status of kidney function.
e. The general health of the patient.

Is any one procedure preferable for removal of the prostate?

No. Each procedure has its definite indications, depending upon the particular findings in any given case.

What is meant by a "two-stage" prostate operation?

In some instances—because of poor general health or impaired kidney function, infection, stones, or associated diseases such as heart trouble or high blood pressure—it is too risky to remove the gland directly. In these cases, a period of preliminary urinary drainage is required; when this is carried out, it is called a first-stage (cystotomy) prostate operation. In this operation, the bladder is opened surgically and is allowed to drain on to the abdominal wall. After a suitable interval of time, when kidney function has returned to normal, infection has subsided, and any bladder stones which are present have been removed, the prostate is then excised by the surgeon, who inserts his finger into the bladder and shells out the gland. This procedure is the second stage of the operation.

Is the entire prostate gland removed when performing a prostatectomy?

In actuality, no. A rim of normal gland tissue usually is left behind.

What is a cystotomy?

It is the first stage of a two-stage prostate operation in which a rubber tube is placed into the bladder through an abdominal incision.

Is it ever necessary to operate upon the prostate gland as an emergency procedure?

Yes, if acute obstruction to the passage of urine develops secondary to an enlarged prostate.

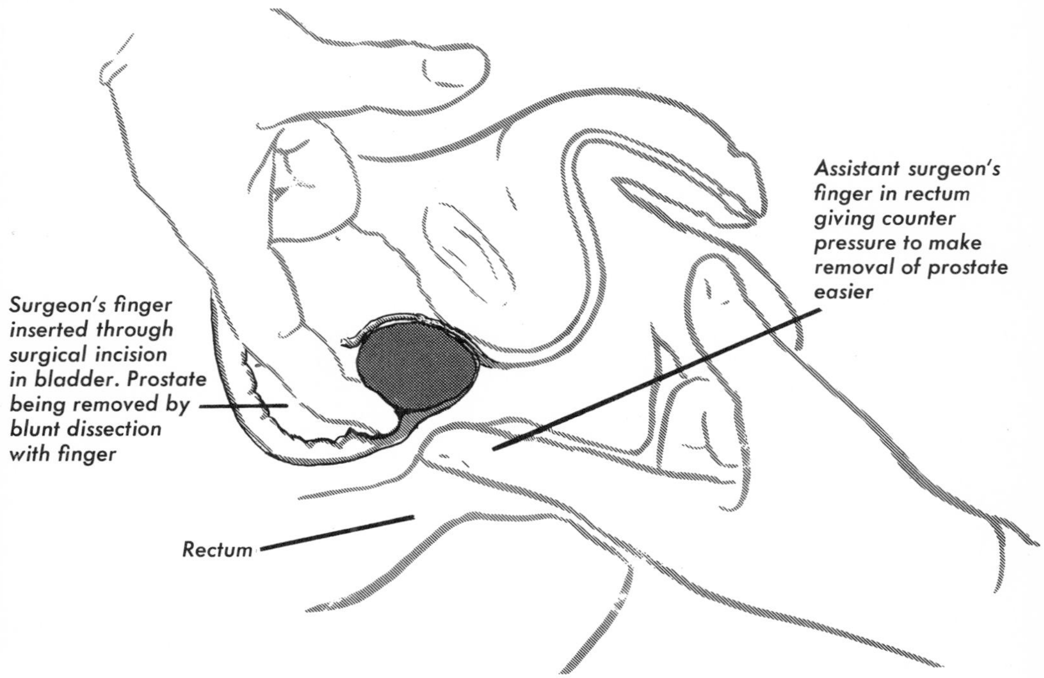
Assistant surgeon's finger in rectum giving counter pressure to make removal of prostate easier
Surgeon's finger inserted through surgical incision in bladder. Prostate being removed by blunt dissection with finger
Rectum

Removal of the Prostate Gland Through the Open Bladder. This demonstrates how the enlarged portion of the gland which surrounds the bladder neck is removed. Today, this operation is not used as often as a one-stage operation for removal of the enlarged prostate.

How long is the period between the two stages of this operation?

This may vary from a week to an indefinite period of time, depending upon the improvement in the general condition of the patient.

Are operations upon the prostate serious?

Yes, but with our present-day knowledge and with the use of better surgical techniques and the aid of antibiotics, the vast majority of patients undergoing prostatic surgery can look toward a safe and satisfactory recovery.

Does the prostate ever enlarge again and cause urinary obstruction after it has once been removed?

Not if a thorough removal has been carried out. Occasionally, after a transurethral resection through a cystoscope, prostatic tissue may grow and cause some obstruction.

CANCER OF THE PROSTATE

How common is cancer of the prostate?

It is generally agreed that somewhere between 10 and 20 per cent of all men past fifty years of age will develop cancer of the prostate, and it becomes increasingly more common with age so that among those who live into the nineties, almost all will have prostate tissue which may be termed malignant. The activity is low, and these men usually succumb to some other more active disease.

At what age is cancer of the prostate most apt to occur?

In the sixties, seventies, and eighties.

What are the symptoms of cancer of the prostate?

Unfortunately, early cancer of the prostate produces few, if any, symptoms. It is only when the disease has become advanced that it makes itself known. The only way to detect early cancer of the prostate is to examine the gland at regular intervals. For this reason, it is important that men over fifty years of age have a yearly examination of the prostate gland.

How is a positive diagnosis of cancer of the prostate made?

a. Cancer of the prostate feels much firmer and more irregular on rectal examination than benign enlargement.
b. It is distinguished from benign enlargement by taking a biopsy of the gland, usually by way of a biopsy needle inserted through the rectum, and submitting it to microscopic examination.

Do all cases of cancer of the prostate cause symptoms?

No. It has been found that in many individuals the tumor may lie dormant for an indefinite period, never causing symptoms nor spreading to other parts of the body.

Is there any medical treatment for cancer of the prostate?

Yes. Some relief may be obtained by giving large doses of *female* sex hormones. In some cases, the growth of the tumor is retarded by the suppression of male hormone secretion that results from the administration of the female sex hormone.

Does simple benign enlargement of the prostate ever become cancerous?

Such a transition is extremely rare.

For how long can the female sex hormones be effective in retarding the progress of cancer of the prostate?

Although this form of treatment is not curative, it may suppress a cancerous growth and prolong life for many years.

Is x-ray therapy or radium helpful in the treatment of cancer of the prostate?

Only insofar as it relieves pain. It cannot cure the disease.

Are there any radioactive substances which are helpful in the treatment of cancer of the prostate?

Yes. The injection of radioactive gold directly into the gland has, on occasion, given promising results. This method of treatment is still in its early stages of development.

What is the surgical treatment for cancer of the prostate?

a. In early cases, the treatment is removal of the entire gland (radical prostatectomy).
b. In more advanced cases, removal of the testicles is also performed.
c. Surgical removal of the adrenal glands or the pituitary gland has been reported as retarding the rate of growth and extension of far-advanced cancers of the prostate. These, however, are drastic procedures used only as a last resort.

* * * *

Will operations for removal of the prostate cause impotence?

Ordinary prostatectomy does not cause impotence. However, a radical operation for removal of the prostate gland usually does cause impotence. Since many of the patients are in the twilight years of their active sex life, this is often not a matter for major concern.

Will operations upon the prostate gland result in inability to control urination (incontinence)?

Temporary loss of control frequently follows extensive surgery upon the prostate. However, this will clear up within several weeks to several months in the great majority of cases.

Does loss of urinary control occur after ordinary prostatectomy for benign enlargement?

Very rarely, and then for a few weeks only.

How long a hospital stay is necessary for prostate operations?

For one-stage prostate operations, twelve to fourteen days. For two-stage operations, three to four weeks.

Are special nurses advisable after operations upon the prostate?

Yes, for a period of three to four days.

Are blood transfusions employed in operations upon the prostate?

Yes, although hemorrhage following these operations is much less likely to occur today than in former years.

How long a period of convalescence is necessary after an operation upon the prostate?

Four to five weeks.

Does enlargement of the prostate ever recur after removal?

Once in a very great while, when the gland has not been completely removed, regrowth of gland tissue may take place. This is treated by reoperation, with removal of more of the gland.

Do stones ever form in the prostate gland?

Yes, this is not an uncommon finding, particularly in glands that have been infected over a period of years.

What is the treatment for stones in the prostate?

They are operated upon only when accompanied by symptoms such as those caused by enlargement of the prostate.

What type of anesthesia is used for a prostate operation?

This will depend upon the general condition of the patient. In some cases, a low spinal anesthesia is used; in others, a general inhalation anesthesia is employed.

Is it common practice to tie off the vas deferens leading from the testicle when performing a prostatectomy?

Yes, this is done as a preliminary measure to prevent inflammation of the epididymis, a structure adjacent to the testicle.

How does urine leave the body after a prostate operation?

If a suprapubic prostatectomy has been performed, a tube is placed from the bladder to an incision in the abdominal wall. When a retropubic prostatectomy is done, or when a transurethral resection is done, a rubber catheter is placed in the urethra to drain the urine.

What is the usual interval of time before the resumption of normal voiding?

Following suprapubic prostatectomy, approximately two weeks; after retropubic prostatectomy, approximately one week; after transurethral resection, approximately five to seven days.

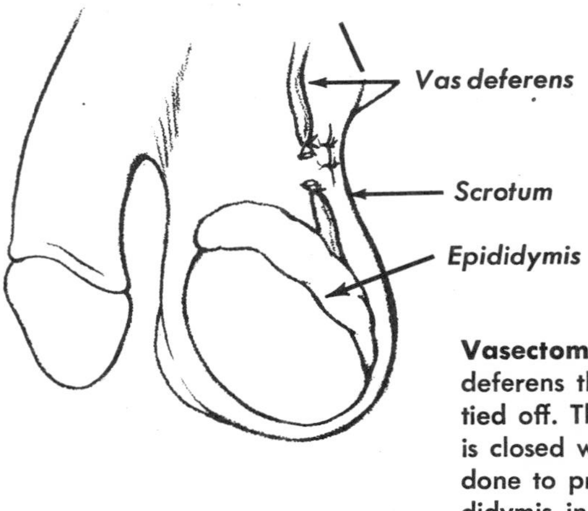

Vasectomy. This drawing shows a vas deferens that has been cut and the ends tied off. The small incision in the scrotum is closed with two stitches. The operation, done to prevent inflammation of the epididymis in prostate surgery, also creates sterility, as sperm from the testicle can no longer be carried through the vas to the seminal vesicles.

HAPTER 57

The Rectum and Anus

(See also Chapter 62 on Small and Large Intestines)

What is the anus?

The last inch or one and a half inches of the intestinal tract.

What is the rectum?

That portion of the bowel extending up from the anus for a distance of six to eight inches.

Is rectal or anal disease common?

Nearly one-third of all adults at one time or another suffer from some local disease of the anus or rectum, such as hemorrhoids, fissures, or fistulas.

Is it necessary for the maintenance of good health to have a bowel movement every day?

No. Bowel habits vary widely among normal people.

Is it normal to have one or two movements daily?

Yes, for some people.

Can a person lead a normal life if he moves his bowels only every other day or every third day?

Yes, providing he has a regular pattern of bowel function.

Does the type of food that one eats affect bowel function?

Yes.

What foods are best avoided when one has acute rectal or anal disease?

a. Highly seasoned spicy foods.
b. Alcoholic beverages.

What determines regularity of bowel movement?

a. The formation of good habits in early childhood.
b. The eating of a well-rounded diet containing plenty of fresh fruits and fresh vegetables.
c. A good general state of health.

Will good bowel habits in childhood usually lead to good habits when one is older?

Definitely, yes.

Is it harmful to take a lubricant such as mineral oil over a prolonged period of time?

No, if it is really necessary for normal function. However, it should not be taken at the same time of day as vitamin-rich foods, as it may interfere with vitamin absorption.

Should a person take a laxative when he has abdominal pain?

Never! This practice can be dangerous—particularly if the cause of the pain is appendicitis or some other inflammatory process in the intestinal tract.

Is a change in one's bowel habits significant of disease?

Yes. Very often it means that there is trouble. Recurrent diarrhea or constipation should lead one to have a thorough medical survey of his intestinal tract.

What abnormalities in bowel function should cause one to seek medical advice?

a. Episodes of diarrhea.

b. Episodes of constipation.
c. Change in the appearance or caliber of the stools.
d. Blood in the stool.
e. Black-colored stool.
f. Mucus in the stool.

Are there any laxatives which are better than others?

The milder the laxative, the better. Lubricants or stewed fruits are preferred for the relief of constipation.

When is it permissible to take laxatives?

Occasionally, when there is a period of constipation in a patient who ordinarily has normal bowel function.

When is it permissible to take lubricants?

When there is a tendency toward chronic constipation in an older person.

When should enemas be taken for constipation?

Only when the patient is otherwise in good health and has no other symptoms referable to the intestinal tract.

Is there any adequate treatment for chronic constipation?

Yes. Eat plenty of fresh fruit and vegetables and develop regular habits. Also, the taking of lubricants or bulk-forming medications may prove helpful.

Is there a tendency for constipation to become more prevalent as one grows older?

Yes. The abdominal muscles (so important in aiding bowel evacuation) tend to weaken.

How does one treat constipation in children?

a. Train the child toward regular bowel habit.
b. Give the child a well-rounded full diet.
c. If necessary, give the child lubricants to aid him until he develops regularity.

What is the significance of a chronic diarrhea?

It may indicate an infection of the bowel, such as dysentery or colitis. Any diarrhea lasting more than a few days should be investigated by a physician.

What is the best treatment for constipation in adults or older people?

a. Make sure there is no underlying disease of the large bowel, rectum, or anus.
b. Improve dietary habits.
c. Establish regular bowel habits.
d. Use bulk-forming medications or, if necessary, lubricants.

Of what significance is blood in the stool?

It may be caused by:

a. Excess straining at stool when constipated.
b. Hemorrhoids or some other anal condition.
c. An acute colitis associated with diarrhea.
d. A chronic colitis.
e. A benign tumor, such as a polyp.
f. A malignant tumor of the rectum or bowel.

What is the significance of a black stool?

It is caused by bleeding high in the intestinal tract, as from an ulcer. Certain iron medications, when taken orally, can also cause black stools.

What is the significance of mucus in the stool?

Mucus does not necessarily signify a disease process, as many people, especially women in middle life, will have mucus in the stool when no real disease exists. However, it should be checked by a physician.

Is it harmful for one to strain at the stool for prolonged periods of time?

Yes. This can lead to hemorrhoid (pile) formations.

Are colonic irrigations helpful in curing disease?

No. Years ago, certain colon conditions were treated by this method but now it has been proved that they are of little, if any, benefit.

Is it true that people who do not have a regular bowel movement are likely to become sluggish, have headaches, and feel weak?

They may develop such symptoms because of the psychological effect upon them. However, there is no sound physical reason why constipation for a day or two should cause these reactions.

HEMORRHOIDS
(Piles)

What are hemorrhoids?

They are varicose dilatations of the veins which drain the rectum and anus.

What causes hemorrhoids?

It is felt that these veins break down and their valves become incompetent because of the strain placed upon them by irregular living habits. Chronic constipation, irregularity of bowel evacuation, and prolonged sojourns on the toilet are thought to be conducive toward hemorrhoid formation. Pregnancy, because of the pressure of the baby's head in the pelvis, also leads toward hemorrhoid formation.

How common are hemorrhoids?

This is the most common condition in the anal region and affects almost 25 per cent of the population at one time or another.

How can one tell if he has hemorrhoids?

There are one or more swellings or bulges about the anus, which become more pronounced on bowel evacuation. There is also a sense of fullness in the anal region, more pronounced on bowel evacuation. Hemorrhoids are frequently painful and may be accompanied by considerable rectal bleeding.

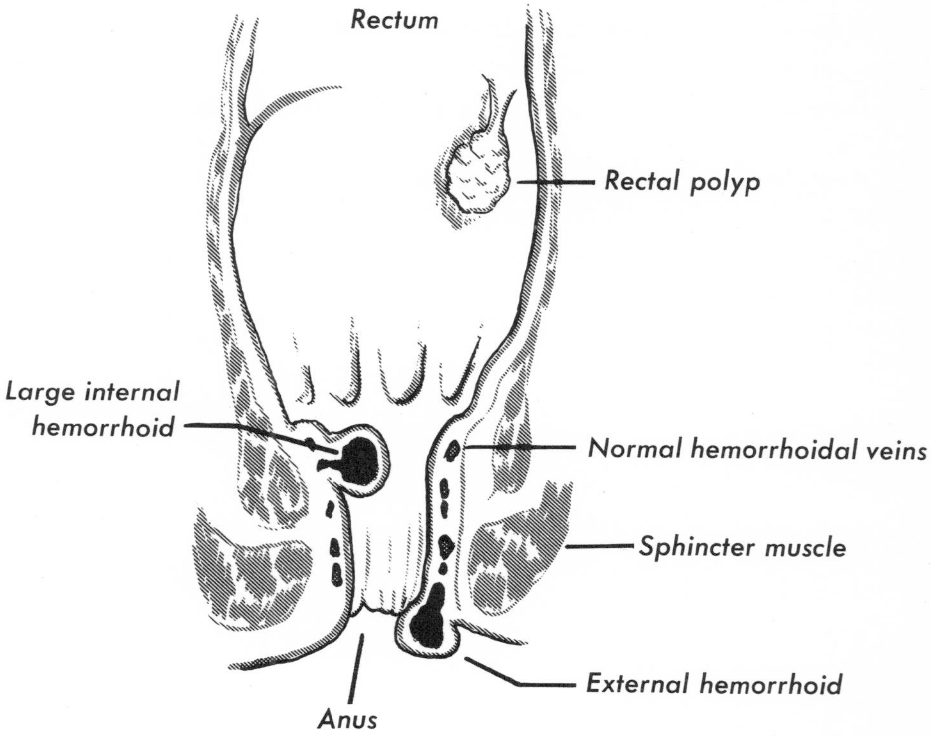

Rectal Polyps and Hemorrhoids. Rectal polyps are benign tumors found within the rectum. They are thought to be the forerunners of cancer, and for this reason they should be removed surgically. Hemorrhoids are varicose veins within the rectum. When they bleed and cause pain, they should be removed surgically.

Is there any way to prevent getting hemorrhoids?

Yes, to a certain extent. Regular bowel evacuation, the eating of a good diet with sufficient roughage, and the avoidance of straining at stool will diminish the chances of getting hemorrhoids.

How can a positive diagnosis of hemorrhoids be made?

Your physician will be able to tell by a rectal examination whether hemorrhoids are present.

What are the various forms of treatment for hemorrhoids?

a. Medical treatment, which includes the taking of lubricants to ensure a regular stool and the use of medicated suppositories inserted into the rectum.

b. The injection treatment, if the hemorrhoids are of the internal type.
c. Surgical removal of the hemorrhoids.

Do all types of hemorrhoids respond to the injection treatment?

No. Only the internal type can sometimes be successfully treated by this method.

What can happen if hemorrhoids are not treated?

a. They may bleed severely and cause a marked anemia with all of its serious consequences.
b. The hemorrhoids may become thrombosed (clotted), producing extreme pain in the region.
c. The hemorrhoids may prolapse (drop out of the rectum and not go back in again).
d. Hemorrhoids may become strangulated and gangrenous.
e. Hemorrhoids may become ulcerated and infected.

Does neglect of hemorrhoids ever lead to the formation of cancer of the rectum?

No, but the abrupt development of hemorrhoids is occasionally secondary to the development of a tumor in the large bowel.

What determines whether or not surgery is recommended for hemorrhoids?

Those cases which do not respond to adequate medical management must be operated upon.

Will the surgeon perform other tests before performing hemorrhoidectomy?

Yes. The surgeon will perform a sigmoidoscopy to make sure there is no disease high up in the rectum above the hemorrhoids.

Can sigmoidoscopy reveal the presence of a cancer in the rectum or lower bowel?

Yes. That is the main value of performing this examination.

How and where is the sigmoidoscopy performed?

It is done in the surgeon's office by the passage of a sigmoidoscope into the rectal canal. A sigmoidoscope is an instrument about ten inches long which allows direct visualization of the entire rectum and the lower portion of the large bowel (the sigmoid).

Is sigmoidoscopy a painful examination?

No. Only slight discomfort accompanies sigmoidoscopy.

Are hemorrhoids sometimes an indication that other disease exists in the lower intestinal tract?

Yes. That is the reason sigmoidoscopy and x-rays are advocated before the decision is made to remove the hemorrhoids.

Is hospitalization necessary when hemorrhoids are to be removed?

Yes. The hospital stay will last anywhere from four to seven days.

Is hemorrhoidectomy a serious operation?

No. The risks are negligible.

What are the chances for full cure following the removal of hemorrhoids?

Well over 95 per cent.

Is there a tendency for hemorrhoids to recur?

Yes, but the number of such instances is small.

Is hemorrhoidectomy followed by much pain?

Yes, for the first week or two after the operation.

What is done when the hemorrhoids are removed?

The varicosed veins are dissected out from the surrounding tissues and are ligated and cut away.

What anesthesia is used?

Usually a low spinal or caudal anesthesia, although occasionally a local anesthesia or a general anesthesia may be given.

How long does it take to perform a hemorrhoid operation?

Approximately fifteen to twenty minutes.

Are any special preoperative measures necessary before hemorrhoidectomy?

No, except to see that the bowel is empty before operation.

What special diet is necessary after hemorrhoidectomy?

The avoidance of highly seasoned foods and alcoholic beverages.

How soon after a hemorrhoid operation will bowel function return to normal?

It may take several weeks before bowel function returns completely to normal.

What special postoperative measures are usually advised?

A lubricant, such as mineral oil, is taken twice a day, and the patient is told to sit in a tub of warm water two or three times a day. Frequent postoperative visits to the surgeon will be necessary.

Is it common to have bleeding at the stool following a hemorrhoid operation?

Yes. This may continue for a few days to a few weeks after operation.

How soon after a hemorrhoid operation can one do the following:

Bathe	Three to four days.
Walk out on the street	Four to five days.
Walk up and down stairs	Four to five days.
Perform household duties	Seven to ten days.
Drive a car	Two to three weeks.
Resume marital relations	Three to four weeks.

Return to work	Two to three weeks.
Resume all physical activities	Four to six weeks.

Should one return for regular checkups after a hemorrhoid operation?

Yes, about every six months.

FISSURE IN ANO

What is a fissure in ano?

It is an ulceration or split in the mucous membrane of the anus.

What causes a fissure?

Chronic constipation, with overstretching of the mucous membrane at the anal outlet. The cracked surface becomes infected and an ulcer forms. The ulcer tends to remain, as it is kept open by the stretching at bowel evacuation.

What are the symptoms of fissure in ano?

Pain on moving the bowels, accompanied by a slight amount of bleeding.

What is the treatment for fissue in ano?

Medical treatment may result in healing in many cases if carried out early. It will consist of taking lubricants such as mineral oil and the placing of medicated suppositories into the rectal canal. Those patients who fail to respond to medical management must be operated upon.

What kind of operation is performed for fissue in ano?

The fissure is removed with a small elliptical incision and the underlying sphincter muscle is cut so as to relax the anus for a period of time.

Are the hospital procedures and the preoperative and postoperative measures the same for fissure in ano as for hemorrhoid operations?

Yes. (See the section on Hemorrhoids in this chapter, for the answers to these questions.)

How long does it take for fissures to heal following surgery?

Three to four weeks.

Do fissures in ano ever recur?

Yes, but only in rare instances.

Does the sphincter muscle heal and will bowel function return to normal after an operation for a fissure?

Yes. Healing takes place within a few weeks and bowel function will return to normal.

ABSCESSES AND INFECTIONS ABOUT THE ANUS

(Perirectal and Perianal Abscess)

Are abscesses in the area about the anus and rectum very common?

Yes.

What causes these abscesses?

It is thought that the infection originates in the lining wall of the anus or rectum and tunnels its way out toward the skin.

What is the treatment for these abscesses?

These abscesses should be incised very early in their course and drained widely.

Do these abscesses always heal completely?

No. Some of them will open and close for several weeks or months, eventually resulting in fistula formation.

Is hospitalization necessary to open these abscesses?

Only the large, extensive abscesses that are accompanied by great pain and high temperature must be opened, under anesthesia, in a hospital. The less severe ones can be opened under local anesthesia in a surgeon's office.

Fissure in Ano and Fistula in Ano. This diagram shows two very common conditions about the anus and rectum. A fissure is much like a split lip, since it is caused by a crack in the mucous membrane lining the anus. As the anus dilates during a bowel movement, the mucous membrane splits, preventing the fissure from healing. A fistula is a tunnel or tract leading from the inside of the anus or rectum to the outside surface of the skin. It tends to become chronically infected, and in order to obtain a cure, it must be removed surgically.

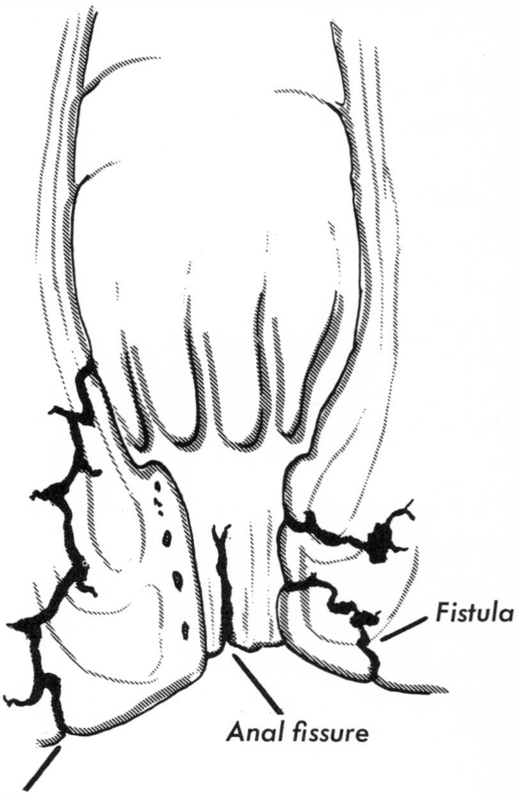

FISTULA IN ANO

What is a fistula in ano?

An abnormal communication between the mucous membrane lining of the rectum or anus and the skin surface near the anal opening. A fistula is therefore a tunnel, or tract.

How common is fistula in ano?

Fistulas comprise approximately one-fourth of all conditions about the anus or rectum.

What causes fistulas?

They represent the end result of an infection that has originated in the rectal or anal wall and which has tunneled its way out to the skin surface.

Are fistulas ever caused by tuberculosis?

A very small percentage of fistulas are associated with tuberculosis of the lungs. However, today this is an extremely rare occurrence.

What are the symptoms of fistula in ano?

The patient usually gives a history of a painful boil or abscess alongside the rectum which opened and discharged pus at some time previously. The abscess closed and opened alternately over a period of several weeks or months, leaving a small discharge but causing relatively little pain.

What happens if a fistula in ano is not treated?

The fistulous tract tends to spread and tunnel about the rectum and may reach the surface at several points alongside the rectum or anus. Also, the sphincter muscle controlling the outlet may be damaged by an untreated fistula.

What is the treatment for fistula?

All fistulas which fail to heal over a period of several weeks should be operated upon.

What kind of operation is performed?

The fistulous tract is removed or laid open widely. This usually includes cutting the sphincter muscle, as in the operation for a fissure in ano.

Are the hospital procedures and the preoperative and postoperative measures similar for fistula in ano to those for fissure in ano and hemorrhoids?

Yes. (See the section on Hemorrhoids in this chapter, for the answers to these questions.)

What are the chances for cure of a fistula after surgery?

Excellent. Only rarely will a fistula recur. Occasionally, a large extensive chronic fistula will recur and reoperation will become necessary in order to effect a permanent cure.

Does bowel function return to normal after a fistula operation?

Yes, within a few weeks.

How long do fistulas take to heal?

This is a more extensive operation than a fissure operation and the tissues may take from six to ten weeks to heal fully.

PRURITUS ANI
(*Itching Anus*)

What is pruritus ani?

It is a chronic itching of the skin around the anus.

What causes pruritus ani?

a. The skin in this area is moist, highly sensitive, and is soiled re-repeatedly by feces.
b. This skin area is often allergic to irritating soaps, clothing, etc.
c. Associated anal conditions, such as hemorrhoids, fissures, colitis, etc., may cause irritation and set up an itching-scratching pattern.
d. Highly neurotic or disturbed people tend to develop pruritus ani much more frequently than others.

What are the symptoms of pruritus ani?

a. Uncontrollable itching, worse during hot weather and at night.
b. Irritation and burning of the skin around the anus.

What is the treatment for pruritus ani?

There have been innumerable treatments carried out, but none have proved completely effective in all cases. If an allergy is present, it must be discovered and treated. If any associated anal condition is present, it must be eliminated. The anus must be kept clean and dry. Soaps must be used infrequently and cautiously. There are many salves which can bring considerable relief when used properly, especially ointments containing cortisone and itch-relieving ingredients.

Can excessive use of soap and water be harmful in pruritus?

Yes. Soap and water may irritate rather than benefit the condition.

How long can pruritus last?

It tends to be chronic and many people have it for years.

Does recovery ever take place spontaneously?

Yes. Often the condition disappears by itself.

Is psychotherapy ever valuable in the treatment of pruritus ani?

Yes, if the patient is an emotionally disturbed person.

PROLAPSE OF THE RECTUM

What is prolapse of the rectum?

It is an extrusion of the mucous membrane lining of the rectum through the anal opening.

When does prolapse occur most often?

When straining at the stool.

Who is most likely to have this condition?

Young children and older people.

What causes prolapse?

Excessive straining at the stool, sometimes associated with diarrhea or constipation, in a person with a weak musculature.

What is the treatment for prolapse of the rectum?

Some cases require no treatment other than improved bowel habits and the eradication of the associated diarrhea or constipation. Others may require some form of surgical bolstering of the muscle supports of the anal canal and excision of redundant mucous membrane.

What kind of operation will be performed?

For the minor type of prolapse, an operation around the rectum will be performed. For the major types, an abdominal operation is carried out, with shortening of the rectum and a reconstruction of the musculature which holds the rectum in place.

Are operations for prolapse more often necessary for older people than for children?

Yes.

Are operations for prolapse successful?

Yes, but there are many failures in advanced cases in older patients.

POLYPS OF THE RECTUM AND ANUS

What are polyps?

Polyps are wartlike growths of the anal or rectal mucous membrane which may vary in size from that of a small pea to that of a golf ball or even larger.

Where are polyps found?

Polyps can be found anywhere in the large bowel, from the anal orifice upward.

What causes polyps?

Polyps are growths, like other tumors. The exact cause is unknown.

How common are polyps?

They are the most common tumor within the intestinal tract.

Who is most likely to develop polyps?

Polyps are seen in all age groups but tend to make their appearance more often during the fourth, fifth, and sixth decades of life.

Do polyps tend to run in families or be inherited?

Only the multiple polyps of the large bowel. This is a distinct disease. It is called multiple polyposis, and should be distinguished from the isolated, individual polyp so often found in the rectum or about the anal region.

How can one tell if he has a polyp?

Polyps near the anal region will sometimes be extruded on bowel evacuation and can be felt. But the most common symptom is painless bleeding from the rectum on bowel evacuation in a patient who has no other anal or rectal disease.

How does the surgeon make the diagnosis of rectal polyps?

Polyps can often be seen by direct visualization through an anoscope or sigmoidoscope.

What harm can polyps do if untreated?

Some polyps will undergo cancerous changes if not removed. Simple removal of polyps can prevent this from happening!

What is the treatment for polyps?

Polyps of the anus and rectum should be removed. If small enough, this can be carried out in the surgeon's office. If the polyps are large or high up in the bowel, they must be removed in the hospital.

What operative procedure is performed?

Through an anoscope or sigmoidoscope a snare is placed around the polyps and the base of the polyp is burned with an electric needle. Thus, through the rectal canal, the polyp is withdrawn along with the tightened snare.

How can one tell if a polyp is becoming malignant?

The excised polyp will be sent to the laboratory and a microscopic examination will be carried out.

How soon will the laboratory report be available?

Within four to seven days.

What is done if the polyp has proved to be malignant?

An abdominal operation is performed for the removal of that segment of involved bowel.

How long a period of hospitalization is necessary?

For the ordinary polyp, only one to three days.

Are any special preparations necessary before performing polyp removal?

No; just the ordinary cleansing of the bowel.

What special postoperative measures are advised after polyp removal?

A lubricant such as mineral oil should be used, and the patient should follow a bland diet.

Do polyps tend to recur?

A polyp, once removed, rarely recurs unless it has proved to show signs of malignant changes within it. However, people who have formed one polyp may develop others.

How often should one return for a checkup following polyp removal?

Approximately every six months.

Is there any way to prevent the formation of another polyp?

No.

How soon after a procedure of this kind can one return to normal activity?

Usually within two to three days.

Will bleeding continue for a few days after polyp removal?

This sometimes occurs and should not occasion alarm.

CANCER OF THE RECTUM AND ANUS

Is cancer of the rectum or anus a common condition?

Yes. It is one of the most frequently encountered malignant growths in the entire body.

What causes cancer of the rectum?

The cause is unknown, but it is a medical fact that many cancers in this region originate from the benign polyps described above.

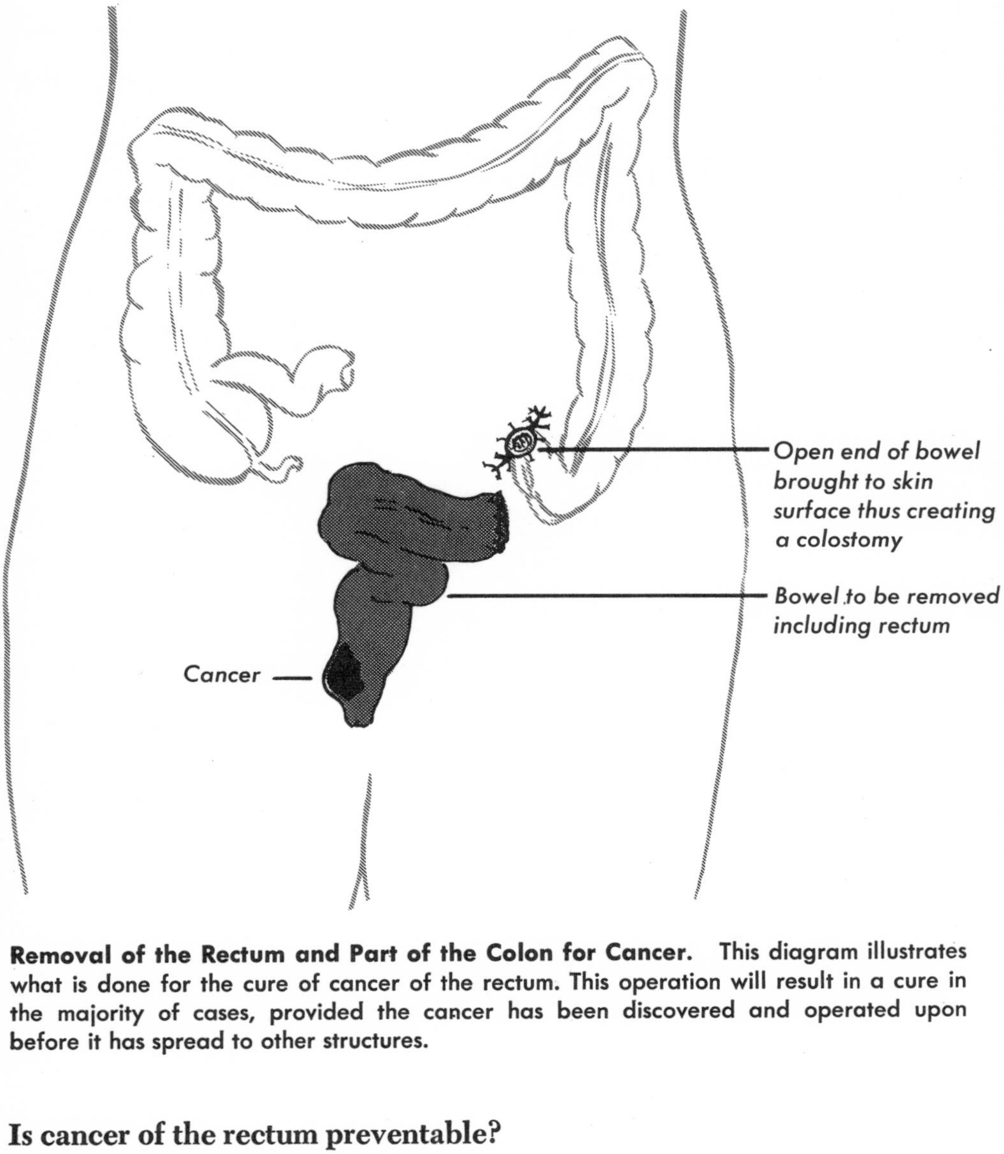

Removal of the Rectum and Part of the Colon for Cancer. This diagram illustrates what is done for the cure of cancer of the rectum. This operation will result in a cure in the majority of cases, provided the cancer has been discovered and operated upon before it has spread to other structures.

Is cancer of the rectum preventable?

To a certain extent, insofar as periodic rectal examinations and sigmoidoscopic examinations may uncover a benign condition which might have resulted in cancerous degeneration if it had not been removed.

How is the diagnosis of cancer of the rectum made?

a. By examination with the physician's finger, which is inserted into the rectal canal.

b. By taking a piece of the tumor tissue and submitting it to microscopic examination. (This is a simple office procedure.)

What symptoms are caused by cancer of the rectum?

a. The outstanding symptom is blood in the stool.
b. There may also be a change in bowel habit.

At what period in life is cancer of the rectum most often seen?

It may come on at any time, but is most usual in middle and later life.

What is the treatment for cancer of the rectum?

Removal of the entire rectum and approximately two to three feet of bowel. An artificial opening for the passage of stool is fashioned on the abdominal wall. This artificial opening is known as a colostomy. In some cases, when the cancer is high up in the rectum, it is possible to remove the cancer-bearing portion of the rectum and to re-establish bowel continuity. In such an instance, an artificial opening is unnecessary.

Is surgery for cancer of the rectum dangerous?

Today surgical recovery takes place in well over 95 per cent of cases. However, it is a major procedure which takes two to three hours to perform and necessitates hospitalization for several weeks.

Is cancer of the rectum ever curable?

Definitely, yes! More than half the cases can be cured if seen at a stage before the tumor has spread to other parts of the body.

Can a patient lead a full, normal existence with the rectum removed?

Yes. There are many thousands of people who engage in all activities despite the fact that they have no rectum. They learn to care for their colostomy in such a manner that the bowel is emptied at a set time each day, permitting them full activity. Various bags are applied over the colostomy opening which seal in any feces or odor while the patient is away from home.

CHAPTER 58

Rheumatic Fever

(See also Chapter 10 on Arthritis; Chapter 14 on Bones, Muscles, Tendons, and Joints; Chapter 27 on Heart; Chapter 42 on Nervous Diseases)

What is rheumatic fever?

Rheumatic fever is a specific disease thought to be bacterial in origin and characterized by attacks of fever lasting anywhere from several weeks to several months. In addition, there may be inflammatory involvement of many tissues and organs of the body, such as the heart, joints, skin, lungs, and nerves.

The disease is most common between the ages of five and fifteen, but may occur at any age.

Attacks of rheumatic fever tend to recur over a period of many years.

What is the cause of rheumatic fever?

The exact manner in which rheumatic fever comes about is still unknown. However, there is abundant evidence to indicate that this illness is closely related to infections by the streptococcus germ.

Rheumatic fever often has its onset shortly after sore throat, tonsillitis, scarlet fever, and other infections caused by the streptococcus. However, it is felt that a peculiar kind of individual susceptibility is necessary in order for this relationship to develop.

Is heredity a factor in the susceptibility to rheumatic fever?

Rheumatic fever has been definitely noted to be more prevalent in certain families than in others. However, it is not known whether this is caused by a hereditary predisposition or because the environment and living habits are predisposing.

Can an individual have rheumatic heart disease without a known previous history of rheumatic fever?

Yes. In most cases, a careful inquiry into the individual's history will uncover significant data to indicate a previous episode of rheumatic fever. However, there are many instances where careful investigation does not bring to light a past episode of rheumatic fever. The characteristic heart symptoms and signs will, nevertheless, permit a diagnosis of rheumatic heart disease to be made, even without such a history.

How does rheumatic fever affect the joints?

In the acute illness, all degrees of joint involvement may occur. These vary from vague discomfort in the extremities to severe pain in one or more joints, with swelling, redness, heat, and extreme tenderness on touch or motion. Commonly affected are the joints of the knees, ankles, elbows, and wrists. However, any other joint may be affected.

A characteristic of rheumatic fever is the "migratory" nature of the joint involvement; that is, the inflammation may settle in one joint and subsequently subside, only to crop up in another joint.

Does rheumatic fever cause permanent joint damage or crippling?

No. Once the acute illness subsides, the joints revert to a perfectly normal condition, without residual damage. Even repeated attacks of rheumatic fever do not permanently damage the joints.

What organs may be permanently injured by an attack of rheumatic fever?

While it is true that during the active stage of this disease many organs may be involved, almost all except the *heart* escape serious permanent damage.

How does rheumatic fever affect the heart?

During the acute stage, rheumatic fever may set up areas of inflammation:

a. Within the heart muscle itself, causing myocarditis.
b. On the inner lining of the heart and on the heart valves, causing endocarditis.
c. On the outer lining of the heart, causing pericarditis.

What is the effect of rheumatic fever upon the heart during the active and acute stage?

The patient may have any degree of heart involvement. It may be so mild as to be undetectable clinically. It may be so severe as to be rapidly fatal. Fortunately, fatalities in the initial attack of acute rheumatic fever are rare and are becoming even more rare with newer methods of detection and treatment.

What are the later effects of rheumatic fever upon the heart?

The most important medical feature of rheumatic fever is the effect it has upon the heart valves. This usually becomes manifest a number of years after the acute attack.

A patient may recover completely from an acute attack of rheumatic fever and, for all practical purposes, appear and feel perfectly normal. However, the initial inflammatory lesion in the valves of the heart may lead to extensive scar tissue formation. As a result of this process, the valves become distorted, damaged, and incapable of performing their duties adequately.

The greater the number of attacks of acute rheumatic fever, the more extensively are the heart valves damaged.

How can one tell if he has rheumatic valvular damage?

By complete examination, supplemented, if necessary, by other procedures, such as electrocardiography, fluoroscopy, and x-ray studies.

What is the significance of valvular damage?

a. As previously described, the heart valves are situated between the various chambers and exits of the heart. Their function is to keep the blood circulating in one direction and to enable the work of the heart to be utilized in the most efficient manner by the circulatory system. Depending upon the manner in which the valves are injured and distorted, they may either cause greater resistance to the natural forward flow of blood or they may permit backward leakage of blood from one chamber to the preceding chamber. Both abnormal processes may occur in the same damaged valve.

Because of the defective valves, the heart must work harder to accomplish its work. Eventually, the chambers of the heart become dilated, the heart muscle becomes strained, and the entire organ becomes less and less capable of performing the job required of it. (See Chapter 27, on the Heart.)

b. Injured heart valves are particularly prone to superimposed bacterial infection. The occurrence of this complication results in a bacterial endocarditis, a most serious disease which, until recently, was associated with an extremely high mortality.

c. Patients with rheumatic valvular disease are also prone to form blood clots on the inner lining of the heart. These may, in time, break loose and be carried by the circulation to various parts of the body, where they will cut off the circulation to vital organs and cause profound tissue damage (embolism).

d. Patients with rheumatic valvular disease may develop disorders in the rhythmicity of the heart contractions, such as fibrillation. This will sharply curtail the efficiency of the heart and may lead to heart failure.

Does one attack of rheumatic fever inevitably lead to heart damage?

Not always.

Can heart valves which have been damaged by rheumatic fever be cured?

The damage to the valves cannot be reversed. However, in certain instances surgery may alter the abnormality so that valve function is greatly improved.

What is the likelihood of recurrence of rheumatic fever?

Prior to present day treatment, the incidence of recurrence was approximately 75 per cent when the first attack occurred during early childhood. If the first attack occurred in an older individual, the possibility of recurrence is much less, and recurrence is found rarely among those whose initial attack takes place in adulthood.

What signs warn of the possible presence of rheumatic fever?

a. Unexplained fever.
b. Unexplained joint or muscle pains.
c. The appearance of nodules over bony prominences such as the elbows, back of the hand, feet, kneecaps, skull, spine, and other areas. (The skin can usually be moved over rheumatic nodules.)
d. Peculiar and unexplained skin rashes.
e. Chorea (St. Vitus dance).
f. Recurrent spontaneous nosebleeds.
g. Recurrent abdominal pains.

How long does an attack of chorea last?

An attack usually lasts from several weeks to several months. It usually terminates in complete recovery.

How is chorea related to rheumatic fever?

It is felt that chorea is one of the manifestations of rheumatic fever.

Is rheumatic fever contagious?

No.

What is the treatment of acute rheumatic fever?

a. Bed rest for as long as the attack lasts. This may be for several weeks.
b. Antibiotic drugs, given regularly for an extended period of time.
c. Aspirin in sufficient doses to relieve fever and inflamed joints.
d. Cortisone and/or related drugs, depending upon the severity of the condition and the individual preferences of the attending physician.

Can recurrent attacks of rheumatic fever be prevented?

Experience over the past few years has shown that recurrent attacks of this disease may be cut down or eliminated by giving daily dosages of penicillin, sulfonamides, and other antibiotics to susceptible individuals while they are well.

Is tonsillectomy of any value in the treatment of rheumatic fever?

Usually not. Tonsillectomy is advised only when there is definite evidence of disease within the tonsils, not as a routine procedure for the sake of helping in the treatment of rheumatic fever.

Is the extraction of teeth of benefit to a patient with rheumatic fever?

Usually not, unless the teeth are infected.

What special precautions are necessary for a patient with rheumatic fever who is undergoing dental treatment?

The patient should receive antibiotics and be carefully supervised by his physician. These precautions are carried out to prevent bacteria from lodging on the heart valves.

Is St. Vitus' dance (chorea) a frequent complication of rheumatic fever?

Yes, especially among children.

What are the symptoms of St. Vitus' dance?

The child gets very irritable and nervous, with periods of elation and depression. Along with this, there are the characteristic purposeless, jerky movements of muscles of the arms, legs and face.

How long does an attack of St. Vitus' dance usually last?

It may last for several weeks or months, but will invariably subside spontaneously.

Does an attack of St. Vitus' dance leave permanent brain damage?

No.

Is recovery complete after an attack of St. Vitus' dance?

Yes.

Is special treatment necessary for St. Vitus' dance?

Some physicians feel that the giving of cortisone or one of the other of the steroid drugs helps in bringing this condition under control. However, St. Vitus' dance will subside by itself even if treatment is not given. All that will be necessary is to keep the child quiet, have him avoid excitement, and sedate him whenever the symptoms are particularly severe.

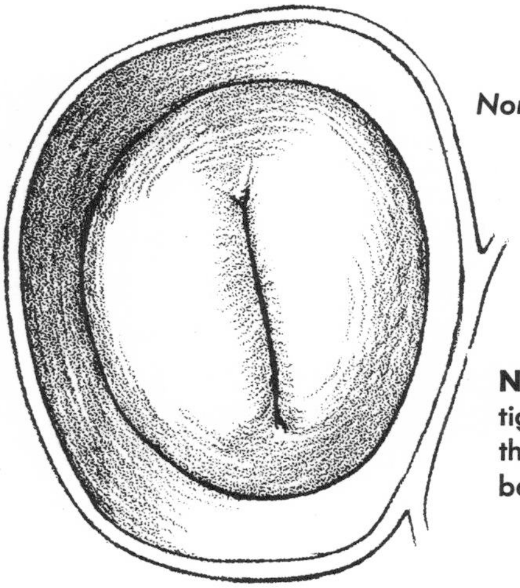

Normal Mitral Valve. This strong, tightly closed mitral valve lies between the atrium and ventricle, the two chambers on the left side of the heart.

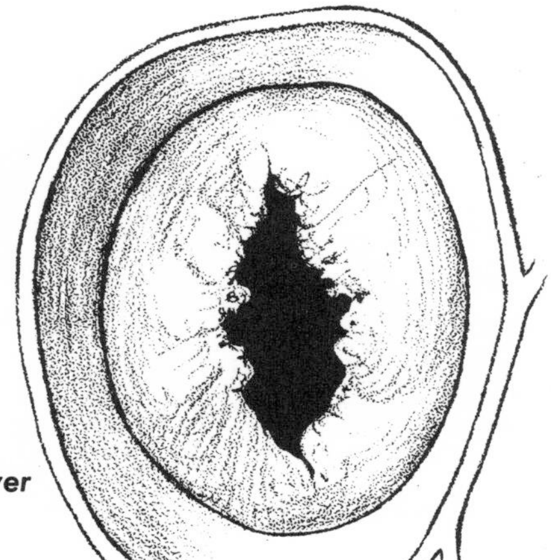

Damaged Mitral Valve. This mitral valve, weakened and distorted by rheumatic fever, is subject to infection, and will cause the heart to work harder.

CHAPTER 59

The Salivary Glands

(See also Chapter 18 on Contagious Diseases; Chapter 36 on Lips, Jaws, Mouth, Teeth, and Tongue)

Where are the salivary glands, and what is their function?

The salivary glands are:

a. The parotid glands, located in front of and a little below each ear.
b. The submaxillary glands, located just about an inch in front of and below the angle of the lower jaws.
c. The sublingual glands, which lie in the floor of the mouth under the tongue.

These glands manufacture and secrete saliva which reaches the mouth through ducts (tubes) leading from the glands to the oral cavity.

Are the salivary glands often involved in inflammatory processes or infections?

The parotid glands are involved considerably more often than the other glands, particularly when mumps—a virus infection—is present. In the days before the liberal use of the antibiotic drugs, pus-forming infections of the parotid gland were seen sometimes as a complication of major surgery or in debilitated patients. Such a condition, acute parotitis, is now a rarity.

Do abscesses or infections ever involve the submaxillary glands?

Occasionally, especially when a stone has blocked the submaxillary duct leading into the mouth. Marked swelling, pain, tenderness, and

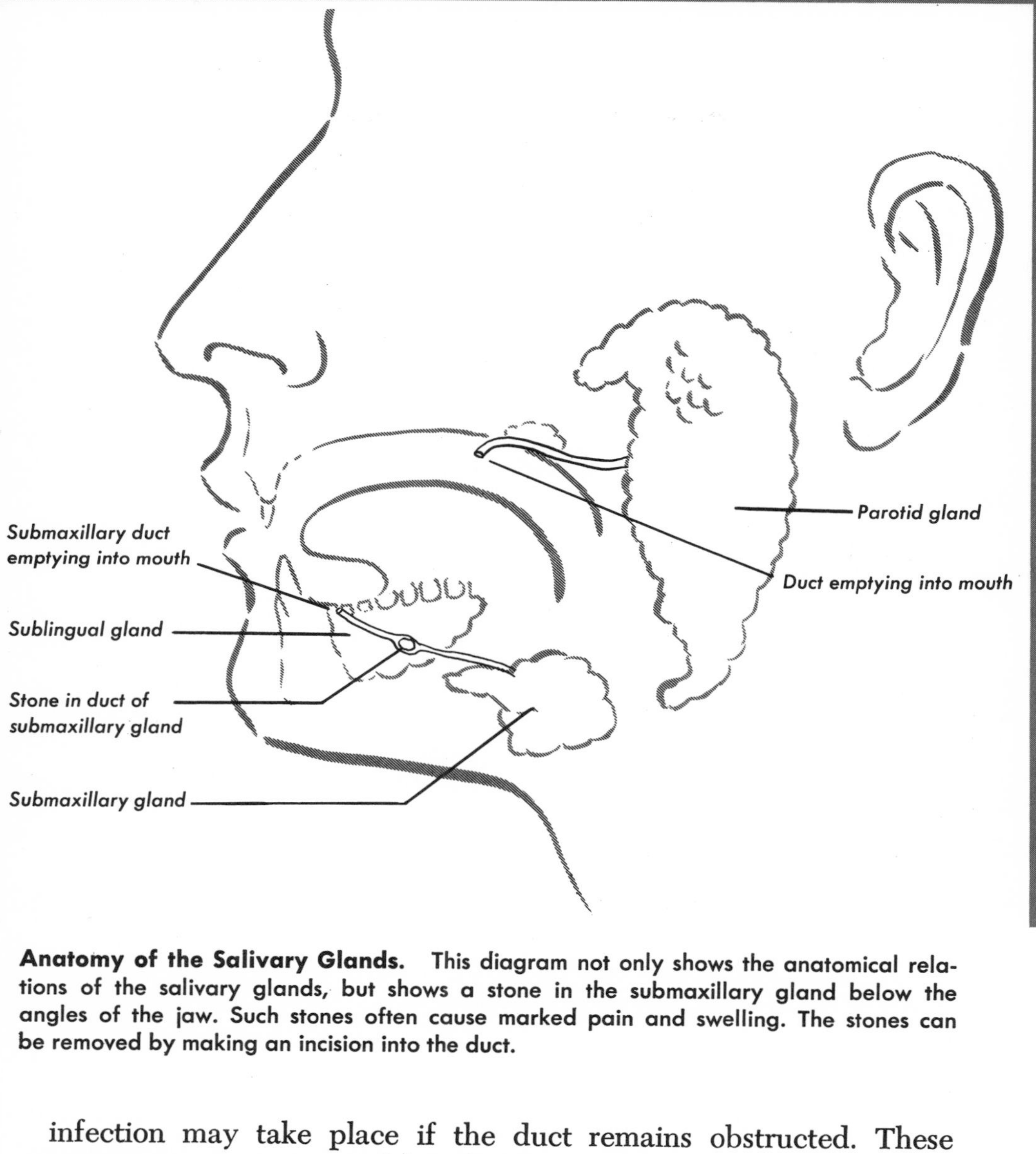

Anatomy of the Salivary Glands. This diagram not only shows the anatomical relations of the salivary glands, but shows a stone in the submaxillary gland below the angles of the jaw. Such stones often cause marked pain and swelling. The stones can be removed by making an incision into the duct.

infection may take place if the duct remains obstructed. These symptoms are aggravated by chewing or eating.

How can one tell if there is a stone blocking the submaxillary duct?

In some instances, the stone can be felt by placing the examining finger within the mouth along the duct. X-ray examination will demonstrate the stone's presence on occasion. In the remainder of cases, the diagnosis must be made by the clinical history and symptoms.

What is done about a stone in one of the salivary ducts?

It should be removed surgically under local anesthesia by making an incision into the duct and lifting out the stone.

Do stones, once removed, have a tendency to recur?

Occasionally.

If an abscess has formed in the submaxillary gland, what treatment is recommended?

Simple incision and drainage of the abscess if it has spread beyond the confines of the gland, or removal of the entire gland if the abscess is localized to the gland itself.

Where is the incision made for the removal of the submaxillary gland?

Beneath the chin and off to the side of the midline. An incision approximately two to three inches long is necessary for the removal of the gland.

Is it ever necessary to remove the parotid gland?

Yes, but only when a tumor has formed, not for abscess formation.

What is the treatment for an abscess within the parotid gland?

Incision and drainage, usually in the hospital under general anesthesia.

SALIVARY GLAND TUMORS

Are tumors of the salivary glands common?

Yes, particularly the so-called "mixed tumors" which involve the parotid gland.

Are tumors of the parotid gland usually malignant?

No. Most parotid tumors are benign, but the gland does often become involved in a cancerous growth.

Do parotid tumors tend to recur once they are removed?

Yes, about one in five may recur even if they are benign.

How can one tell if a salivary tumor is benign or malignant?

The benign tumors grow slowly and usually are surrounded by a capsule. Many of them are freely movable beneath the skin. Malignant tumors of the salivary glands grow rapidly and become adherent to the skin and surrounding tissues. Of course, following removal, microscopic examination will result in a conclusive diagnosis.

Does the removal of one of the salivary glands interfere with digestion or adequate production of saliva?

No.

Are operations upon these glands dangerous?

No, but operations for the removal of parotid tumors are long and tedious to perform. Great care must be exercised to avoid injury to the nerve filaments of the facial nerve which course through the parotid gland. Injury to this nerve will result in a certain amount of facial paralysis.

What anesthesia is used for operations upon the salivary glands?

General anesthesia for the major surgical procedures; local anesthesia for minor operations.

Where is the incision made for operations on the parotid gland?

In front of the ear and down along the angle of the jaw on to the neck.

Are the operative scars disfiguring following surgery on the parotid or submaxillary glands?

No. Fine thin lines are usually obtained several months later when these wounds have healed completely.

Is it always possible to avoid injury to the facial nerve when operating to remove a tumor of the parotid gland?

No. It is sometimes necessary to disturb or even cut a branch of the nerve when removing an extensive growth of the parotid gland. However, this is not a frequent occurrence, and when it does happen it is excusable on the grounds that the most important consideration is the total removal of the offending tumor.

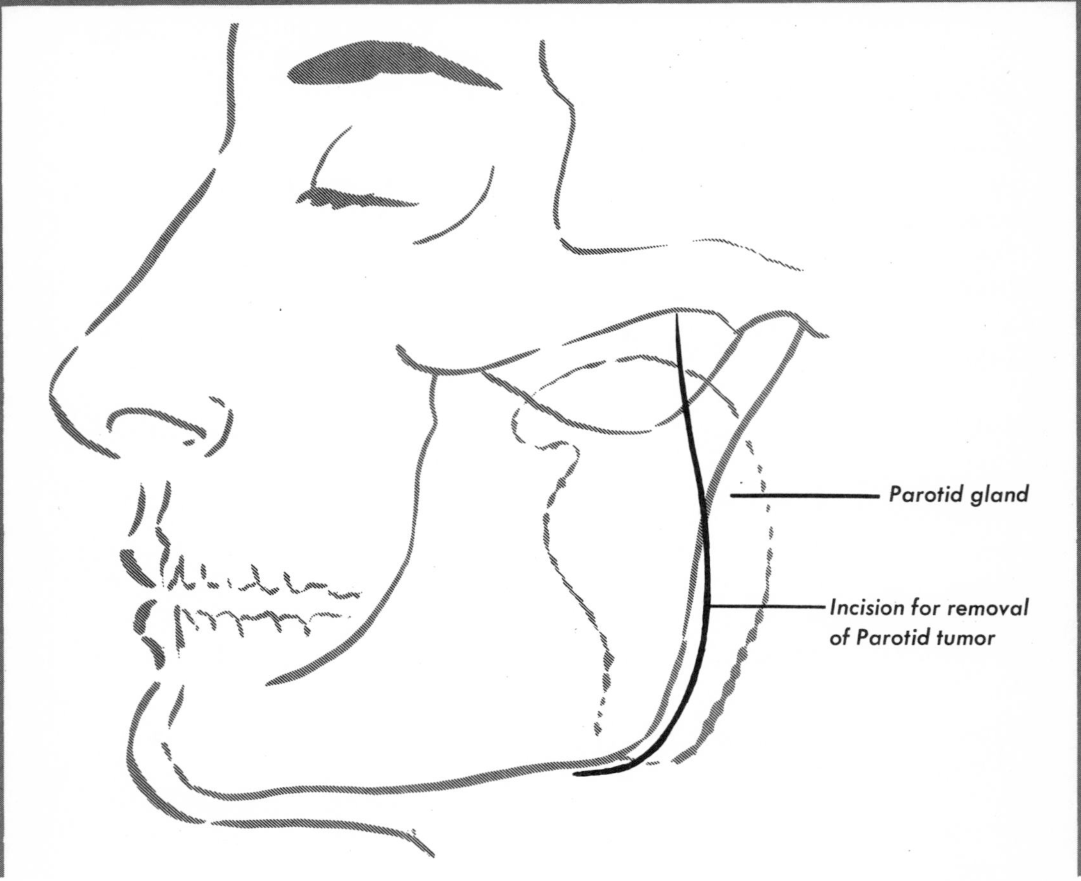

Incision for Operation upon the Parotid Gland. The parotid gland is often the site of tumor formation, and such tumors should be removed. Most cases of parotid tumor can be cured, since these growths are not usually of a high degree of malignancy. While performing the surgery, great care must be exercised not to injure the facial nerve which courses through the gland.

What happens if the facial nerve is injured during the removal of a parotid tumor?

The face becomes partially paralyzed and distorted with a drooping and twisting of one side of the mouth. In rare cases, a branch of the nerve to the eyelid may be injured, and this will interfere with the patient's ability to close his eye completely.

If the facial nerve has been injured, is the face deformity permanent?

More or less, although the deformity tends to become less prominent as time passes.

Can these nerves be repaired successfully once they have been cut?

They are very small in diameter, some being no wider than ordinary sewing thread. It is therefore most difficult to find their ends and sew them together again.

Recently, by means of ingenious muscle and nerve transfers, it has become possible to restore the face to near-normal appearance. To accomplish this, the services of an expert plastic surgeon will be required.

Do the wounds from these operative procedures have a tendency to drain?

Yes. They may drain saliva on to the skin for many days or weeks postoperatively. However, the drainage will eventually subside and the wounds will heal completely.

How soon after the salivary glands are operated upon can one resume eating?

Fluids are taken for the first few days after surgery; then a normal diet may be resumed.

How long a hospital stay is necessary following surgery upon these glands?

Most patients can leave the hospital within a week after surgery.

If a parotid tumor recurs, is it possible to get a cure by reoperation?

Yes. A more extensive removal of parotid tissue will bring about a cure in the great majority of cases.

What is the treatment for a tumor of the submaxillary or sublingual glands?

Complete removal of the gland.

Are operations for tumors of the submaxillary or sublingual glands successful?

Yes, unless the procedure has been carried out for a rapidly growing cancer of these structures. Such malignant involvement is, fortunately, a rare occurrence.

CHAPTER 60

Sex

(See also Chapter 3 on Adolescence; Chapter 17 on Child Behavior; Chapter 24 on Female Organs; Chapter 39 on Male Organs; Chapter 41 on Mental Health and Disease; Chapter 73 on Venereal Disease)

What determines the sex of a child?

The presence or absence of a particular chromosome within the male sperm. The female egg has nothing to do with the determination of sex.

Can sex be predicted before birth?

Only by a rather complicated and somewhat dangerous test, and then only in about three out of four cases. Some of the fluid surrounding the embryo is withdrawn and is submitted to hormone studies. At present, this test is in its experimental stage and is not advocated.

Is there such a thing as changing a person's sex?

No, despite the many newspaper reports to the contrary.

What is a hermaphrodite?

A person born with development of sex organs bearing some of the characteristics of both male and female. It is often necessary to perform an operation to remove a piece of glandular tissue and submit it to microscopic examination to determine whether it is of ovarian or testicular origin. There are also certain examinations of blood cells and skin which will help indicate whether the person is predominantly male or female.

What is a pseudohermaphrodite?

A person who possesses the sex gland (ovary or testicle) of one sex, but whose secondary sex organ (penis or vagina) has been modified by excesses or deficiencies of certain hormones.

At what age should children be told the "facts of life"?

There is no special age, but when they ask questions they should be answered honestly and without signs of embarrassment. It is unwise to avoid their questions, and it is equally unwise to give them more information than they seek or to give them incorrect information.

If children touch their genitals repeatedly, should it be stopped or should it be ignored?

It is natural for children to touch themselves in this area, but if it becomes an excessive habit, consult your physician. It may indicate an emotional disturbance; or it may be due to local irritation. Do not threaten or punish your child because of this habit, as it may create neurotic guilt feelings.

What should be the parent's attitude toward the child who masturbates?

It is perhaps wisest for the parent to ignore this practice unless it occurs in a child who is emotionally disturbed or unstable. In such event, the parent should seek medical advice. It is unwise to threaten or punish children for masturbation.

Does masturbation cause sexual difficulties in adult life?

No, but unhealthy and erroneous attitudes about it may interfere with healthy sexual expression.

Does any physical or mental harm of a permanent nature result from masturbation?

No, unless the practice is accompanied by an excessive sense of guilt. Then it may lead to emotional disturbance.

Is sexual contact essential for normal living?

No. It is a common belief that sexual intercourse is a necessary component of normal adult living. Some people live happy, fruitful lives in a completely celibate state. However, in many cases, lack of sexual contact is part of, or the result of, an emotional disturbance.

Can physical or mental harm result from a lack of sexual contact?

Many maladjusted people erroneously attribute their unhappiness to lack of sex contacts, when in fact the lack of sexual contact may be the product of the maladjustment.

What part do the hormones play in one's sexual desires?

Hormones, along with the psychological attitude, play a significant role in conditioning an individual toward sexual experiences; that is, hormones stimulate desire.

Is it true that the early development of sexual attitudes will determine, to a great extent, the subsequent patterns of adult sexual behavior?

Definitely, yes!

Physiologically, what is the age of maximum sexual activity for the male and the female?

According to some investigators, the teen years constitute the period of greatest activity for males, whereas the late thirties and early forties are the years of greatest sexual urge in females.

Do men normally have a greater sexual desire than women?

Not biologically, but women are inhibited by social dogmas and therefore tend to suppress their desires more than men.

Does a person's desire for sex vary from time to time, or does a person who is uninterested tend to remain uninterested throughout life?

No. Sexual desire may vary greatly from time to time.

Is there a change in sexual desire in women after menopause?

There may be considerable increase in libido (sex desire) after menopause.

Does the removal of the uterus and tubes and ovaries alter a woman's sexual desire or ability?

No. As a matter of fact, it frequently results in increased desire.

What is nymphomania?

A neurotic form of behavior in women in which there is excessive sexual desire and activity without actual gratification.

What is the significance of the erotic dream?

It is a normal phenomenon, occurring most often in adolescence and early adulthood.

Should someone with a serious heart condition limit sexual activity?

Yes, as it may place too great a physical strain on the heart. People who have had recent attacks of coronary thrombosis should consult their physician before resuming marital relations.

What diseases can be transmitted through sexual contact?

(See Chapter 73, on Venereal Disease.)

What is meant by the term "oversexed"?

This is a neurotic form of behavior in certain women or men, and is often typified by those who have relations indiscriminately and excessively without accompanying feelings of love or affection. (The word "oversexed" is not a medical or psychiatric term.)

What is meant by the term "undersexed"?

There are many people whose interests in life include little desire for physical relations. The term "undersexed" is, therefore, a purely relative term, of little meaning.

What is frigidity?

Lack of sexual desire and lack of sexual responsiveness.

What causes frigidity?

It is almost always an emotional phenomenon which has its origin in neurotic attitudes toward sex. Many of these attitudes begin in early childhood, and as one matures they lie deep in the individual's unconscious memories, where they continue to exert an important influence upon his or her emotions and behavior.

Does frigidity have any influence on one's ability to bear children?

None whatever. It is a common misconception that women must attain climax in order to conceive.

Is there a satisfactory treatment for frigidity?

Psychotherapy may be helpful, but the therapy must be intensive and prolonged.

What is impotence?

The inability of the male to consummate the sex act.

Is impotence caused by physical or mental disturbance?

In the great majority of cases, it is caused by an emotional or mental disturbance. However, it is important that possible physical causes be ruled out by a thorough medical examination.

At what age in life do men usually become impotent?

This varies markedly. Many men are potent and fertile in their seventies and eighties.

What is the treatment for impotence?

In the vast majority of cases, psychotherapy is indicated. Only rarely is impotence of physical or glandular origin, except in men in their later years of life.

Is the use of hormones successful in the treatment of impotence?

Usually not, unless the patient is quite advanced in age or unless there is a definite hormone deficiency. By far the greatest cause of impotence in men under sixty to seventy years is psychological or emotional, and will not respond to hormones or medication.

What is the difference between impotence and sterility in men?

Impotence is the inability to have sexual relations. Sterility means the inability to fertilize an egg. Some men may be potent but sterile; others may be fertile but impotent.

What causes homosexuality?

It is generally conceded to be a neurosis arising from emotional problems and attitudes within the home during early childhood. The development of homosexuality hinges upon the relationship of the child to the parents and to brothers and sisters.

Is homosexuality a physical defect?

No. People are not born homosexuals. It is essentially an environmentally determined abnormality and is classified as a neurosis.

Are homosexual tendencies inherited?

No.

How early in life can one detect a homosexual tendency?

It sometimes can be detected during early adolescence.

What should be done if homosexual tendencies appear in a young person?

Such a person should be referred to a competent psychiatrist for intensive treatment.

Is homosexuality a curable condition?

Yes, in certain cases, after intensive and prolonged psychiatric treatment. Results are better with the young patient.

Can a normal person be persuaded to become a homosexual?

Only if the neurotic tendency has existed in a latent form. Also, if circumstances are such as to deprive him of normal sexual outlets for prolonged periods.

Is homosexuality on the increase today?

It is not thought to be. However, homosexual individuals hide their attitudes today much less than heretofore. Thus, the public gets the impression that homosexuality is on the increase.

MARITAL RELATIONS

Is it wise to seek medical advice on sex matters before marriage?

Yes. All couples should consult with their family doctor before marrying. Many young people harbor erroneous information and ideas about sex which cause unfounded fears and which interfere, at times, with healthy marital adjustment.

Can a doctor tell, on physical examination, whether a young couple will be physically suited to one another?

It is exceedingly rare that two people are anatomically or physically "unsuited" to one another. Almost all incompatibility is psychological in origin, not physical!

Can prolonged sexual inhibitions and sexual misinformation during youth and early adulthood be harmful to a mature marital relationship?

Yes. Children and adolescents should be as well informed on sex matters as they should be about any other important phase of living. Failure to educate them properly in sex matters may lead to unhappy marriages and sexual maladjustment in adult life.

Where can one obtain information of a reliable nature on sexual subjects?

Write to the American Medical Association Information Service in Chicago. They will send you excellent material on the subject.

Is the first sex act always very painful for a woman?

No. There may be some pain, but a tender attitude on the part of the man and proper premarital instruction may avoid a great deal of pain.

Do virgins always bleed upon first contact?

No. This is a common misconception.

What is the most common cause of sexual incompatibility?

Psychological disturbance in either or both of the partners.

Can sexual incompatibility be effectively treated?

Yes, by psychotherapy.

Is a simultaneous climax necessary for a well-adjusted marital relationship?

No, but it is desirable. Many young couples can learn, over a period of time, to attain this state.

Does the failure of a wife to reach climax indicate that she does not love her husband?

No.

Is it natural for men to reach a climax more rapidly than women?

Yes, usually.

Is it harmful for people to have incomplete sexual relations?

Yes, because it interrupts a process which normally should reach completion.

Can excessive marital relations be harmful to general health?

It depends on one's definition of "excessive." Harm may arise when one or both parties to the marriage is maladjusted. If both are happy and content, there is no such thing as "too much love."

Is there a normal frequency of marital relations?

No.

Is there a normal pattern of sexual behavior for married people?

There is no definite pattern. Whatever gives the two people the most happiness is appropriate and normal for them. This involves wide variations in sexual practices and frequency of lovemaking.

Can a man and wife be incompatible because of physical differences in anatomical structure?

No.

Can marital relations be consummated during menstruation without harmful effects?

Yes. However, it is often considered unpleasant.

Is it possible to become pregnant without actually having intercourse?

This occurs only in exceedingly rare instances. When it does take place, sperm must of necessity be deposited in large numbers in and around the vaginal orifice. (Of course, it does *not* take place from kissing, or from bathing in the same tub that a man has recently used.)

What is dyspareunia?

Painful intercourse.

Is painful intercourse a physical or psychological condition?

It is usually psychological, but sometimes may have physical components if the female has an inflammation or abscess or mechanical pelvic abnormality.

Is there any effective treatment for dyspareunia?

Yes. Psychotherapy, if the condition is emotional in origin; medical treatment of the physical condition, if physical factors are present.

What constitutes sexual abnormality in a marital relationship?

This is most difficult to answer. What is considered perverse in one society is considered normal in another society. The primary gauge should be the happiness of the couple and their mutual agreement on sex practices. Most physicians agree that if a couple is happy in their life together, their practices fall within that broad but poorly defined classification of "normal."

CHAPTER 61

Skin and Subcutaneous Tissues

(See also Chapter 2 on Abscesses and Infections; Chapter 7 on Allergy; Chapter 16 on Cancer; Chapter 18 on Contagious Diseases; Chapter 25 on First Aid; Chapter 47 on Parasites and Parasitic Diseases; Chapter 73 on Venereal Disease)

Does diet influence complexion?

Yes. Certain foods may aggravate existing skin conditions. However, this does not always apply. People can be guided best by their own experience and by medical advice.

Are cosmetics harmful to the skin?

When used judiciously on a normal skin they are not harmful and, in fact, may even be helpful. However, in certain skin conditions, cosmetics can do harm, particularly when they produce plugging of the skin pores or when people are allergic to certain cosmetics.

Does massage help skin tone?

In some conditions massage is helpful, in others it may be harmful. It is important to secure medical advice before submitting to skin massage.

Are skin creams ever beneficial?

Yes, in certain skin conditions characterized by dryness. However, skin creams should be prescribed by a physician, as there are ingredients in some of the commercial products which may be harmful to certain skins.

Are the "hormone" creams ever beneficial to the skin?

In some instances. However, these medications should be used only on a doctor's prescription.

Is sun-tanning beneficial to one's skin and health?

Not particularly. As a matter of fact, more harm than good comes from overexposure to the sun.

What harm can come from overexposure to the sun?

An actual burn may result. Also, certain tendencies toward development of skin tumors may be aggravated by repeated *overexposure* to the rays of the sun. Then, too, there are skin diseases which can result directly from sun sensitivity.

What can be done to prevent skin wrinkles?

Nothing. Wrinkles can be treated by plastic surgery in certain cases, but the benefit is usually of a temporary nature.

Are the commercial products safe and useful in the treatment of cracking skin and chapped hands?

Yes; some are quite efficient.

Can one prevent the formation of "brown spots" which appear on the face as one grows older?

No, but some of these can be removed easily without leaving any blemishes.

Is there any relationship between the condition of the hair, fingernails, and skin?

Yes. The nails and hair are actually part of the skin, in the general sense of the term.

Are clay packs and mud baths beneficial to the skin?

Psychologically, they give many people a feeling of improved skin and well being.

Is the careful use of ultraviolet rays beneficial to people without skin difficulties?

Only insofar as being sun-tanned gives them a sense of improved health. Actually, there is no physical benefit, and care must be exercised not to produce a severe burn!

Are skin conditions ever caused by a lack of vitamins in the diet?

Occasionally. Consult your physician for a general checkup and he will tell you if vitamins need be taken.

Is there any specific treatment for excessively large pores in the skin of the face?

No, except that the face should be kept clean so that the pores are less noticeable.

ACNE

What is acne?

A condition characterized by the appearance of blackheads and pimples on the face and frequently the chest and back. It occurs most often in adolescents and young adults.

Is it normal for adolescents to have a mild degree of acne?

Yes.

What causes acne?

To the best of our knowledge, the condition represents a disturbance in glandular function in the skin due to changes in certain hormone secretions.

Does acne always require treatment?

Many mild forms require no treatment. If the pimples and blackheads are numerous and the patient is physically and psychologically disturbed by their presence, treatment is very important.

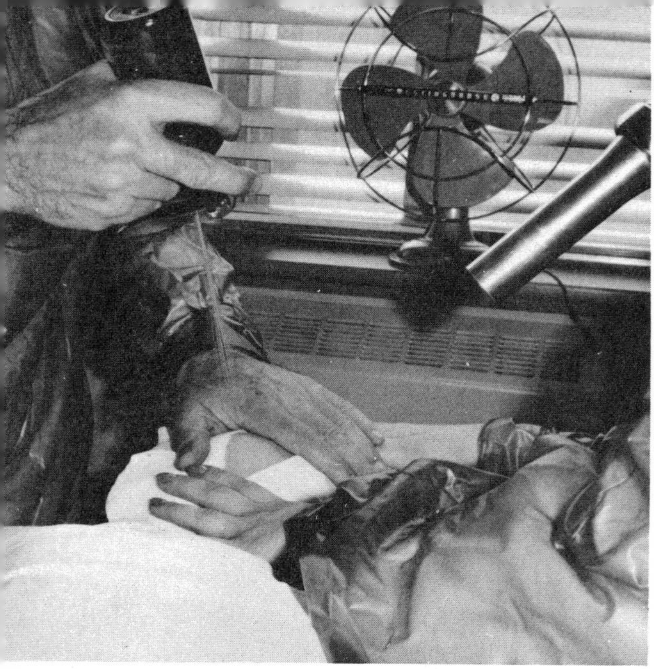

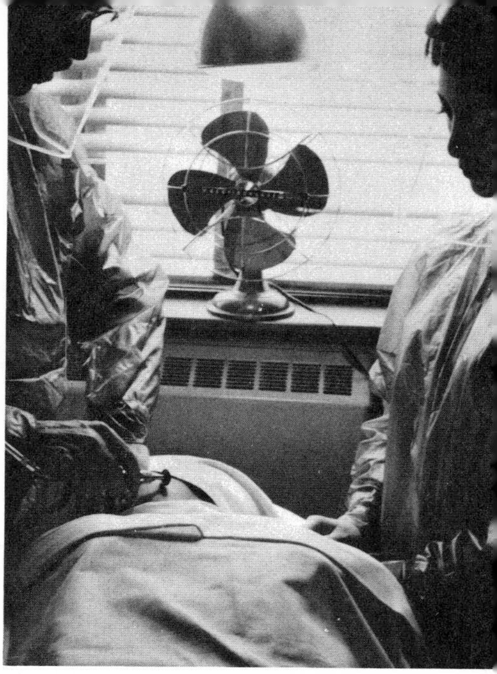

Application of Skin Anesthetic (Ethyl Chloride) Prior to Skin Planing. Skin planing or dermabrasion is a new method for treating the scars left by acne. In many cases, the skin can be smoothed out.

Skin Planing. In this photograph, (above right) the patient is about to have the abrasive wheel applied to the skin surface.

Below: Close-up View of Skin Planing. Several treatments are usually necessary to get the desired result, and it will take the skin anywhere from a few days to a few weeks to heal.

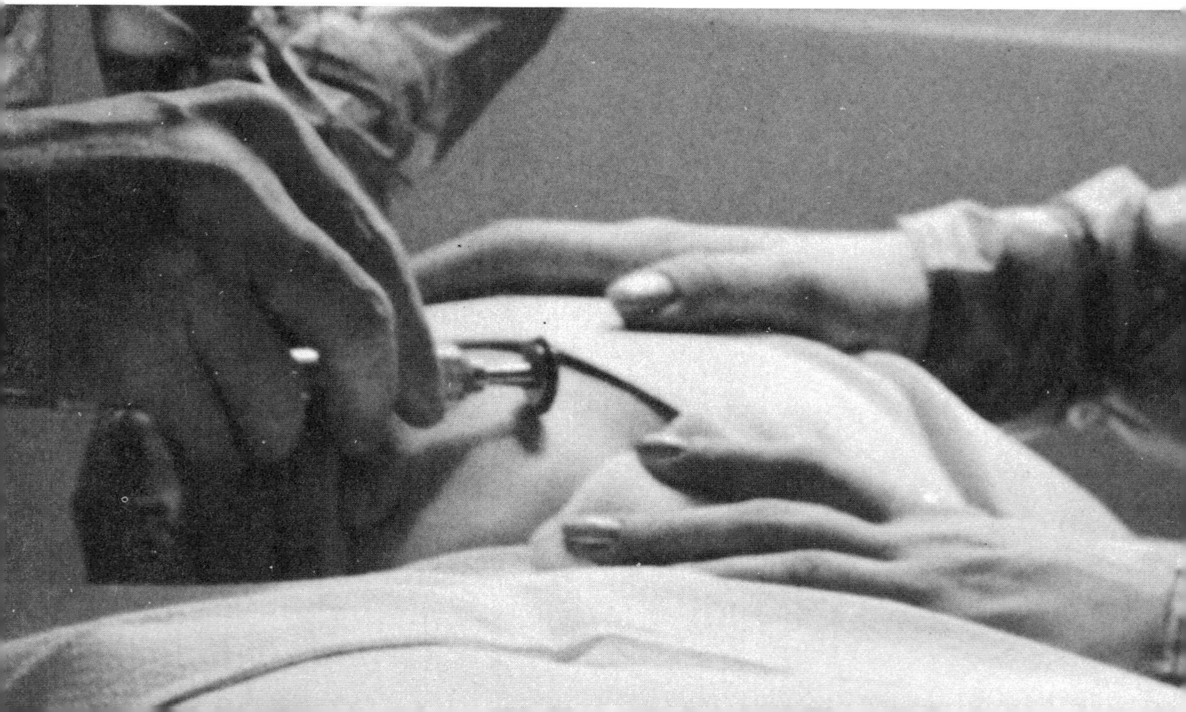

Is acne curable?

Proper management can, in the great majority of cases, produce either a marked improvement or complete cure.

Is it dangerous to squeeze blackheads?

Yes, if done improperly. Your physician should give instructions as to the exact method of carrying out this procedure.

Is it important for the patient with acne to wash his face frequently with soap and water?

Yes. The regular use of a proper cleansing agent three to four times a day is very helpful. However, some skins are extremely sensitive and care must be exercised not to cause irritation.

Is sunlight helpful for acne?

Yes. The condition improves considerably during those months in which exposure to sun is increased.

Are ultraviolet treatments beneficial?

Yes. Such treatments should be carried out under a doctor's supervision.

Are x-ray treatments beneficial in the treatment of acne?

X-ray treatment is very effective in certain resistant forms of acne but is used conservatively today by most dermatologists because of their increasing concern with unnecessary exposure to x-ray radiation. Patients with acne should be treated with other methods first, with x-ray therapy reserved as a last resort for those who do not respond to other methods.

Does acne leave scars on the skin?

In many cases, when treated properly, little scarring remains. However, in some patients scarring may be a very serious problem, particularly because of the bad psychological effect upon the patient.

What is the treatment for acne scars?

In the last few years, a technique of *skin planing* (dermabrasion) has been developed. This consists of grinding away the superficial layers of the skin down to the bottom of the scar. When the skin heals, either the scar is gone or the pitting of the skin is diminished, so that the general appearance is considerably improved.

How is skin planing carried out?

With an abrasion machine which revolves and scrapes off the superficial layers of skin.

Is skin planing a painful procedure?

No, because the skin is anesthetized with a local anesthetic while the planing is being performed.

IMPETIGO

What is impetigo?

Impetigo is a contagious infection of the skin which occurs most often in children, but may also occur in adults.

Is it very contagious?

Yes.

What does impetigo look like?

It begins as a blister which rapidly changes to a crust. The spots are seen, as a rule, on the exposed parts of the body, such as the face and hands.

How is impetigo treated?

With ointments containing one of the antibiotic drugs.

Are these ointments effective in curing impetigo?

Yes. Cure will result within a few days.

What precautions should be taken to avoid spread of impetigo to other members of the family?

Each individual should use his own towel, his own eating utensils, and should sleep in a bed by himself.

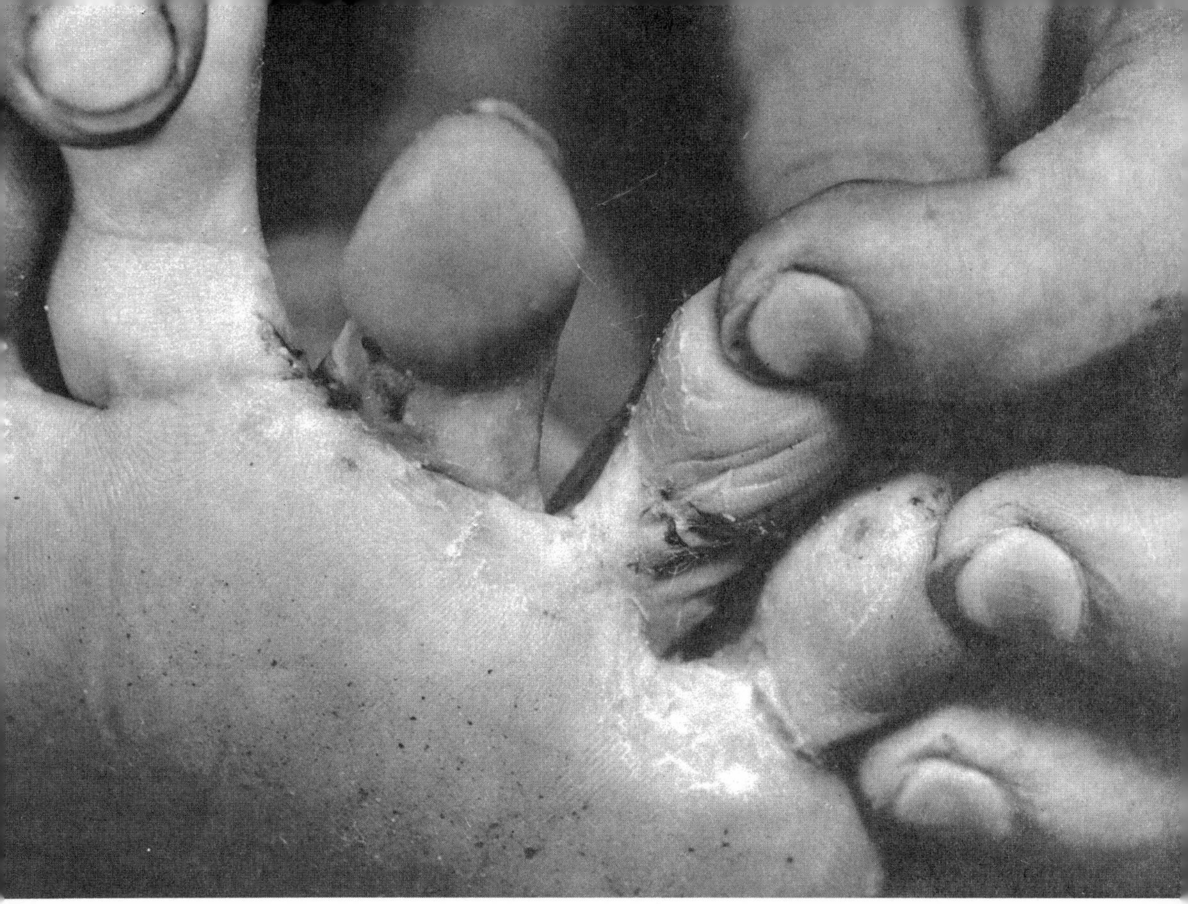

Typical Athlete's Foot Infection (Tinea Pedis). This picture demonstrates how the fungus of athlete's foot grows in between the toes. This particular picture shows a mild case.

ATHLETE'S FOOT

What is athlete's foot?

A fungus infection of the skin of the feet.

What is a fungus?

A fungus is a very small, microscopic type of plant cell which may grow on the skin and, under certain conditions, may produce an infection.

Is athlete's foot a common condition?

Yes. It is one of the most frequently encountered of all skin conditions.

Is athlete's foot contagious?

Yes, but not highly so.

How can athlete's foot be prevented?

By keeping the feet clean, cool, and dry. This means changing shoes and socks daily. Dry the skin between the toes thoroughly after bathing. Make sure soap between the toes is thoroughly rinsed out before completing the bath.

Why do some people have repeated attacks of athlete's foot?

This is usually due to poor foot hygiene. However, there may be a focus of infection in one of the toenails. Unless such a focus is cleared up, recurrences (particularly during warm weather) may be anticipated.

Does athlete's foot ever spread to other parts of the body, such as the hands or groin?

Yes.

What is the treatment for athlete's foot?

There are several highly effective fungicidal preparations which will control athlete's foot. Some fungus infections can be cured by internal medication which, of course, should be given only under the doctor's supervision.

ECZEMA

What is eczema?

This is a general term used to describe an itching, oozing inflammation of the skin.

What part of the body is most often affected?

The hands, but other parts of the body may also become involved.

What is housewife's eczema?

This is an irritation of the hands, usually due to the excessive or careless use of detergents and other chemicals used in the routine of housework.

Acne. Acne is perhaps the most commonly encountered of all skin conditions and is seen most frequently in adolescents and young adults. The characteristic lesions show small abscesses and infected sebaceous cysts.

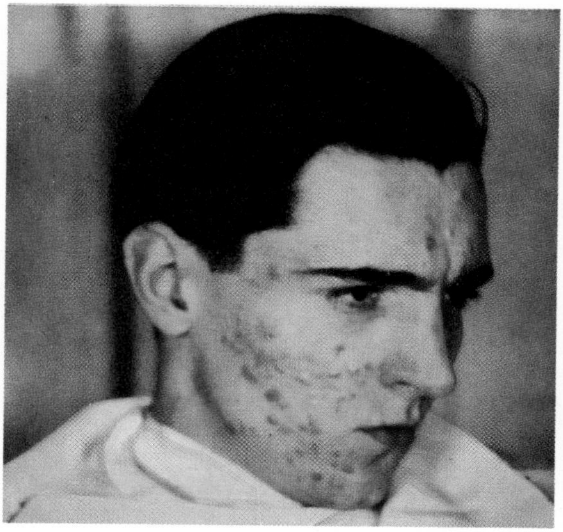

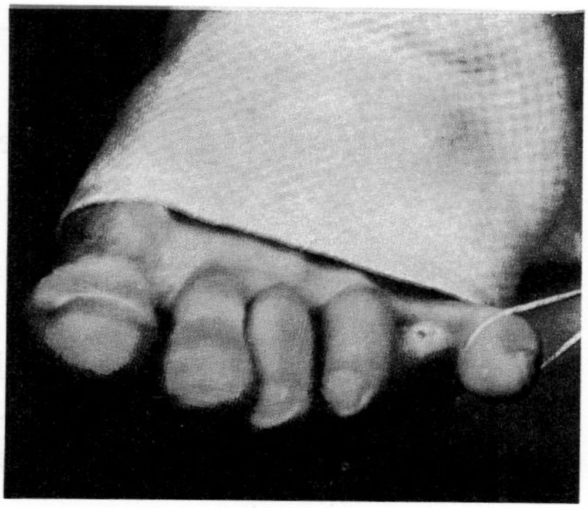

Athlete's Foot. This photograph demonstrates a somewhat more severe case of athlete's foot. There are many preparations today which can relieve this condition, but it has a tendency to recur even after it has been eradicated.

Impetigo. The characteristic lesion shows superficial crusts, which often separate and leave a raw base. Impetigo often occurs on the face but also affects other parts of the body. It can be cured quite quickly now with the application of antibiotic ointments. Impetigo is very contagious and has often caused epidemics in infant nurseries.

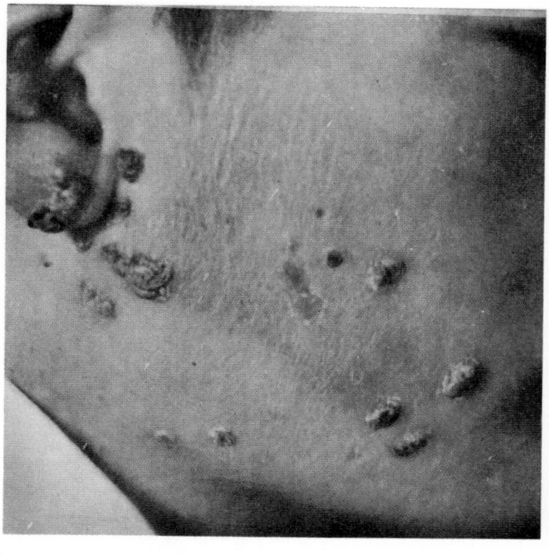

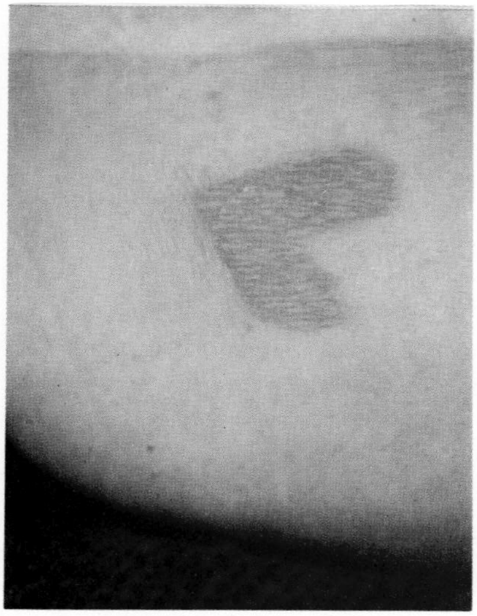

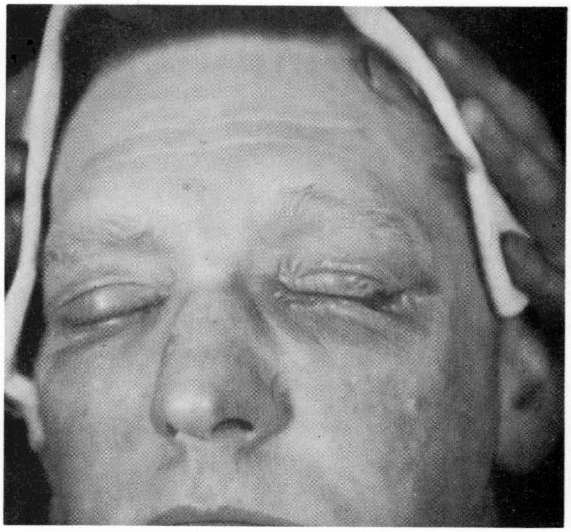

Contact Eczema. The reaction (above left) is due to sensitivity to lipstick which has been applied, as a test, to the skin of the arm; the reaction (above right) is due to sensitivity to an eye lotion. If the offending medication or substance is withdrawn, most contact eczema disappears spontaneously within a few days.

Shingles (Herpes Zoster). Herpes Zoster or shingles is a skin eruption thought to be due to a virus infection of a nerve. It is seen commonly on the chest or abdomen and may cause sufficient pain and discomfort in its early pre-eruptive stages to be mistaken for a more serious disease.

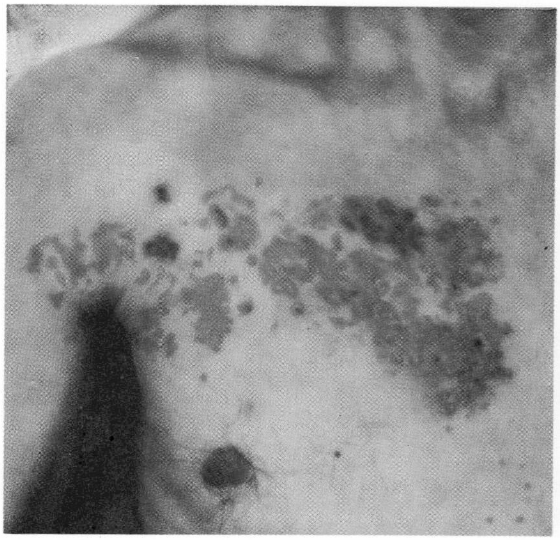

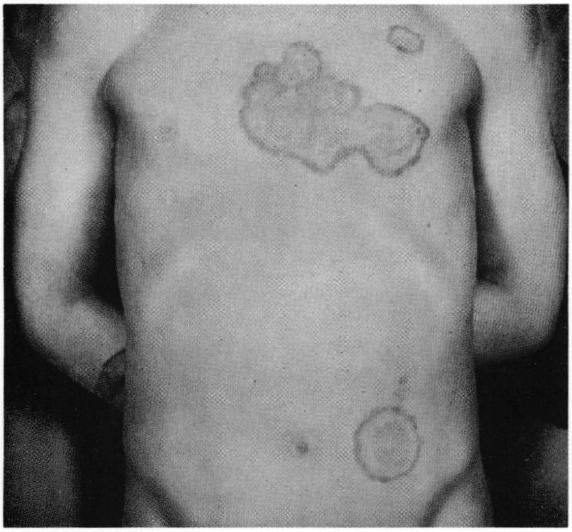

Typical Ringworm Infection (Tinea Corporis). Ringworm is a rather common skin condition, especially in children. The lesion is caused by a fungus. One of the favorite sites for ringworm is the groin.

Alopecia Areata. The bald area in alopecia is perfectly smooth, clean, shiny, and contains no stubble of hair. Alopecia comes on rather abruptly, lasts for several months, and then may disappear spontaneously. Treatment is sometimes of value.

Psoriasis. Psoriasis is a very common skin disease, and it tends to last off and on for many years. Characteristically, the rash is seen on the knees and elbows, but it also affects the trunk. Fortunately, itching is not a marked feature in this condition. Some of the newer drugs are helpful in causing a remission or disappearance of the rash for lengthy periods of time, but recurrence is the general rule.

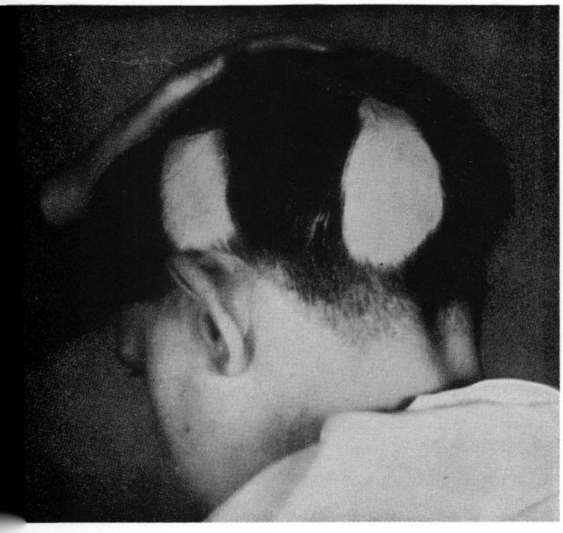

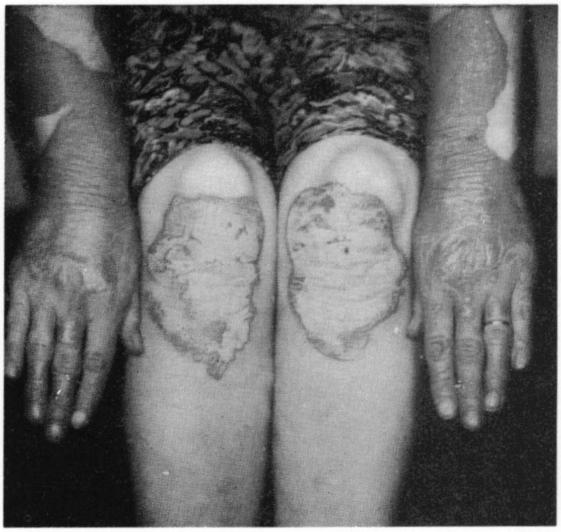

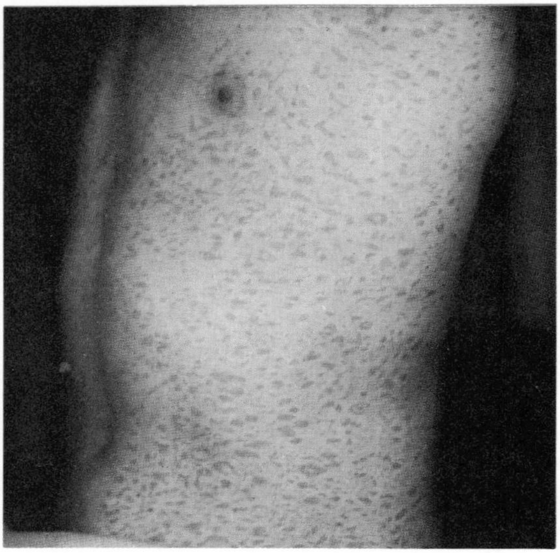

Pityriasis Rosea. This is a common skin eruption which lasts four to six weeks and then disappears by itself. It affects the trunk, the upper arms and thighs. Although its cause is unknown, it may be a systemic disease because it is often accompanied by temperature rises and a feeling of malaise.

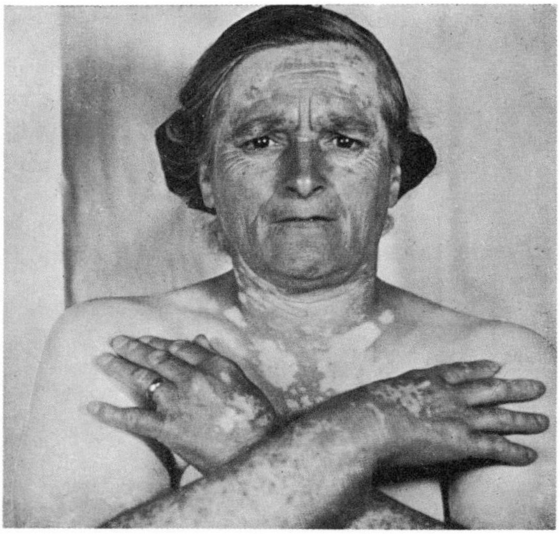

Vitiligo. This condition is characterized by spotty loss of pigment in the skin. Skin texture remains perfectly normal. Women with vitiligo upon exposed surfaces often use cosmetics to make the skin tones blend more naturally.

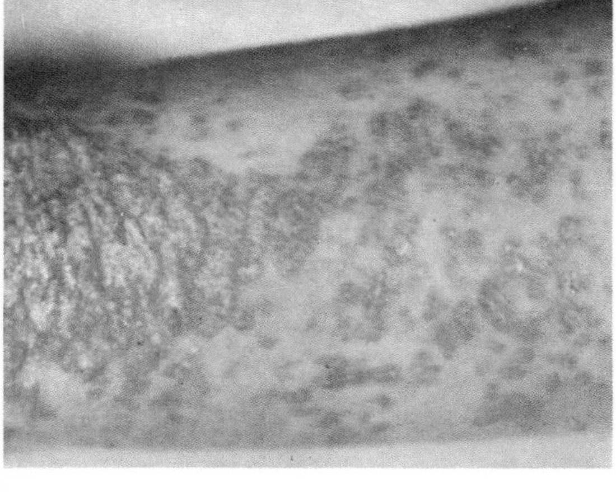

Lichen Planus. This disease often affects the limbs and is characterized by discrete, reddish, plaque-like areas with normal skin in between. There may also be milky white spots in the lining of the mouth.

Do the majority of women develop eczema from detergents?

No. Most women have a skin which is resistant to the irritative effects of the common detergents.

What precautions should one take to avoid housewife's eczema?

a. If the hands are known to be sensitive, it is a good idea to use rubber gloves with a cotton lining while doing work involving contact with these chemicals.
b. Do not wear gloves more than fifteen minutes at a time.
c. Avoid the use of excessive hot water while wearing gloves.
d. Turn the gloves inside-out every two or three days to allow them to dry thoroughly.

Is the use of protective creams important or helpful in the prevention and management of this condition?

Yes, but it is advisable that the creams be prescribed by a physician. No two skins are exactly alike, and certain creams which may be helpful for one person, may be harmful for another.

BATHING AND THE SKIN

How often should people bathe?

People with dry skin will find that excessive bathing may irritate their skin and cause unnecessary itching during cold weather. Such people rarely should bathe more than once or twice a week. However, if one's occupation involves exposure to excessive dirt, more frequent bathing will, of course, be necessary.

What can those with sensitive skins do to cut down on skin irritation resulting from bathing?

Special soaps can be used which may prove very helpful.

How can those who must restrict their bathing to once or twice a week keep their bodies clean?

Simple water baths, without soaping, may be taken more frequently.

Is the skin less sensitive to bathing during warm weather?

Yes.

PERSPIRATION AND BODY ODORS

What causes excessive sweating?

This is usually a manifestation of an unstable circulation or a nervous overactivity of the sweat glands in the skin. It is very common in adolescents and young adults.

Does excessive sweating require treatment?

As a rule, no. However, if the skin shows signs of being irritated or damaged by the excessive sweating, then certain preparations may be used to offset it.

Are the patented advertised deodorants helpful in stopping perspiration and perspiration odors?

Yes, but people with sensitive skins must guard against irritation from these preparations.

What causes body odors?

Certain bacteria, acting on sweat, form substances which are odoriferous. Some detergents contain a chemical which destroys these bacteria and thus does away with the offensive odor.

"COLD SORES"

(*Herpes*)

What are "cold sores"?

Cold sores (herpes) represent a virus infection of the skin. They occur usually on the face, particularly around the lips.

What causes repeated attacks of this type of infection?

Some people seem to get recurrences whenever the skin of the face is overheated. This may occur following exposure to wind or sun, during the course of other infections with fever, or in association with a menstrual period. When there is excessive exposure to sun or wind, cold sores may be prevented by applying protective ointments.

"SHINGLES"

(*Herpes Zoster*)

What is shingles?

A virus infection of the skin which appears along the course of one of the nerves—most often around the chest.

Is this condition very painful?

Yes. Several days after the onset of pain, a rash appears along the line of the nerve. It is the combination of the pain and the appearance of a typical rash which makes the diagnosis apparent.

How long does shingles usually last?

The rash usually lasts two to four weeks. However, the pain may last longer—for several weeks or more.

Is shingles contagious?

No.

Is this condition serious?

Not as a rule. However, in some cases the pain may last for several weeks or months after the rash has gone and may be very severe.

What is the treatment for shingles?

There is no specific treatment for this condition. Relief of pain with appropriate drugs is the most important measure to be taken.

Does shingles eventually disappear by itself?

Yes.

RINGWORM

What is ringworm?

A fungus infection of the skin due to a small microscopic plant.

Are there different types of ringworm?

Yes. When ringworm involves the scalp it is known as tinea capitis; when it involves the feet it is known as athlete's foot; when it occurs on the body it is known as tinea corporis; in the groin it is known as tinea cruris.

Is ringworm contagious?

Yes, to a certain extent. It is not as communicable as some of the contagious diseases, such as measles, chickenpox, etc. However, in a family where one person has ringworm, certain simple precautions like the use of one's own towels, slippers, etc., is advisable.

Is there an ointment which will cure all types of ringworm?

No. The treatment of ringworm depends entirely upon the particular type as well as the individual in whom it occurs.

Can ringworm be cured?

Yes. Medication given by mouth, especially in scalp ringworm, has been able to shorten the treatment considerably. This, however, must be done under the doctor's supervision.

How is scalp ringworm recognized?

As a rule, it occurs only in children. Small spots on the scalp where the hair has fallen out or broken off should arouse one's suspicions. There is a special lamp (Wood's light) which causes infested hairs to light up or "fluoresce," thus helping to establish the diagnosis.

Is ringworm a very serious condition?

No, inasmuch as it does not endanger life, but every attempt should be made to clear it up and to prevent recurrences.

THE HAIR

Is there any satisfactory treatment for baldness?

Baldness may be of several different types. A proper diagnosis as to the type of baldness is important, as certain types cannot be helped. Your physician can advise you if you have the kind of condition which will respond to treatment. Don't waste money on advertised patent medicines or so-called "cures"!

Is baldness inherited?

Not directly, but one does inherit a tendency toward becoming bald.

Do the medicines so widely advertised to the public actually help in growing hair on bald heads?

No.

Does scalp massage help baldness?

The cause of the baldness determines whether such massage will be beneficial, and only your doctor can advise you accurately.

What is alopecia?

Alopecia is a technical term used to describe loss of hair.

Are there different types of alopecia?

Yes. One type, alopecia areata, is a patchy loss of hair which is unrelated to the usual types of baldness.

How does one treat the ordinary type of baldness occurring in young men?

Examination of the scalp is the first important step. If there is any disease of the scalp itself, correction of such a condition may often prevent the further loss of hair.

Does the appearance of premature gray hair or premature baldness have any significance as to general health?

None whatever. It is often a family trait and has nothing to do with premature aging or length of life.

Does cutting or shaving the hair make it grow in heavier?

No. This is a common misconception.

How often should the hair be shampooed?

This varies with the individual. Some people require frequent shampooing, two to three times weekly. Others, because of the structure of their hair, would do well to shampoo it no more than once every two weeks.

Can anything be done for excessive growth of hair on a young woman's face or body?

Yes. It can be removed by electrolysis. In some cases, excessive growth of hair is due to a disordered functioning of one of the endocrine glands. For this reason, it is important before embarking upon treatment to investigate the patient's general health.

How is excessive growth of hair on a normal person treated?

Depilatories, if used carefully, may be helpful. However, the most effective method of removing excessive hair is by electrolysis.

What is electrolysis?

A procedure whereby a small needle is introduced into the hair follicle and an electric current is passed through the needle, thus destroying the root of the hair. The hair is then removed by the operator. If done accurately, electrolysis will result in permanent removal.

Is electrolysis dangerous?

Not if performed properly upon skins which can tolerate it.

Does one have to see a physician for electrolysis?

No. There are many competent electrologists who can remove hair properly.

Is it safe to treat hairy moles by electrolysis?

No. A physician's advice is essential before electrolysis is used on moles.

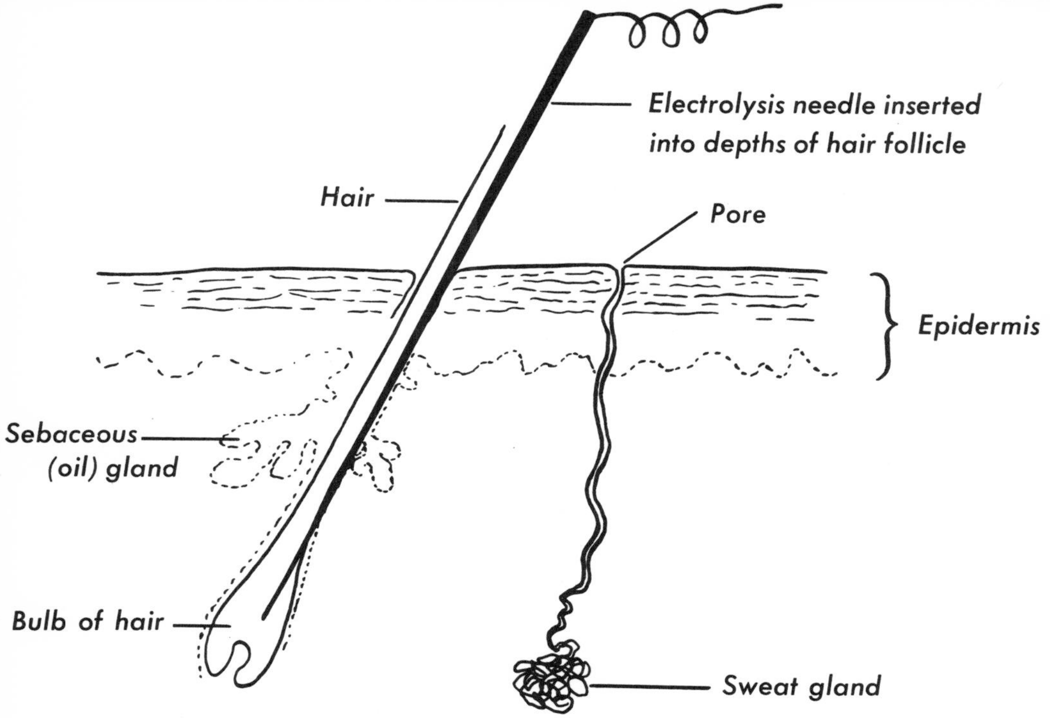

Technique for Electrolysis (Hair Removal). The needle electrode is placed deep into the hair follicle and an electric current is passed through it to destroy the hair and the hair follicle, so that regrowth will not take place.

Is it dangerous to dye the hair?

When the preliminary patch test has been satisfactorily completed to make certain that there is no allergy or sensitivity to the chemicals used, and when the dyeing is done by trained, skilled operators, then it is harmless.

SEBORRHEIC DERMATITIS AND DANDRUFF

What is seborrheic dermatitis?

A skin condition which causes dandruff when it involves the scalp.

What is dandruff?

Dandruff is a term used to describe the appearance of flakes and scales in the scalp. It is due, as a rule, to a disordered functioning of fat glands which nourish the hair.

Is dandruff contagious?

No.

Is there any effective treatment for dandruff?

Yes. Your physician can prescribe certain preparations which will either cure or control this condition.

CHILBLAIN

What is chilblain?

Chilblain is a sensitivity reaction to cold manifested by characteristic red and bluish, blotchy skin changes which appear most frequently on the anterior surface of the legs.

Is chilblain essentially the same as frostbite?

Yes.

Is it necessary to seek medical advice for chilblain?

Yes, because sometimes it is an indication of disturbance in the blood vessels and circulation of the skin.

KELOID

What is a keloid?

A reaction of the skin following a laceration, abrasion, or wound, in which there is excessive scar formation. Instead of a flat, thin white line of healing, there is marked thickening, elevation, and redness of the healed scar.

What causes keloid scar formation?

The cause is unknown. Some people have a type of skin which heals in this manner.

What is the treatment for keloids?

Surgical removal, followed within 24 hours with intensive x-ray radiation to the wound area. This method has resulted in cures in more than 50 per cent of cases. In the remainder, the keloid forms again.

When is a patient most likely to get a good result from the removal of a keloid?

The longer the interval between the development of a keloid and its surgical removal, the better will be the result. It is wise not to remove a keloid until it has been present for at least two years.

Is there any way of knowing in advance whether one will develop keloids following an operation?

No, unless previous operations have been followed by such scars, or if they have appeared following injuries or other conditions.

SCABIES

What is scabies?

A skin condition due to infection with a small parasite or insect.

How does one recognize scabies?

An itching and eruption develops over most of the body. It is worse at night.

Does scabies often affect children?

Yes. It is one of the most common conditions of the skin affecting children. It is usually caught from a schoolmate or playmate.

Does scabies often affect more than one member of a family?

Yes.

Is scabies contagious?

Yes.

Is scabies curable?

Yes. There are medications which can bring about prompt cure.

LICE

What types of lice affect humans?

There are three different forms of lice infestation:

a. Head lice. b. Body lice. c. Genital lice.

How can one recognize head lice?

There are small nits which are seen clinging to the hairs themselves. These nits look like dandruff. However, when one tries to remove them, it becomes apparent that they are tightly adherent to the hair and will not come away like dandruff.

Are there other ways of diagnosing head lice?

Yes. In many cases, in addition to the nits, lice can be seen moving around the scalp and among the hairs.

Is the treatment of head lice difficult?

No. Today there are several preparations which make treatment very simple. Shaving the head is no longer necessary, nor does one have to soak the scalp with some of the old-fashioned foul-smelling preparations which were popular many years ago.

How can one recognize the presence of body lice?

There are scratch marks on the backs of people who have body lice.

Where do body lice live?

Usually in the seams of dirty clothing or underwear, not actually in the skin.

What is the treatment for body lice?

Sterilization of all garments and frequent bathing.

What are "crabs"?

A form of louse infestation which involves the hair around the genitals.

What is the treatment for "crabs"?

There are several ointments which, when applied properly, will bring about prompt cure.

Is this condition contagious?

Yes. It is contracted either by wearing clothing worn by one already infected with the disease, by sexual contact, or by sleeping in the same bed with an individual who is infected.

Must the hair be shaved, in treating "crabs"?

No.

PSORIASIS

What is psoriasis?

A chronic skin disease characterized by reddish, silvery patches and plaques appearing anywhere on the body but having a predilection for the elbows, knees, and scalp.

Can psoriasis be inherited?

There is some evidence that certain families show a higher frequency of this disease than others.

Can psoriasis be cured?

Treatment may be effective in causing the spots to disappear, but they have a tendency to recur from time to time.

Is psoriasis contagious?

No.

Is psoriasis a common skin condition?

Yes. It is one of the most prevalent.

Is there a standard form of treatment for psoriasis?

No. Treatment varies with the individual case and many different methods may be used over a period of months or years.

Does psoriasis tend to get better by itself as one grows older?

No.

Does psoriasis ever shorten or endanger life?

No.

LUPUS

What is lupus?

Lupus is a term used to designate certain skin diseases which are seen on the face but often involve other parts of the body. Lupus is sometimes associated with involvement of the internal organs.

Are there different forms of lupus?

Yes. One type, called lupus vulgaris, is a form of skin tuberculosis.

What is lupus erythematosus?

A disease usually occurring on the central part of the face in what is called the "butterfly area," extending across the nose to both cheeks.

Is sun exposure dangerous in lupus erythematosus?

Yes. It may aggravate the condition considerably.

Is lupus erythematosus serious?

Yes. Some forms of this condition remain localized in the face and can be treated effectively by certain medications. Other forms are associated with involvement of other parts of the body and are so serious that they do not respond to treatment.

Is lupus erythematosus ever fatal?

In rare instances. However, newer forms of treatment, particularly with the cortisone group of medications, have been very effective in controlling it.

PITYRIASIS ROSEA

What is pityriasis rosea?

A relatively common skin disease occurring, as a rule, in the spring and autumn of the year.

How can pityriasis rosea be recognized?

It begins with a reddish patch on the chest, back, arms, or legs. This patch may look similar to ringworm and is called the "mother" or "herald" patch. Within a few weeks after its appearance, a rash suddenly appears on the entire body and may be accompanied by fever, itching, and a feeling of malaise.

Is pityriasis rosea contagious?

No.

What is the treatment for pityriasis rosea?

There is no treatment other than medication to relieve itching.

Does pityriasis tend to clear up by itself even if untreated?

Yes. It will disappear in approximately six weeks.

VITILIGO

What is vitiligo?

Loss of pigment in the skin in patchy areas.

What causes vitiligo?

The cause is unknown.

Is there any treatment for vitiligo?

There are new drugs which are sometimes effective, but these are not without danger and careful medical supervision is necessary while taking them.

POISON IVY

Is poison ivy a skin allergy?

Yes. It is due to hypersensitivity to a substance present on the leaves of the poison ivy plant.

Is the skin ever allergic to plants other than poison ivy?

Yes. Certain people may be allergic to other plants such as primrose, sumac, poison oak, etc.

Poison Ivy Vine. Contact with poison ivy often causes a marked irritation of the skin, with itching that can last for several weeks. At present there is no one specific treatment that will cure this extremely annoying condition, although there are several remedies which can bring about temporary relief.

Close-up of Poison Ivy Plant. Everyone, including young children, should be taught to recognize the typical appearance of the poison ivy plant so as to avoid it. A good rule is, "Leaves three, let it be!" Many people who have thought they were immune to poison ivy suddenly break out with a severe case of sensitivity.

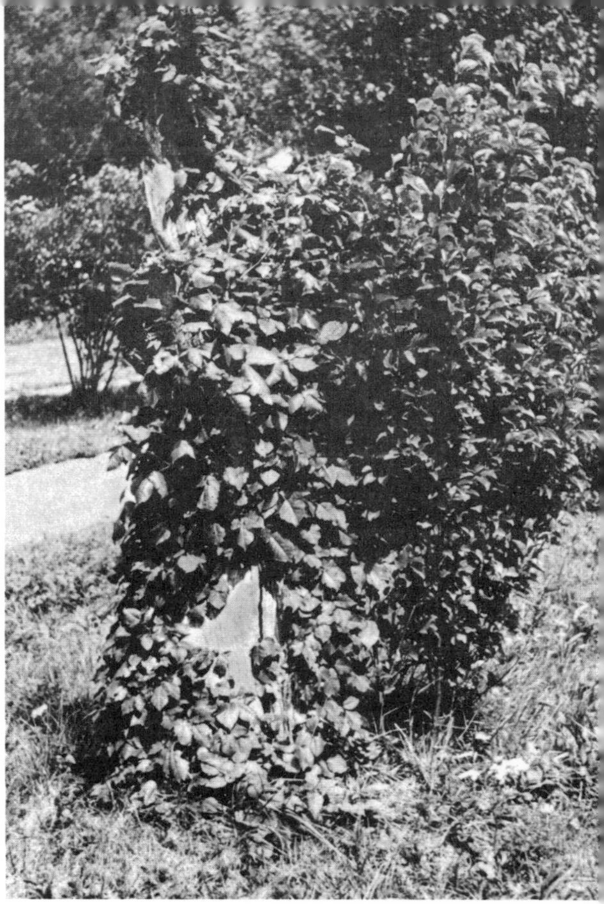

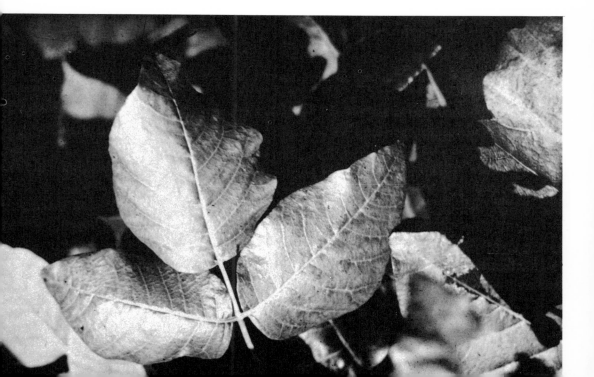

Is poison ivy contagious?

No.

Can poison ivy be prevented?

There is as yet no injection or medication which will prevent attacks of poison ivy with any degree of certainty.

How can one avoid getting poison ivy?

By learning to recognize the plant and avoiding it.

Is it necessary to have direct contact with the poison ivy plant to contract it?

Yes. It is not gotten merely by being in the vicinity of the plant, although the smoke of burning ivy leaves can cause the condition.

What is the best treatment for poison ivy?

There are many simple "anti-itch" preparations which have a soothing effect. The new cortisone drugs are effective in shortening the course of the disease, but they must be used under careful medical supervision.

How long does poison ivy last?

It may last from one to six weeks.

Does one attack of poison ivy give any immunity against future attacks?

No.

SURGICAL CONDITIONS OF THE SKIN AND SUBCUTANEOUS TISSUES

How frequently do people develop tumors or cysts of the skin or tissues directly beneath the skin (subcutaneous tissues)?

Very few people go throughout life without developing a tumor or cyst of the skin or subcutaneous tissues.

What are the common conditions of the skin or subcutaneous tissues which may require surgery?

a. Sebaceous cysts. These cysts or sacs may form when the pores of sebaceous glands become plugged and the secretions accumulate and cannot gain exit.

b. Moles (nevi). Almost all people have moles somewhere upon their bodies. They may be non-pigmented, brownish, or blue-black in color. They may be extremely small or may grow to large size. Most people are born with these moles, but some moles may develop later on in life.

c. Warts (verrucae). These, too, occur in most people at one time or another during their lives.

d. Blood vessel tumors of the skin (hemangiomas). These may occur at any time from birth to old age, and are recognized as red spots on the skin. They vary in size from that of a pinhead to several inches in diameter. At birth, they are known as "wine stains."

e. Fibrous tumors (fibromas). These appear as hard lumps in the skin or beneath the skin and are usually the size of a cherry pit.

f. Fatty tumors (lipomas). These occur directly beneath the skin in the fatty tissues. They may vary in size from that of a pea to that of a grapefruit or even a watermelon.

g. Ganglions. These are thin-walled cysts of the tendons or joints and are most commonly seen on the back of the wrists of children and young adults.

h. Cancers of the skin (epitheliomas). This is found most often upon exposed portions of the body in people in middle or older age. Epitheliomas are very common but do not tend to spread or kill the patient.

Do all sebaceous cysts, warts, moles, blood vessel tumors, fibromas, lipomas, etc., have to be removed surgically?

No. They should be operated upon when they show increase in size, when they are in an area subject to repeated irritation, when they become infected, when they become painful, or when they bleed repeatedly.

Where are procedures for removal of these tumors and cysts usually carried out?

Small sebaceous cysts and warts are often removed in the surgeon's office. Moles, blood vessel tumors, ganglions, fibrous or fatty tumors and cancers are removed in the hospital.

What anesthesia is used for the removal of these lesions?

Most can be removed with the use of local novocaine anesthesia.

Is it necessary to remain in the hospital after these operations?

Often, it is permissible to go home the same day as the operation. If a large tumor has been removed or if the surgery has been extensive, it may be advisable to stay for two to three days.

SEBACEOUS CYSTS

Are sebaceous cysts known by any other name?

Yes. They are also called wens or dermal cysts.

What are the common sites for sebaceous cysts?

They may appear anywhere on the body but are more commonly seen on the scalp, face, and back.

If a sebaceous cyst gives no pain must it be removed?

Yes, if it begins to enlarge. These cysts have a great tendency to become infected if left in place over a prolonged period of time.

Are sebaceous cysts dangerous?

No.

Can a sebaceous cyst be removed when it is infected?

Usually not. At this stage, it can only be opened surgically and the pus drained out. Removal is performed at a later date, when all of the infection has subsided.

MOLES

Are moles (nevi) dangerous?

The great majority are not dangerous.

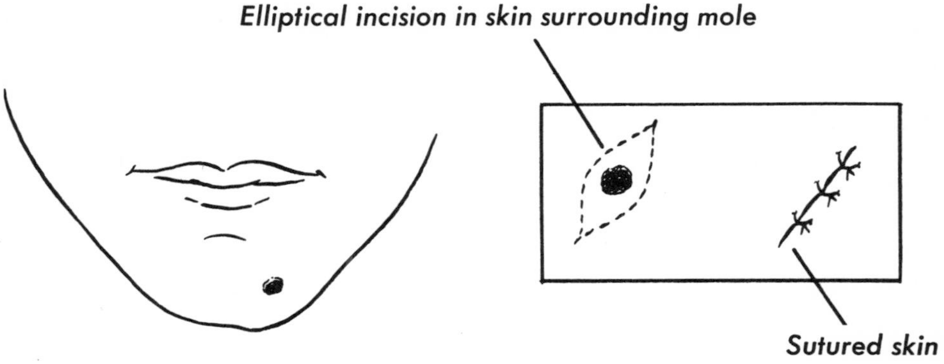

Excision of a Mole. Most deeply pigmented moles should be treated by surgical removal rather than by electric needle fulguration. Certain moles, especially the bluish-black type, have a tendency to undergo malignant changes. For this reason, any mole which starts to grow or change color should be removed.

How does one know whether a mole is malignant or is likely to become malignant?

A mole, or birthmark, which suddenly begins to increase in size or change in color, or one which bleeds or is irritated by clothing, should be examined carefully to see if it is potentially malignant. Most of these moles prove to be benign, but early removal may be instrumental in preventing them from developing into cancer at some future date.

Will the surgeon or dermatologist know which mole should be removed and which can be safely let alone?

Yes.

Do moles always originate in childhood?

No. They frequently appear later in life.

What is the proper treatment for a mole which has suddenly undergone changes?

Wide surgical removal including normal skin and subcutaneous tissue around the mole. If a mole happens to be large, it may be necessary to put a skin graft in its place to cover the skin defect remaining from its removal.

Is it wise to cauterize brown or blue-black moles with an electric needle?

No. Surgical removal is the best treatment.

WARTS

What causes warts?

Warts are thought to be caused by a filtrable virus.

Do warts ever come from handling frogs?

No. This is a common misconception.

Must all warts be removed?

No. Sometimes the removal of one large wart will result in the others disappearing by themselves.

Is there any effective way to prevent warts from forming?

No, except that existing warts should not be picked at or irritated, as this may lead to the formation of others.

Do warts disappear when untreated?

Yes, in some people.

What are the standard treatments for most warts?

If they are to be removed at all, the most frequent way to do it is with an electric needle. Other warts are removed with surgical excision. Some warts are removed with x-ray radiation and still others are burned off with chemicals.

Do all of these methods prove successful in curing warts?

Yes, in almost all cases.

If a wart is properly removed, is there a tendency for it to re-form?

No, but new ones may develop elsewhere in the body.

Do warts on the soles of the feet (plantar warts) produce many symptoms?

Yes. They may be very painful and should be removed.

BLOOD VESSEL TUMORS

What is the significance of a blood vessel tumor of the skin (hemangioma)?

The smaller tumors have no significance at all. Larger ones should be surgically removed or destroyed with an electric needle or by freezing with carbon dioxide snow.

Do blood vessel tumors often turn into cancer?

No. This is an exceedingly rare occurrence.

Do blood vessel tumors tend to bleed?

If they are located superficially in the skin and if they happen to be injured, active bleeding may take place.

What is the treatment for bleeding from a blood vessel tumor?

Direct, firm pressure over the bleeding point until a physician can treat it.

FIBROUS TUMORS

(Fibromas)

Where are fibrous tumors (fibromas) most frequently located?

In the skin of the arms or legs, but they may occur anywhere on the body.

What is the treatment for fibromas?

If they grow or if they cause pain, they should be removed by surgical excision.

Do fibromas tend to form cancer?

No. This is exceedingly rare.

Do fibromas tend to recur once they have been removed?

No.

FATTY TUMORS

(Lipomas)

Are fatty tumors (lipomas) very common?

Lipomas are about the most common of all benign tumors occurring in the human body.

Where are lipomas usually located?

They occur anywhere in the body within the subcutaneous tissues or between muscle bundles.

Are lipomas painful?

Usually not.

Do lipomas tend to turn into malignant tumors?

This occurs extremely rarely and is characterized by sudden, rapid growth of the tumor.

When should a lipoma be removed?

When it shows evidence of growth, when it is irritated or subject to injury because of its location, or when it becomes painful or unsightly.

GANGLIONS

What is a ganglion?

A cyst of a tendon or a joint, most commonly appearing about the wrist area. Ganglions are also seen on other parts of the body, particularly on the fingers and foot.

What is the treatment for a ganglion?

Surgical removal, if it tends to grow or to become painful.

Is it wise to break a ganglion by hitting the wrist with a book or other object?

No. This is bad treatment and may be followed by recurrence.

Do ganglions ever recur once they have been removed?

Yes, in about 10 per cent of the cases.

What is the treatment for a ganglion which recurs?

Surgical removal a second time.

SKIN CANCER

Is cancer of the skin curable?

Practically every cancer of the skin, if treated early enough, is completely curable.

What are some of the early signs of skin cancer?

It is rarely possible for a patient to make a diagnosis himself. However, a good principle to follow is that a person should consult his physician whenever he has a localized sore which fails to heal within a month's time.

What is the treatment for skin cancer?

a. It can be removed with a surgical excision, including surrounding healthy skin and underlying subcutaneous tissue.
b. Certain skin cancers can be burned away with an electric needle.
c. Other skin cancers can be obliterated by x-ray radiation or other radioactive substances.

Where does skin cancer occur most frequently?

On the exposed surfaces of the body, around the nose and eyes or on the back of the hands.

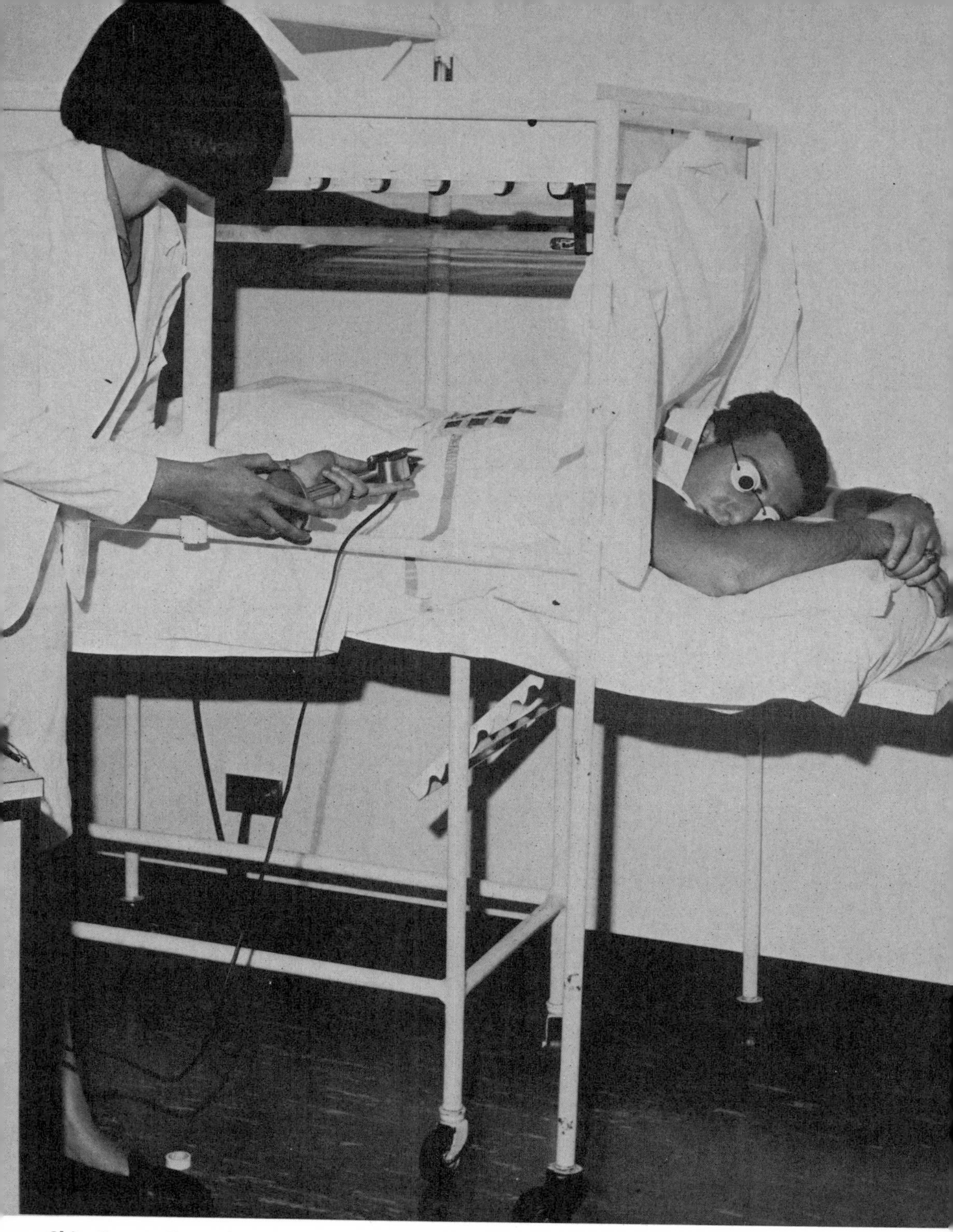

Skin Cancer Test. The effect of ultraviolet light on different substances on the skin of a patient who has had a skin cancer is noted in this test.

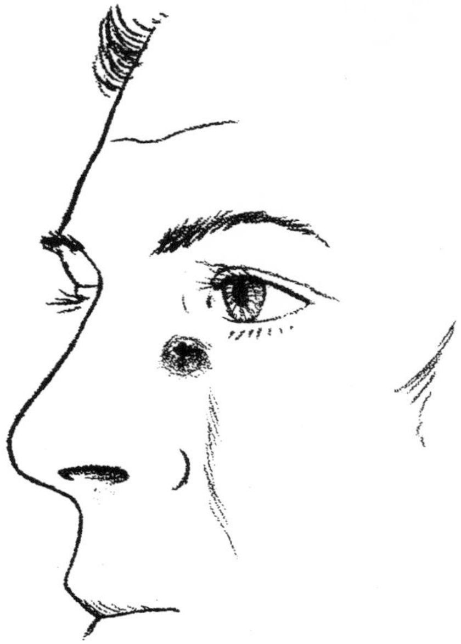

Basal Cell Cancer. This common type of skin cancer is frequently found on the side of the nose. It is curable by surgery or x-ray treatment.

Is the cause for skin cancers known?

In certain instances, the cause can be attributed to repeated or constant irritation. Some skin cancers can be caused by the irritation of petroleum or petroleum products, phosphorus, or other substances which have repeated contact with the skin of the hands over a period of many years. It has been noted that those who have been repeatedly overexposed to sunlight during the course of their lives are more prone to the development of skin cancer.

HAPTER 62

The Small and Large Intestines

(See also Chapter 16 on Cancer; Chapter 46 on Pancreas; Chapter 57 on Rectum and Anus; Chapter 65 on Stomach and Duodenum)

What is the small intestine?

It is that part of the intestinal tract extending from the duodenum (immediately beyond the stomach) to the junction with the large intestine at the ileocecal valve located in the right lower part of the abdomen.

How long is the small intestine?

If its coils were straightened out, it would extend for approximately twenty feet.

What is the main function of the small intestine?

By secretion of certain chemicals, called enzymes, it breaks down various foods into their basic components, thus permitting their absorption through its mucous membrane. The food elements enter into the lymph and bloodstream and travel to the liver, where they are further altered for eventual use by the tissues of the body.

In what form are foods absorbed through the wall of the small intestine?

As carbohydrates (sugars), fats and proteins. Also, chemical components of foods such as potassium, sodium, chlorides, calcium, iron, phosphorus, etc. are absorbed through the small intestinal lining.

Is water absorbed through the small intestinal lining?

Yes.

Is the small intestine essential to life?

Yes, since it is the main area from which foods and chemicals are absorbed. However, at least half of it can be removed when necessary in cases of disease, and the remaining portion will be capable of sustaining normal nutrition and digestion.

What is the large intestine?

It is that portion of the intestinal tract arising at its junction with the small intestine at the ileocecal valve, located in the right lower portion of the abdomen and ending with the anal orifice.

Are there other names for the large intestine?

Yes. It is referred to as the colon or as the large bowel.

How long is the large intestine?

Approximately five to seven feet.

What is the main function of the large intestine?

Contrary to common belief, a large proportion of the stool is made up of bacteria, not of food waste or leftover undigested food particles. It is the function of the large bowel to absorb the water from this fecal stream which has come to it from the small intestine and to propel it forward toward eventual evacuation through the anal opening.

Does the large intestine play a major role in the digestion and absorption of food?

No. Its main function is water absorption, although certain essential chemicals are absorbed by the first portion of the large bowel.

Is the large intestine essential to life?

No. In cases of advanced ulcerative colitis, it is sometimes necessary to remove the entire large intestine, including the rectum and anus. This state is compatible with active living.

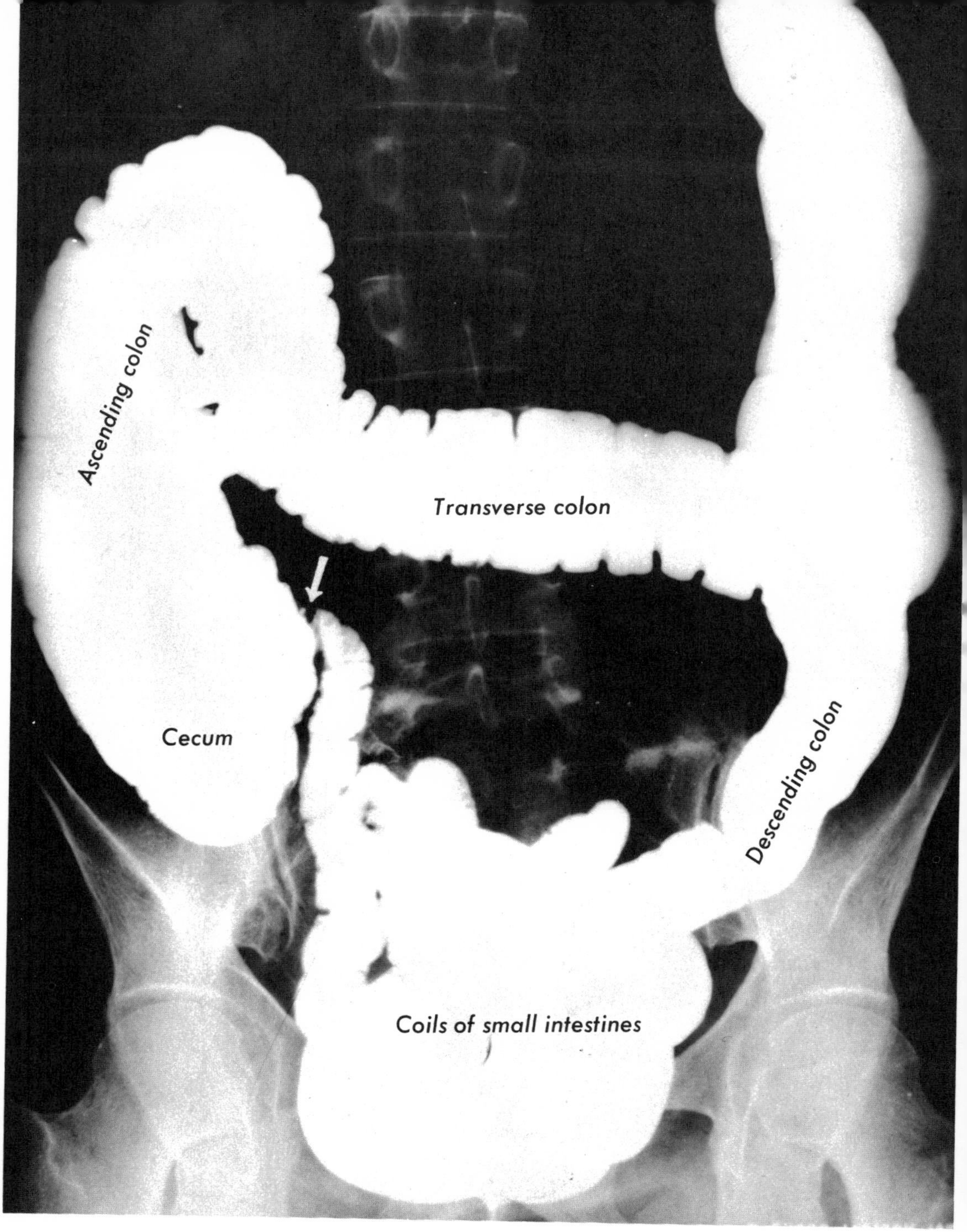

X-ray of Small and Large Intestine. The small intestine can be seen emptying into the large intestine (arrow). The ascending colon travels up the right side of the abdomen, the transverse crosses the abdomen, and the descending colon goes down the left side of the abdomen toward the rectum.

What takes over the function of the large intestine when it is removed?

The terminal few feet of the small intestine. The end of the small intestine is brought out onto the abdominal wall and serves in place of an anal opening. This is called an ileostomy.

CHRONIC CONSTIPATION

What is constipation?

Difficulty in having a bowel movement or irregularity and infrequence of bowel movements.

What are the most common types of constipation?

a. Functional constipation, caused by poor bowel habits, improper eating habits, irritable colon, spastic colitis, or emotional disturbances.

b. Organic constipation, caused by paralytic or mechanical obstruction to the passage of stool. Such things as adhesions, tumors of the bowel, stricture of the anus or rectum, or inflammatory conditions may produce organic constipation.

Is there a certain type of person who is more apt to develop constipation?

Yes. Neurotic, highly strung people may develop spasm of the bowel with consequent constipation. Also, the indolent, slovenly type of person, whose habits are irregular, may develop chronic constipation.

Is it necessary to have a bowel movement every day?

No. Many people normally move their bowels only every second or third day.

Does failure to move the bowels for a day or two cause symptoms such as headache, logyness, etc.?

If these symptoms are produced, they are usually of emotional origin, for there are no real physiological ill effects from constipation of such brief duration.

How many days can one safely go without a bowel movement?

If a normal pattern of regularity exists, it is within the bounds of normal health to have a movement every second or third day.

What are common causes of constipation in children?

a. Functional disorders, with poor bowel training.

b. Organic disorders, such as celiac disease or Hirschsprung's disease (megacolon).

How important is diet in the causation or cure of constipation?

Very important. Foods with high roughage content, such as fresh fruits, fresh vegetables, and bran, aid normal bowel function. Starches and fatty foods have relatively little residue and do not aid in relieving constipation.

Is a change in one's bowel habits and a change in the usual character of the stools of any significance?

Yes. If repeated, it should be an indication to have a thorough physical examination including a survey of the intestinal tract.

Is the presence of blood in the stool significant?

Yes. It should *always* be investigated.

How does one distinguish between ordinary chronic functional constipation and that which is caused by a serious disease within the large bowel?

The two most significant changes that occur when organic disease is the cause for the constipation are:

a. Blood in the stool.

b. A change in one's usual bowel habits and in the ordinary character of the stool.

Is it harmful to take laxatives over a long period?

Yes. They will upset the regular normal function of the bowel and may, in some cases, cause an irritation of the mucous membrane lining of the bowel.

Is it harmful to take enemas frequently?

Yes, as they may disrupt the normal rhythmic action of the bowels. Also, too frequent enemas, or improperly administered enemas, may injure the lining membrane of the large intestine.

Is it harmful to take lubricants, such as mineral oil, for long periods of time to relieve constipation?

No, if it is really necessary. Mineral oil is not a laxative and serves merely to lubricate the stool and thus aid bowel evacuation. Mineral oil does not significantly interfere with the absorption of vitamins from the intestinal tract, especially when it is taken just before going to bed at night.

What is the treatment for chronic constipation?

a. For functional constipation, the patient must be told to discontinue the use of laxatives, enemas, irrigations, etc. He must be placed on a good diet and made to develop regular habits. Psychotherapy is necessary so that the patient stops relating physical complaints to his bowel function.

b. Organic constipation must be treated actively to remove, through either surgical or medical methods, the disease causing the obstruction and constipation.

What is "auto-intoxication"?

There is no such thing. People erroneously think that symptoms such as headaches, dizziness, dullness, etc., are due to constipation. This is rarely true.

Is constipation curable on a permanent basis?

Yes, if one adheres permanently to the advice of the physician.

Should a patient with chronic constipation be examined rectally?

Yes. It is always a good idea to rule out the possibility of an organic cause for the constipation.

Should a patient with chronic constipation submit to x-ray examination of his intestinal tract?

Yes, particularly if there is a change in the character of the stool or if blood is noticed.

Are colonic irrigations helpful in treating chronic constipation?

Usually not. They should be taken only upon a physician's advice.

DIARRHEA

What is diarrhea?

The passage of frequent loose, unformed stools.

What are common causes of diarrhea?

a. The simplest cause is gastroenteritis, caused by eating spoiled or infected foods or a food to which one may be allergic.

b. Other common causes include the diarrheal diseases, such as dysentery, ulcerative colitis, regional ileitis, diverticulitis, etc.

c. Some of the infectious diseases, such as typhoid fever and cholera, will cause severe diarrhea.

d. The taking of large doses of laxatives or purgatives will cause temporary diarrhea.

e. Diarrhea is often encountered as a functional disturbance among nervous, highly strung, neurotic people.

Is there a certain type of person who is more apt to develop diarrhea?

Yes. The nervous, highly sensitive individual seems to be more prone to develop diarrhea as a reaction to an upsetting or tension-creating situation.

When should one consult his physician because of diarrhea?

a. When it continues unabated for more than a few days.

b. When it is accompanied by other symptoms, such as high fever, aches and pains, and a general feeling of being ill.

c. When there is blood in the stool.

How can one distinguish between functional diarrhea and that caused by serious disease within the bowel?

Functional diarrhea subsides spontaneously within a few days. Diarrhea caused by serious disease may continue for weeks, may be associated with generalized symptoms elsewhere in the body, and may be accompanied by blood in the stool. In addition, stool examination by a competent laboratory may reveal a germ or parasite which is causing the diarrhea.

Should examination of the rectum be performed on people who have prolonged diarrhea?

By all means—both a digital and sigmoidoscopic examination.

Should x-rays of the intestinal tract be performed on those who have prolonged diarrhea?

Yes, if other means of investigation fail to reveal the cause.

Is it important to have the stools examined in determining the cause for prolonged diarrhea?

Yes. A thorough search for parasites, eggs of parasites, and bacteria must be made.

What is the treatment for diarrhea?

This will depend entirely upon the cause. Most diarrheas due to eating spoiled or infected food will subside spontaneously. Other diarrheas will demand the specific treatment required to kill the particular causative agent.

Are medications which bind the bowels helpful in the treatment of prolonged diarrhea?

No. They merely delay treatment.

Are laxatives ever given to end diarrhea?

Not usually. Certainly, they should not be given unless advised by the physician.

Will the taking of antibiotic drugs ever cause diarrhea?

Yes! Many of the mycin group of antibiotics will cause a serious and prolonged diarrhea. This condition is called pseudomembranous enterocolitis and is one of the main reasons why people should take antibiotics only upon the explicit recommendation of their physician.

How do antibiotics sometimes cause diarrhea?

By destroying certain necessary bacteria which should normally grow within the intestinal tract. When these bacteria are destroyed, others which are not sensitive to the particular antibiotic being given (usually staphylococci germs), grow in large numbers and produce an irritation of the mucous membrane lining of the bowel.

GASTROENTERITIS

(See Chapter 65, on the Stomach and Duodenum.)

What is gastroenteritis?

An acute inflammation of the lining of the small intestine and the stomach.

What causes acute gastroenteritis?

There are several causes:

a. A virus, as in intestinal grippe.
b. Allergy to certain foods or drink.
c. Eating spoiled foods.
d. Food poisoning.
e. Taking certain medications which produce overactivity of the small intestine.
f. Taking poisons.
g. Overindulgence in alcohol.
h. A true inflammation caused by a germ, such as typhoid fever, dysentery, or cholera, etc.

What are the symptoms of acute gastroenteritis?

Gastroenteritis usually begins suddenly with loss of appetite and nausea, followed by abdominal cramps, vomiting, and diarrhea. This is followed by excessive weakness and a feeling of prostration. Fever is present if gastroenteritis is of infectious origin. The abdomen becomes distended and tender, usually in the midabdominal region or in the lower abdomen over the region of the small intestines.

How long does acute gastroenteritis usually last?

Two to three days.

How can one distinguish between acute gastroenteritis and other conditions?

By carefully noting the history of the signs and symptoms and by noting the absence of other more serious signs, such as muscle spasm and rigidity of the abdominal wall.

Does one have to be operated upon for acute gastroenteritis?

No, but differential diagnosis between this condition and other conditions which do require surgery, such as appendicitis or rupture of the bowel, etc., must be made.

What is the treatment for acute gastroenteritis?

a. Absolute bed rest.
b. Abstinence from food for twenty-four to forty-eight hours.
c. Sedatives to calm the patient.
d. Medications to diminish bowel activity.

Does recovery from gastroenteritis usually take place?

Yes, unless the enteritis is caused by an overwhelming dose of a true poison or severe food poisoning caused by a specific organism, the botulinus germ.

REGIONAL ILEITIS

What is regional ileitis?

An inflammatory disease affecting the lower portion of the small intestine.

What causes regional ileitis?

The cause is unknown, although it is thought to be caused by a germ or virus which has not yet been isolated.

Are there any other names for this condition?

Yes. It is also called terminal ileitis or regional enteritis.

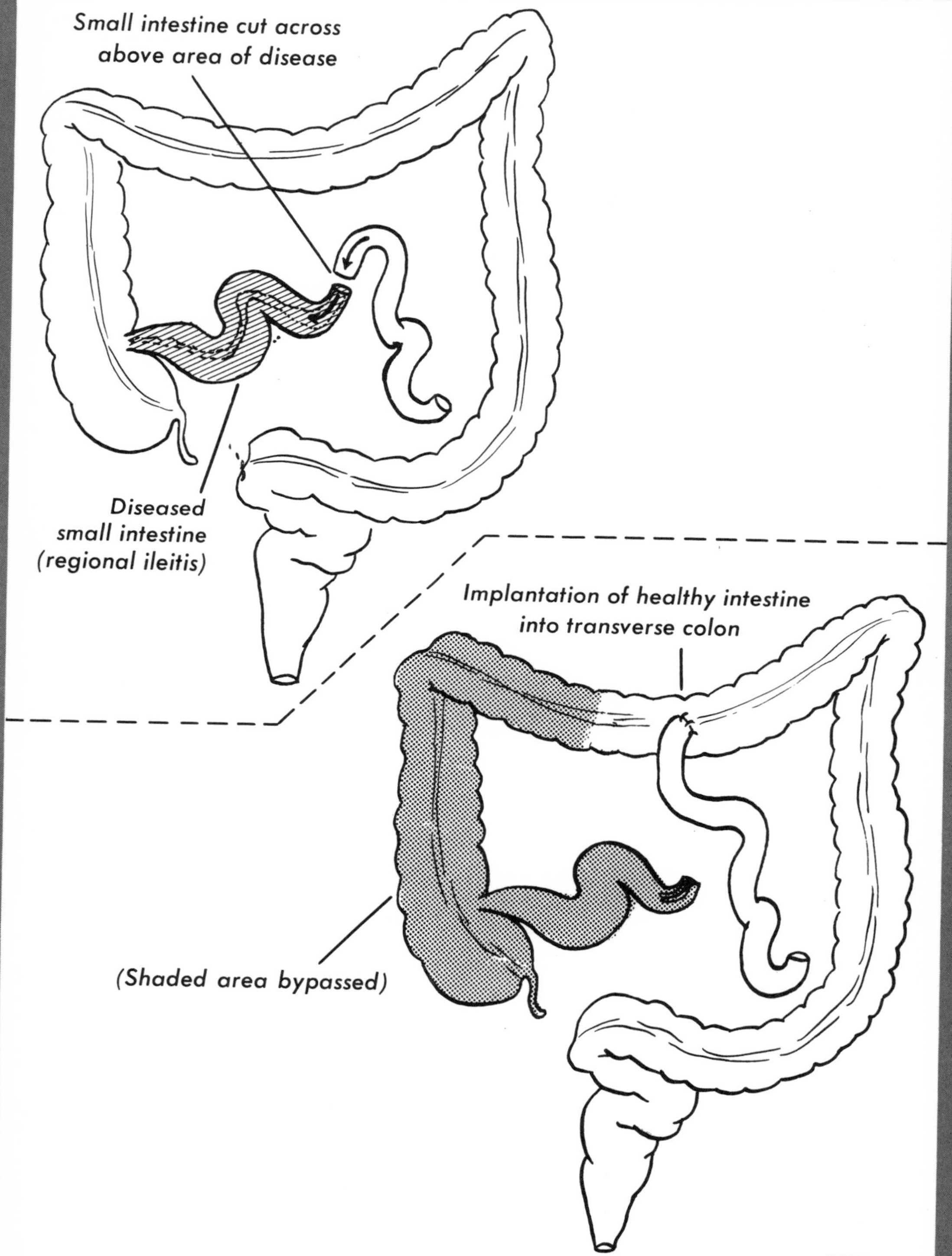

Operation for Regional Ileitis. This diagram shows how the small intestine is cut across above the diseased area and the healthy small bowel is sutured to the transverse colon, thus short-circuiting the inflamed portion.

What are the signs and symptoms of this disease?

It may have its onset with acute attacks of lower or midabdominal cramps, several loose stools per day, loss in appetite, and a mild fever. The condition often subsides after a few days but recurs at intervals over a period of weeks. Eventually, the inflammation of the small bowel may cause obstruction to the passage of stool. There will then be marked abdominal distention, nausea, vomiting, and inability to move the bowels.

Is regional ileitis a common condition?

Yes. It is most often seen in people in their thirties and forties.

How is the diagnosis of regional ileitis made?

It is usually established by characteristic x-ray findings.

What is the course of this disease?

a. In the mild form, an attack may last just a few days and disappear, never to return again.

b. In the more severe form, there are repeated attacks of fever, abdominal cramps, and loose stools. Eventually, there may be abscess formation within the bowel and small intestinal obstruction.

What is the treatment for regional ileitis?

a. In the milder cases, bed rest, a bland diet excluding spices and alcohol, and the administration of antibiotic drugs. Emphasis is laid upon avoidance of excessive work and emotional strain. Some of the newer steroid (cortisone) drugs have been found to give remarkable relief in acute cases.

b. When the disease is far advanced, surgical treatment is necessary. This may involve removing the inflamed portion of the small bowel and joining normal bowel above it to the transverse colon (ileo-transverse colostomy). In certain cases, the inflamed bowel is not removed, but the normal small intestine above the inflammation is joined to the large bowel, thus by-passing the inflamed bowel. The inflammation subsides in the great majority of cases, because the fecal stream does not course over the inflamed intestine.

What is the outlook for recovery in a patient with regional ileitis?

Excellent.

Is there any way to prevent regional ileitis?

Unfortunately, since the cause of this condition is not known, recommendations to avoid it cannot be given.

Is there a type of individual who is more prone to develop regional ileitis?

It is thought that the overworked, fatigued, highly strung individual is more likely to develop this condition. However, well-adjusted people also may develop regional ileitis.

Does regional ileitis, once subsided, have a tendency to recur?

Yes, in a small number of cases.

Can one lead a normal life after part of the small bowel has been removed or by-passed?

Yes. There are some twenty feet of small intestine, and less than half are necessary for the maintenance of normal intestinal function.

Does regional ileitis tend to run in families or to be inherited?

No.

Should special diet be followed after an episode of regional ileitis?

Yes. A bland diet should be followed for a period of months, or even years.

MECKEL'S DIVERTICULUM

What is a Meckel's diverticulum?

It is an outpouching, or finger-like projection of the small intestinal wall, occurring occasionally within the terminal twelve inches or so of the small intestine. It is present from birth and represents a defect in development.

Is this a common condition?

No. It is rare.

What is the significance of Meckel's diverticulum?

It sometimes becomes inflamed, in much the same way as an appendix becomes inflamed.

How can a diagnosis of an inflamed Meckel's diverticulum be made?

The patient, usually a child, will have abdominal pain, tenderness in the midabdominal region, slight fever, and a bloody diarrhea.

What is the treatment for this condition?

When the diagnosis has been made, surgery should be performed promptly, as the inflamed or infected diverticulum may hemorrhage or rupture. Surgery will involve the removal of the diverticulum, a procedure quite similar to the removal of the appendix.

Is this a serious operation?

It is a major operation, but complete recovery is the usual outcome.

How long will it take before recovery from an operation for Meckel's diverticulum?

Approximately the same postoperative course ensues as that following appendectomy.

INTUSSUSCEPTION

What is intussusception?

It is a condition in which one part of the bowel telescopes through another part.

What causes intussusception?

Usually, an inflammation or tumor interferes with normal bowel contraction. The normal intestine above the region of inflammation or tumor continues to contract with force greater than the intestine below, thus producing a telescoping of the bowel above into the bowel below.

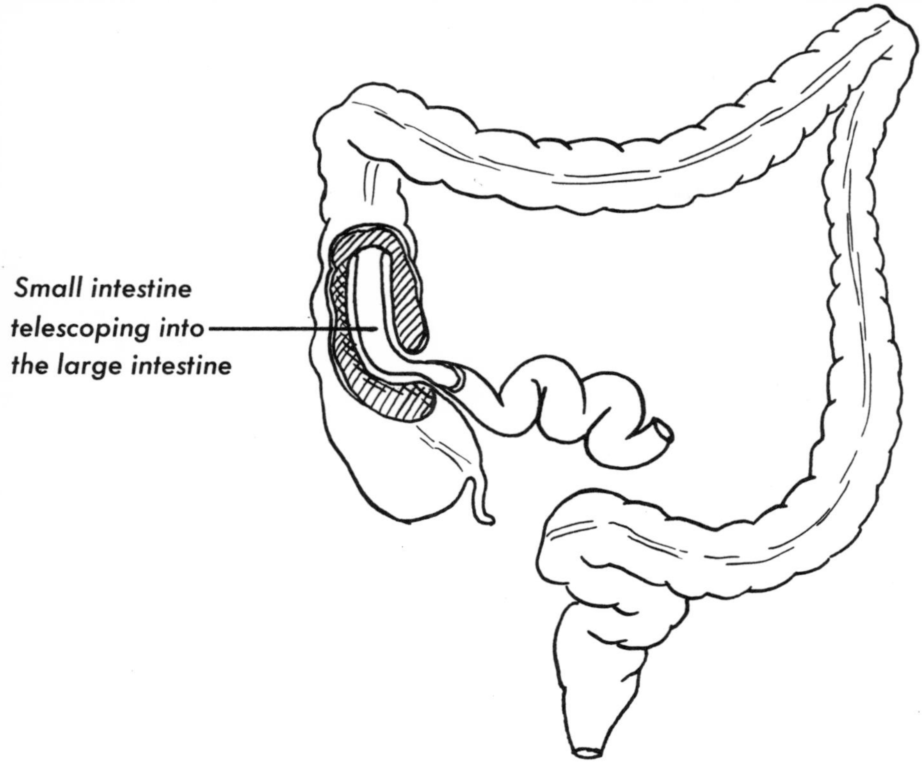

Intussusception of the Small Bowel. Intussusception is a condition in which one portion of bowel telescopes into another. In this diagram the small bowel intussuscepts into the large intestine. This condition occurs most often in children and demands surgery within a few hours in order to avoid gangrene of the bowel.

What is the most frequent site for intussusception?

The small intestine telescopes through into the large intestine at the point where they join, that is, in the right lower portion of the abdomen.

Who is most likely to develop this condition?

Most cases occur in children in their second, third, or fourth year of life.

How is the diagnosis of intussusception made?

By noting the presence of abdominal pain, the feeling of a mass (lump) in the right lower portion of the abdomen, and by characteristic x-ray findings. Bloody diarrhea is also a frequent occurrence in this condition.

What is the treatment for intussusception?

a. In most cases an abdominal operation is performed and that portion of the bowel which is telescoped is gently pulled out into its normal position.
b. In certain cases the condition can be relieved medically by instilling under pressure a barium mixture into the rectum. This must be done by one who is completely familiar with the technique. Under fluoroscopic viewing the barium is permitted to fill the large intestine and is allowed to exert pressure upon the telescoped small bowel until it retracts into a normal position.

Is the medical treatment successful in most cases of intussusception?

At the present time, only a small percentage of cases can be relieved by this technique and it is necessary to operate upon the majority of those children who have this condition.

Once the telescoped bowel has been withdrawn, does it tend to telescope again?

Once this condition has been corrected surgically, it is highly unlikely that it will occur again.

What are the chances for recovery from intussusception?

Excellent, providing the diagnosis has been made within the first day or two.

What are the dangers of intussusception?

The bowel which is telescoped may become gangrenous because of strangulation of its blood supply. This may result in peritonitis and death, if undiscovered.

VOLVULUS

What is volvulus?

It is a rotation or twist of a segment of small or large bowel upon its stalk (mesentery). Such a twist may cut off the blood supply to this segment of the bowel and thus produce gangrene.

Where is volvulus most likely to take place?

In the large bowel, most often in the sigmoid colon in the lower left side of the abdomen.

What causes volvulus?

It is frequently caused by a tumor of the large bowel or by adhesions secondary to a previous inflammation or operation. In some cases it is attributed to an abnormally long mesentery (stalk).

Who is most likely to develop volvulus?

It is seen more often in elderly people or those who have lost large amounts of weight.

What are the symptoms of volvulus?

Acute abdominal pain, nausea and vomiting, obstruction of the intestine, fever, tenderness of the abdomen, and characteristic x-ray findings.

What is the treatment for volvulus?

Prompt surgery, in which the twisted bowel is untwisted and any cause for the abnormal rotation, such as adhesions or a tumor, is removed.

Once a twisted bowel has been untwisted, is it likely to recur?

Not if the cause for the volvulus has been removed.

Will recovery take place?

Yes, in the majority of cases, if the diagnosis is made soon enough. In cases where the diagnosis is made late, gangrene may have set in and peritonitis may already have developed. If this has occurred, the chances for recovery are markedly diminished.

DIVERTICULITIS AND DIVERTICULOSIS

What is diverticulosis?

A condition, usually present since birth, in which there are pouches of mucous membrane that poke out through the muscle wall of the large bowel.

What is the cause of diverticulosis?

It is thought that there is a weakness in the bowel wall at various points where blood vessels pierce it.

What is the difference between diverticulitis and diverticulosis?

Diverticulitis is a disease in which there is an inflammation of one or more of these pouches or protrusions.

Is diverticulosis a common condition?

Yes. It is thought that approximately one in ten people have such diverticula. The great majority, however, have no symptoms secondary to this condition.

Volvulus. In volvulus, the bowel undergoes a twist which may cut off its circulation and lead to gangrene. Treatment is surgical and involves straightening out the bowel and removing the cause for the twist.

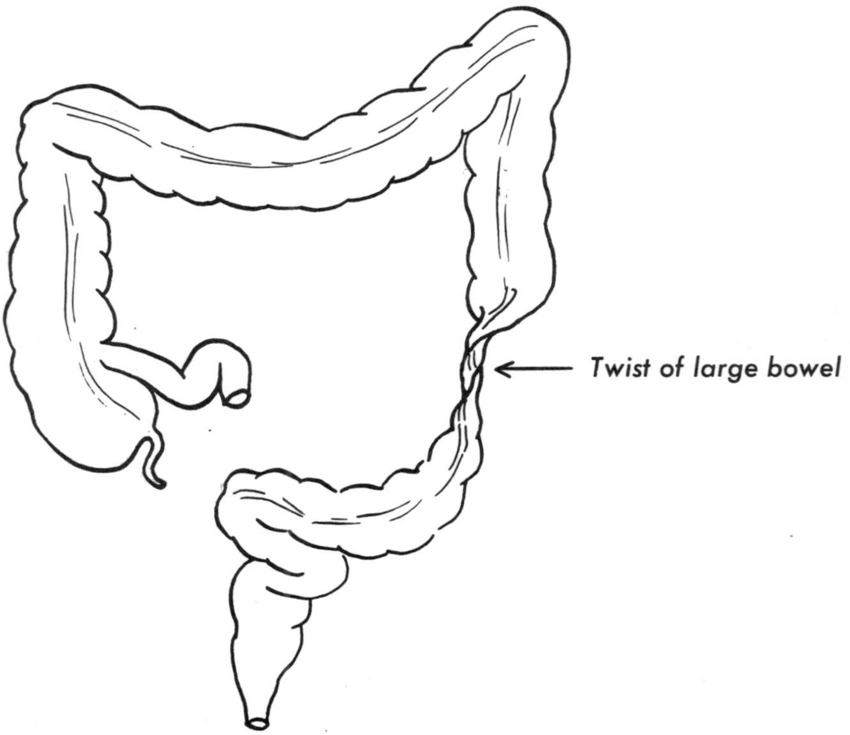

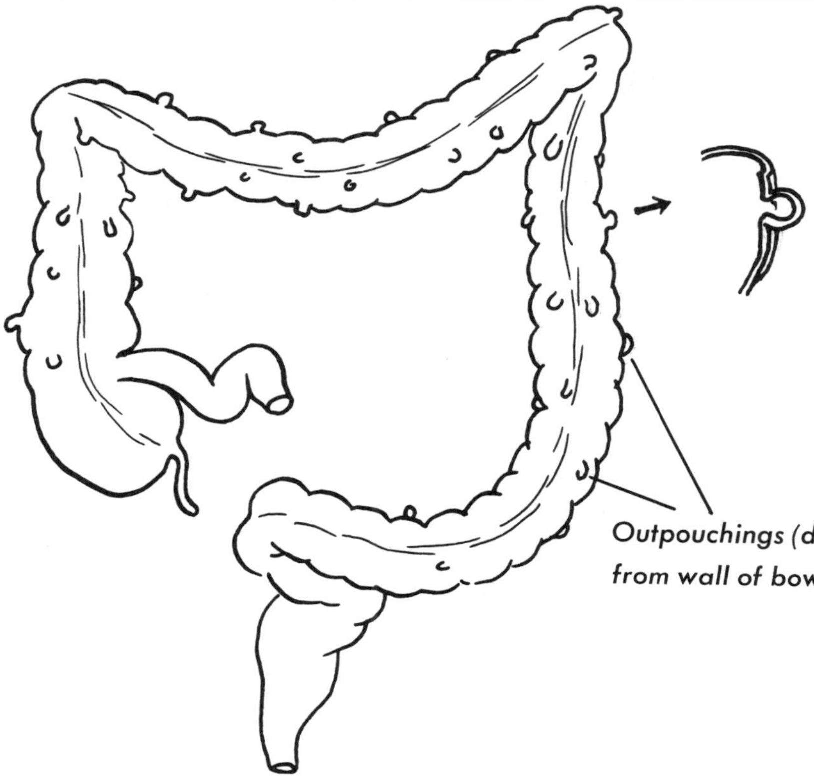

Diverticulosis. This is a condition in which there are many small outpouchings or blisters on the wall of the large bowel. These blisters cause no harm unless they become inflamed (diverticulitis), or unless one of them ruptures, causing peritonitis.

If the majority of people with diverticulosis have no symptoms, how is the existence of the condition discovered?

It is usually discovered by characteristic x-ray findings that are seen when a routine gastro-intestinal x-ray series is taken.

What are the chances of developing diverticulitis if one has diverticulosis?

The great majority of those people who have diverticulosis never have any symptoms whatsoever. Only about 10 per cent will develop inflammation or diverticulitis.

If one has diverticulosis, is there any way to avoid getting diverticulitis?

To a certain extent, yes. This is done by eating foods low in roughage, avoiding spicy foods, and developing regular bowel habits.

What is the treatment for diverticulitis?

In the mild cases, medical treatment is all that is required. This will include:

a. Bed rest.
b. Bland diet.
c. Intensive antibiotic treatment to control the inflammation.

Can most cases of diverticulitis be brought under control with medical management?

Yes. Only one in ten of those people suffering from an initial attack of diverticulitis will require surgery.

When is surgery necessary for diverticulitis?

a. When there have been recurring attacks.
b. When the diverticula threaten to rupture, or actually do rupture, causing a peritonitis.
c. When the inflammation is so bad that it forms localized abscesses or fistulas which extend from the bowel into adjacent organs such as the bladder.
d. When there is repeated massive hemorrhage from the diverticula.

What operations are indicated in the treatment of diverticulitis?

a. If the inflamed diverticula have ruptured and formed abscesses, the abscesses must be drained. In such cases, it may be necessary to perform a colostomy (an opening from the bowel onto the abdominal wall) in order to divert the fecal stream from the diseased area.
b. The ideal treatment for an area of localized diverticulitis is to remove the diseased portion of bowel and to join the healthy bowel above to healthy bowel below.

Are operations for diverticulitis dangerous?

They are serious operations, but complete recovery is general.

Does diverticulitis often recur after surgery?

Only if diseased loops of bowel have been left behind.

How long a period of hospitalization is necessary for diverticulitis?

If one waits for the acute inflammation to subside without surgery, several weeks of hospitalization may be necessary. If surgery is performed, the patient may be ready to leave the hospital within two to three weeks.

Is it often necessary to perform several operations in order to cure this condition?

Yes. The first operation may consist merely of drainage of the abscess secondary to a ruptured diverticulitis; the second-stage procedure may involve a colostomy to divert the feces; the third stage may be carried out to remove the segment of bowel; and a fourth-stage operation may be required to close the opening in the bowel and restore the normal course of the fecal stream.

Are operations for diverticulitis always done in stages?

No. Whenever possible the surgeon will attempt to remove the diseased bowel and restore continuity all in one operation. Unfortunately, this is not always possible.

Can the patient return to a normal existence after an attack of diverticulitis?

Yes, except that he must be careful about his diet and his bowel function.

COLITIS

What is colitis?

Colitis should be classified as functional or organic:

a. Functional colitis includes the so-called "spastic colitis" and "mucous colitis." These are not instances of true inflammatory colitis but represent merely an irritable colon.

b. Organic colitis is caused by true disease processes which are very serious indeed. Ulcerative colitis, amebic colitis, typhoid fever colitis, etc., fall into this category.

SPASTIC OR MUCOUS COLITIS

What is spastic or mucous colitis?

These are conditions in which the large bowel contracts violently and goes into spasm on the slightest provocation. Such bowel often secretes large quantities of mucus which appears in the stool.

What causes mucous or spastic colitis?

They are functional disorders which are thought to be caused by emotional instability and as a reaction to undue stress.

Who is most prone to develop functional colitis?

Young women and men who have deep-seated, unsolved emotional problems.

What are the symptoms of mucous or spastic colitis?

a. Abdominal discomfort, flatulence, and vague crampy pains.
b. Irregular bowel habits, with alternating diarrhea and constipation.
c. Passage of large amount of mucus in the stool.

How does one make a diagnosis of spastic or mucous colitis?

It is very important to rule out more serious conditions, such as ulcerative colitis or a tumor of the bowel. This can be done by taking careful note of the symptoms, by examining the lower bowel through a sigmoidoscope, and by x-ray examination.

What is the treatment for these conditions?

a. It is important to treat the patient psychologically, and in certain cases psychiatric help should be obtained.
b. It is important to discontinue the use of laxatives or enemas, as this will interfere with return to normal bowel function.
c. The patient must be instructed to develop regular eating habits and regular bowel habits. He must avoid highly seasoned foods and alcohol in large quantities.

Do people get well from spastic or mucous colitis?

Yes, but they tend to have recurrences under mental stress, when they have gone off their diet, or when they return to the use of laxatives or enemas.

Are spastic or mucous colitis dangerous conditions?

No. People with these conditions can lead active normal lives despite their irritable colons.

Does mucous colitis or spastic colitis lead to the formation of cancer?

No.

Are the antispasmodic or tranquilizing medications helpful in the treatment of this condition?

Yes. These drugs often relieve the spasm and permit the patient to develop regular bowel habits. The new tranquilizing drugs have also proved somewhat helpful in relieving emotional stress.

CHRONIC ULCERATIVE COLITIS

What is chronic ulcerative colitis?

A very serious inflammatory disease of the large bowel, sometimes involving the small bowel. It is accompanied by bouts of fever, bloody diarrhea, weakness, and a characteristic set of generalized symptoms, including joint aches and pains.

What causes ulcerative colitis?

The cause is not definitely known, but many investigators feel that the disease is bacterial in origin. Emotionally disturbed people in their twenties or thirties are more prone to develop this condition than emotionally stable and older individuals.

What are the symptoms of this condition?

Ulcerative colitis often has its onset in early youth or adulthood, with continuing diarrhea, abdominal cramps, and the appearance of blood and mucus in the stools. There may be as many as fifteen to twenty or even thirty movements a day. If this keeps up, the patient becomes markedly dehydrated, and develops high fever and a prolonged anemia.

What is the usual course of ulcerative colitis?

The condition may continue for several weeks and then subside, only to appear again at a later date within the next few months or years.

How is the diagnosis of ulcerative colitis made?

a. By noting the characteristic symptoms.
b. By examining the large bowel through the sigmoidoscope and noting the characteristic signs of inflammation and ulceration.
c. By noting characteristic x-ray findings.

What is the treatment for ulcerative colitis?

a. In mild cases, medical management is advised. This will include a bland diet, antibiotic drugs, and the prescribing of cortisone or a similar medication. The majority of early cases will subside under this regime.
b. In advanced or recurrent cases, surgery is often necessary. This may invoke the removal of the entire large bowel. When this procedure is carried out, the small bowel (ileum) is brought out onto the abdomen in the form of a permanent ileostomy.

What are the chances for recovery from a severe case of ulcerative colitis?

The chances are excellent, provided surgery is performed at an appropriate time on those patients who do not respond to medical treatment after a thorough trial.

When the entire large bowel has been removed, will the patient always have an ileostomy opening on his abdomen?

Yes, but the great majority of patients learn to manage their ileostomy effectively.

Is it ever possible to save the rectum when operating upon a case of ulcerative colitis?

In a small number of cases of ulcerative colitis, the rectum is not involved in the disease process and can be preserved. In some cases, although they are unfortunately not very many, the small bowel (ileum) can be stitched directly to the rectum at the time of the initial surgical procedure. In other cases, an ileostomy is performed at the initial procedure and the patient is permitted to make an operative recovery. Then, some months or years later, if it is discovered that the rectum is completely free of the disease process, the ileostomy can be taken down and the ileum can be stitched to the rectum. It must be emphasized that this procedure cannot be performed on the great majority of those who must undergo surgery for ulcerative colitis.

Will the patient with an ileostomy be able to lead a full life?

Yes. There are literally thousands of people with permanent ileostomies who go to business and perform all the functions that normal people perform.

Is psychotherapy helpful in treating ulcerative colitis?

Yes, but only when the patient is seen early in the course of the disease.

Is there any way to prevent ulcerative colitis?

No, but if prompt and early treatment is carried out, a great deal can be done to prevent the disease from getting worse.

What may happen if surgery is not performed upon a patient with severe chronic ulcerative colitis?

a. Eventually, death may ensue from an acute attack that involves fever, dehydration, and uncontrollable diarrhea.
b. Cancer of the bowel will develop in a large percentage of those patients who have an active ulcerative colitis for more than ten years.

COLITIS
DUE TO BACTERIA OR PARASITES

What types of colitis are caused by bacteria or parasites?

Dysentery may be caused either by bacteria (bacillary dysentery) or by an amoebic parasite (amebic dysentery).

How is dysentery contracted?

By drinking water or eating foods infected with the specific germs or parasites which cause the disease.

Is there any way to prevent dysentery?

Yes, by avoiding improperly prepared foods when visiting foreign countries and by avoiding inferior restaurants where hygienic supervision of the employees is inadequate.

Is there any effective treatment for dysentery?

Yes. Cure can be brought about by the administration of specific medications, provided they are given early in the course of the disease.

Is dysentery a common form of colitis?

It is seen much more often within recent years because of increased travel to tropical countries. Also, members of our armed services who have seen overseas duty have contracted dysentery and have brought it back to this country.

Can people recover completely from amebic or bacillary dysentery?

Yes, when treated early and intensively. If permitted to go untreated, there is a tendency toward the development of chronic dysentery and serious complications, including the formation of amebic abscesses within the liver or other organs.

Is there a tendency for dysentery to recur?

If inadequately eradicated, recurrent attacks do take place.

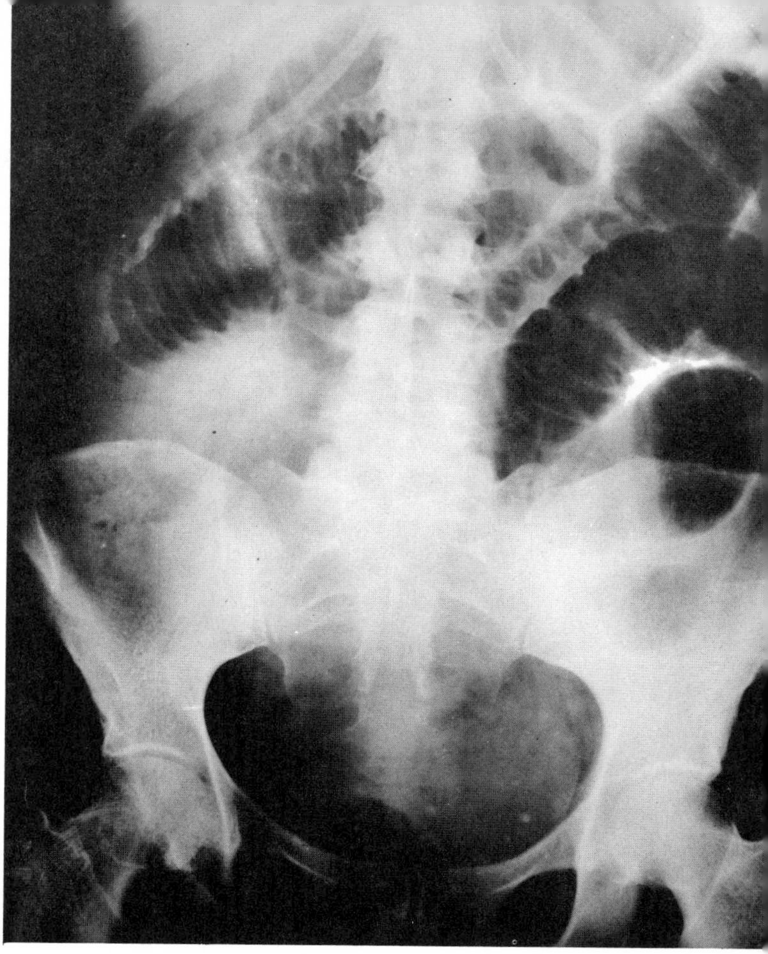

Intestinal Obstruction. This x-ray shows markedly distended loops of intestine secondary to obstruction of the bowel. Intestinal obstruction is a most serious disease and demands prompt treatment, usually surgical.

INTESTINAL OBSTRUCTION

What is acute intestinal obstruction?

It is one of the most serious of all surgical conditions within the abdomen. Intestinal obstruction is caused by an interference with the progressive advance of intestinal contents through the intestinal canal.

What are the most common conditions which produce intestinal obstruction?

a. A tumor either inside or outside the bowel, which presses upon and blocks the passageway.

b. Adhesions causing constriction of the bowel.
c. A twist of the large bowel, as in volvulus.
d. A loop of bowel becoming caught and obstructed within a hernia sac (strangulated hernia).

What are the symptoms of intestinal obstruction?

a. Distention of the abdomen.
b. Inability to move the bowels and complete inability to pass gas.
c. Repeated episodes of vomiting.
d. Colicky abdominal pains.
e. Typical x-ray findings showing obstruction.

Is intestinal obstruction always complete?

No. Partial obstruction takes place first. This will be evidenced by increasing constipation and abdominal distention over a period of several days.

What happens when intestinal obstruction is not relieved?

The abdomen becomes greatly distended and vomiting becomes progressive, until eventually the patient may vomit feces. Chemical balance is upset because of loss of intestinal juices, and death may result from overwhelming toxemia. In other instances, an overdistended bowel may rupture, causing a rapidly fatal peritonitis.

Does intestinal obstruction ever disappear without surgery?

Yes, occasionally, if it is caused by a twist, kink, the telescoping of one segment of bowel in another, or by an inflammation of the lining of the bowel. These conditions sometimes subside spontaneously, thus relieving the obstruction.

What is the treatment for partial intestinal obstruction?

Rubber tubes are inserted through the nose and down through the stomach into the small intestine. By attaching this tube to a suction apparatus, the bowel is deflated and much of the fluid and gas is removed. To sustain the patient, fluids, sugar, and other necessary chemicals are given by intravenous injection.

How is a definite diagnosis of intestinal obstruction made?

By noting the symptoms and by taking x-rays. Intestinal obstruction of mechanical origin is suspected when one notes a scar on the abdomen from a previous operation. This may suggest that a loop of bowel is obstructed by a kink which has formed secondary to an adhesion.

What type of operation is performed to cure intestinal obstruction?

If it is caused by an adhesion or kink, the obstructing tissue is severed with a scissors. If the obstruction is due to a tumor, that segment of the bowel must be removed.

Is it ever necessary to perform more than one operation for acute intestinal obstruction?

Yes. The most important consideration is to relieve the obstruction as soon as possible. This often requires a preliminary colostomy, a procedure in which the bowel is brought out onto the abdominal wall, a small opening made into it, and feces permitted to drain from it.

Is a permanent colostomy necessary following intestinal obstruction?

Usually not. After the obstruction has subsided, the surgeon will investigate the patient more thoroughly to discover the exact cause and the precise location of the obstruction. He will then reoperate, remove the underlying cause for the obstruction, and, at a subsequent date, close the colostomy and re-establish normal bowel continuity.

What are the chances for recovery from complete intestinal obstruction?

The great majority operated upon within twenty-four to forty-eight hours after onset will recover. If the process has gone on for several days, many will die no matter what is done for them.

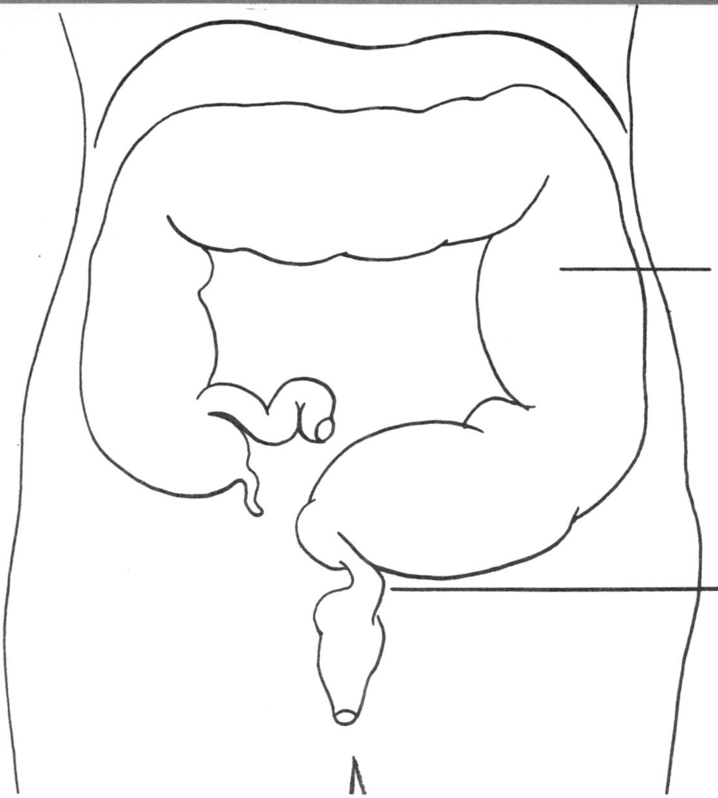

Hirschprung's Disease. This is a condition present since birth, in which a constricted portion of the bowel prevents passage of stool in a normal fashion. As a result of this, the bowel above becomes markedly distended and enlarged. This disease can now be cured surgically by removing the constricted portion of bowel.

HIRSCHSPRUNG'S DISEASE

(*Megacolon*)

What is megacolon or Hirschsprung's disease?

A condition, present since birth, in which the large bowel is tremendously enlarged and distended. A contracted portion, usually only a few inches long, is found in the sigmoid part of the left colon and is thought to be the cause for the enlarged and distended bowel above.

Why is a portion of the bowel constricted in megacolon?

It is thought that certain nerves, which give the bowel the ability to relax and dilate, are missing in this area of the bowel wall.

In whom is megacolon seen?

In young children.

What are the symptoms of megacolon?

a. Inability to move the bowels. Some children never have a normal bowel movement and can evacuate only when they receive an enema.

b. The abdomen in these children is tremendously distended due to the enlarged bowel.

How is the diagnosis of megacolon made?

By noting the symptoms and by taking x-rays which will reveal the characteristic picture of huge distention of the bowel above an area of constriction.

What is the treatment for Hirschsprung's disease?

The great majority of cases require surgery. The constricted segment of bowel is removed and the bowel above is sutured to the rectum below.

Is megacolon curable?

Yes, in almost all cases.

Is this a dangerous operation?

No, but it is a very serious operation, as it involves removal of a segment of bowel.

Is there a tendency for the condition to recur after surgery?

No. Almost all cases are cured permanently.

Can a child lead a normal life after an operation for Hirschsprung's disease?

Yes. The physical and mental development following cure of this condition is astonishingly rapid.

TUMORS OF THE SMALL AND LARGE INTESTINE

Where are most tumors of the intestinal tract located?

The great majority occur in the large bowel. Small intestinal tumors are rare in comparison to large bowel tumors.

What types of tumors exist in the intestinal tract?

a. The benign, non-cancerous tumors, such as polyps or muscle tumors (myomas).
b. Cancer of the bowel.

Do the benign tumors of the bowel ever turn into cancer?

Definitely, yes! This is one of the main reasons why people with intestinal symptoms should consult their doctors promptly.

How can one tell if he has a tumor within his bowel?

Bleeding from the rectum and a change in one's normal bowel habits are the two most reliable warning signs.

Is there any way to prevent tumor formation?

No, but regular physical examinations, including a rectal examination and a sigmoidoscopic examination, are advisable whenever symptoms develop.

What are some of the more common tumors of the bowel?

The most frequently encountered tumor is a benign polyp.

How can one tell if he has a polyp?

Painless rectal bleeding is the most characteristic sign. Larger polyps high in the large bowel may cause intermittent colicky pain or temporary episodes of obstruction.

What is the treatment for polyps?

Those that are located within ten inches of the anus can be removed through a sigmoidoscope, either in the surgeon's office or in a hos-

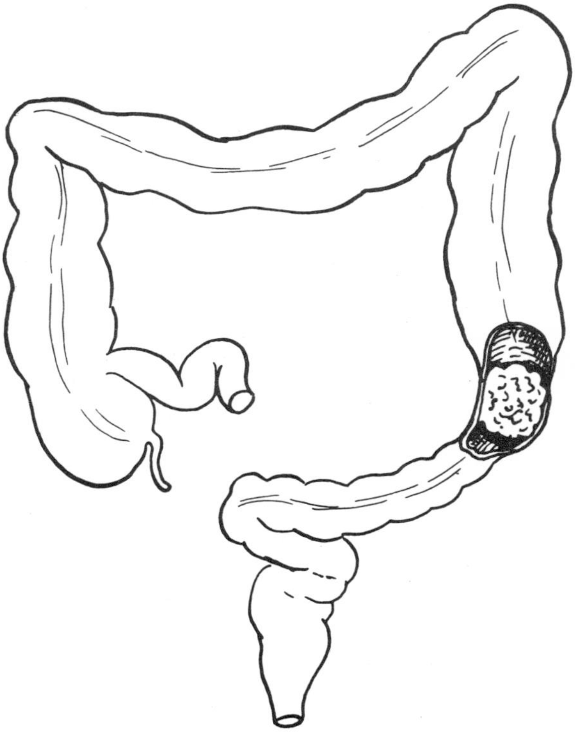

Cancer of the Bowel. This diagram shows how a cancer grows within the passageway of the bowel. It is one of the most common forms of cancer, but fortunately, if it is discovered early, the majority of these patients can be saved.

pital. Those located higher up in the colon are operated upon abdominally. The bowel is opened and the polyp removed.

What is the incidence of cancer of the bowel?

It is one of the most common of all cancers!

Does cancer of the bowel occur more frequently in men than in women?

The distribution is about equal.

When is cancer of the bowel most likely to take place?

During the sixth and seventh decades of life.

Does cancer of the bowel tend to run in families or to be inherited?

No, but a tendency toward the development of polyps and other pre-cancerous lesions may run in families.

How reliable are x-rays in making a diagnosis of cancer of the bowel?

These tests are very accurate and will show a deformity of the lining of the bowel at the site of the tumor.

What is the proper treatment for tumors of the bowel?

Surgery, as soon as the diagnosis is established definitely.

What kind of operations are performed for tumors of the bowel?

a. For the benign, non-cancerous tumors, simple removal of the tumor at its base is all that is necessary.
b. Whenever possible, a malignant tumor, along with a generous portion of bowel above and below, is removed. The ends of normal bowel are then joined to one another above and below. If the passageway cannot be re-established, an artificial opening (colostomy) is made on the abdominal wall. The surgeon's main goal is to remove the entire tumor even though this sometimes necessitates making a permanent artificial opening.

Are operations for removal of bowel tumors serious?

Yes, but surgical recovery takes place in well over 95 per cent of all cases.

How often can a permanent cure be effected through surgery for cancer of the bowel?

The latest results show that more than 50 per cent of all people will live for a period of five or more years after successful surgery for cancer of the bowel.

Is there a tendency for growths within the bowel to recur?

The one that has been removed does not often recur, but in about 5 to 10 per cent of cases, people will develop a tumor elsewhere within the bowel.

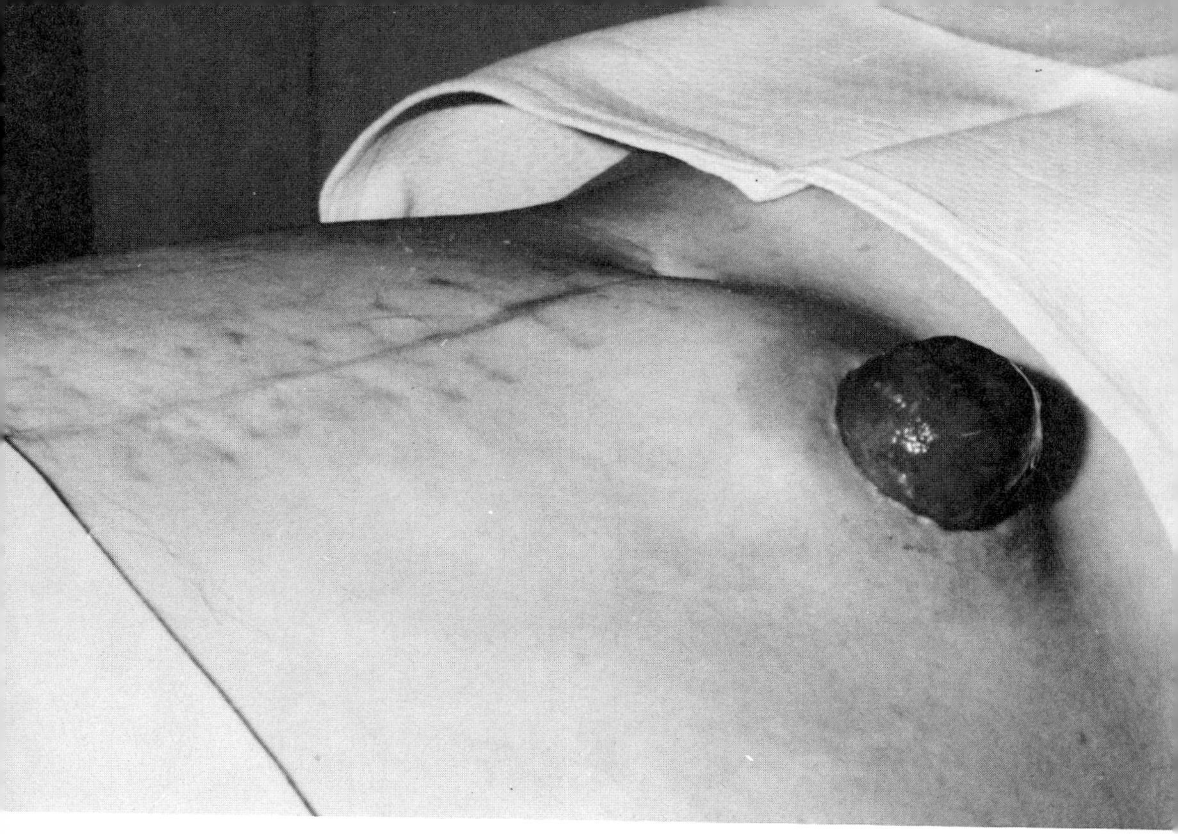

Colostomy. This photograph shows a colostomy, or opening of the bowel on the abdominal wall. It has been performed for a patient who has had the rectum removed because of cancer.

How often should one go for a checkup after removal of a bowel tumor?

At least once every year, or at any time when new symptoms develop.

How does the surgeon decide whether or not to make an artificial opening (colostomy)?

Whenever the bowel continuity can be re-established, the surgeon will do so. However, he will never leave any tumor tissue behind if he can help it.

Are all colostomies permanent?

No. Some are made merely to relieve the obstruction caused by a tumor of the bowel.

When will a surgeon decide to close the colostomy?

When he knows that he can re-establish the normal passageway. This may take place several weeks or months after the original operation.

Can one lead a normal life with a permanent colostomy?

Yes. The great majority of people learn how to control their colostomy so that it functions with almost the same kind of regularity as their normal rectum.

Do people who have colostomies have an odor?

No. They learn how to keep their colostomies clean most of the time. Also, specially constructed bags are often placed over the opening to trap and destroy any odors, should the bowels move while one is out of the house or at work.

Can other people detect that a patient is wearing a colostomy bag or that he has a colostomy?

No. There are many thousands of people who enjoy all activities without discomfort to themselves or anyone around them.

Can a patient live a normal life with a large portion of his bowel removed?

Digestion and nourishment can be normal even when the entire large bowel has been removed. Also, at least half of the small bowel can be removed and still permit normal nutrition.

How can the surgeon distinguish between a benign tumor of the bowel and a malignant one?

The general appearance is important, but tumors of the bowel are always subjected to microscopic examination. Such examination will reveal the exact nature of the growth.

Can the examining surgeon always tell when a patient has a tumor of the bowel by examining the abdomen?

No. This is why it is so important to have x-rays of the intestinal tract taken as a routine procedure whenever there are intestinal symptoms. Also, all people over forty-five years of age, whether they have symptoms or not, should undergo a gastro-intestinal x-ray examination.

Do tumors of the bowel ever take place in young people?

Yes. Occasional cases are seen in adults in their twenties or thirties.

How long a hospital stay is necessary for surgery upon the large bowel?

These operations are among the most complicated of all surgery and may require several weeks of hospitalization. Very specialized preoperative and postoperative care is necessary, including preparation of the bowel with frequent cleansing enemas and the administration of antibiotic and chemotherapeutic drugs. These medications will prevent peritonitis from developing postoperatively.

Is peritonitis a common complication of surgery upon the bowel?

It used to be years ago, but today, with the sulfa and antibiotic drugs, the inside of the intestinal tract can be brought almost to a state of sterility. This permits the surgeon to operate in a clean field and relieves the fear of the development of postoperative peritonitis.

Tumor Removal. The tumor shown in the drawing at the left will be removed along with the part of the intestine indicated between the dotted lines. The severed ends of the intestine are then sewn together as shown on the right.

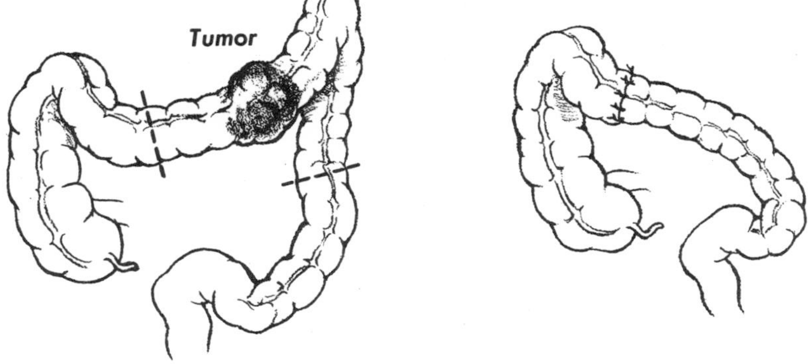

CHAPTER 63

The Spleen

(See also Chapter 12 on Blood and Lymph Diseases; Chapter 69 on Transplantation of Organs)

What is the spleen?

The spleen is a solid purple-colored gland which is soft and elastic in consistency, located in the posterior portion of the abdomen on the upper left-hand side beneath the rib cage. It measures approximately five inches in length, three inches in width, and two inches in thickness.

What is the function of the spleen?

It is a blood-lymph gland concerned with iron metabolism, blood cell storage, and the manufacture and destruction of blood cells. During development of the embryo, the spleen manufactures both red and white blood cells. After birth, this function is taken over by the bone marrow and the spleen confines its activity to the manufacture of certain kinds of white blood cells and to the destruction of old, worn-out red blood cells. It also destroys bacteria and any inert particles which are brought to it by the bloodstream. It stores great quantities of blood, which it discharges into the bloodstream during times of strain or stress.

What are some of the common diseases and disorders of the spleen?

a. Congenital hemolytic anemia (hemolytic jaundice). This condition is characterized by an enlarged spleen, anemia, and mild

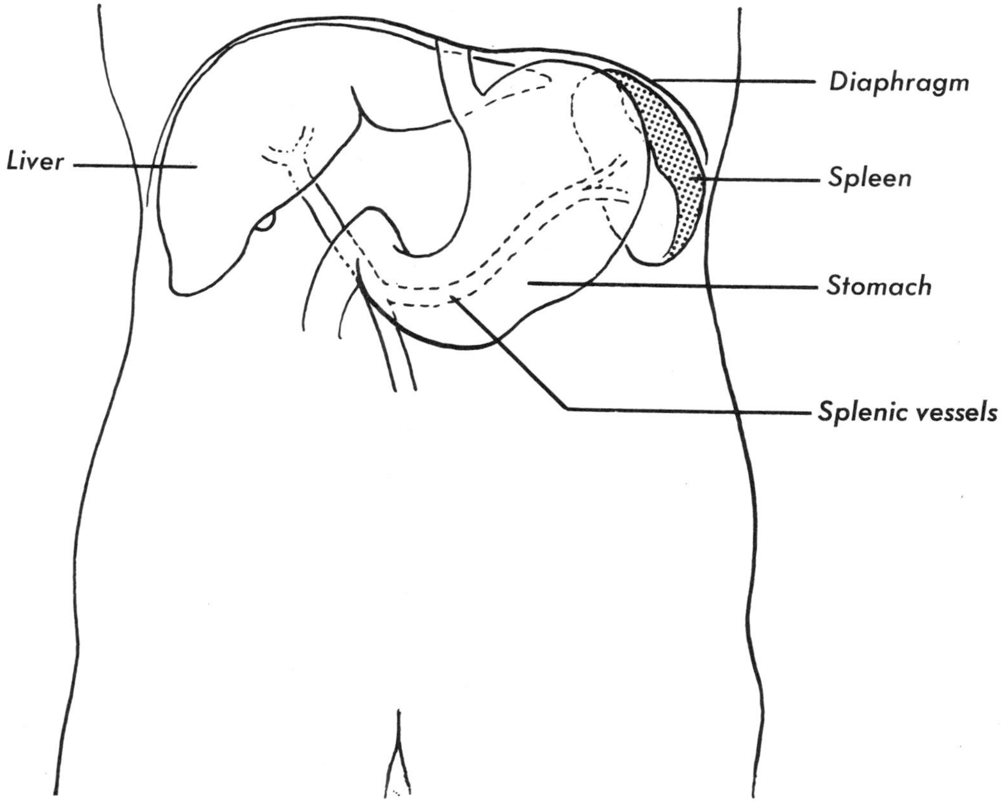

Anatomical Relations of the Spleen. The spleen is an organ located in the upper left portion of the abdomen, beneath the ribs. During the life of the embryo, the spleen manufactures blood cells. After birth, it is concerned with the destruction of old, worn-out blood elements.

jaundice. It is thought to be the result of a defect in the structure of the red blood cells which makes them particularly susceptible to damage. Hemolytic anemia tends to run in families and makes its appearance during childhood.

b. Thrombocytopenic purpura. This is a common disease seen in young adults. It is diagnosed by the appearance of hemorrhagic areas in the skin which appear like bruises, along with bleeding from the nose, gums, or vagina. This type of purpura is caused by a deficiency in blood platelets and by a prolongation of the bleeding time of the blood. (Platelets are necessary for normal blood clotting.)

c. Hypersplenism. This is a general classification for many disorders in which there is overactivity of the spleen, as evidenced by excessive destruction of blood elements. In this classification are six to eight different abnormal conditions.

d. Tumors of the spleen. Benign tumors, cysts, or malignant tumors in the spleen are quite rare but they do, nevertheless, occur.
e. Sickle cell anemia. This is an inherited anemia seen chiefly among Negroes. Diagnosis is made by noting that some of the red blood cells are sickle-shaped.
f. Gaucher's disease. This is a chronic disease, running in families, accompanied by huge enlargement of the spleen. It is seen most often in young women.
g. Cooley's anemia, or Mediterranean anemia. This type is seen in childhood and manifests itself by a large hard spleen and by deformed red cells. There are also characteristic x-ray findings in the bones.
h. Rupture of the spleen. This is a common accident caused by a sudden, severe blow to the abdomen in the region of the spleen. Rupture of the spleen is accompanied by shock, evidences of hemorrhage, and tenderness in the left upper part of the abdomen.

In what other conditions is the spleen found to be enlarged?

a. Leukemia.
b. Hodgkin's disease.
c. Malaria.
d. Cirrhosis of the liver.
e. Thrombosis (clot) of the splenic vein.

Does an enlarged or diseased spleen cause any symptoms?

If the enlargement is very great, it may cause pressure on other abdominal organs. Sometimes the spleen can grow to the size of a watermelon, and when this happens it produces a dragging, heavy sensation in the abdomen.

How does an overactive spleen harm the patient?

It will result in excessive destruction of blood elements, with resultant anemia.

How does one know if he has trouble with his spleen?

The first symptom is usually anemia. When investigating the cause for the anemia, the physician may discover the enlarged spleen on abdominal examination.

How does one distinguish between the various causes for diseases of the spleen?

a. By the familial history of the existence of splenic diseases.
b. By characteristic appearance of the blood on microscopic examination.
c. By other blood tests, such as the bleeding time and clotting time tests, by the appearance of the clot, and by noting the fragility of the red blood cells.
d. By characteristic x-rays which appear in certain splenic conditions.

What are the harmful effects if diseases of the spleen are not treated?

In certain of the splenic diseases which are associated with anemia, the patient can become so markedly anemic that he may succumb to a superimposed infection, such as pneumonia. In other cases, where the blood-clotting mechanism is interfered with, fatal hemorrhage may ensue.

Is there any satisfactory medical treatment for diseases of the spleen?

It is usually necessary to remove the spleen surgically to relieve these conditions.

Does an enlarged spleen always mean that surgery is necessary?

No. Other factors, as determined by blood studies, are necessary to make this decision. Certain conditions, such as Hodgkin's disease, leukemia, Gaucher's disease, and cirrhosis of the liver are seldom benefited by removal of the spleen.

What conditions *are* benefited by removal of the spleen?

a. Thrombocytopenic purpura.
b. Congenital hemolytic jaundice.

c. Certain cases of hypersplenism.
d. Primary tumors of the spleen.
e. Rupture of the spleen.

What conditions may occasionally derive some benefit from removal of the spleen?

a. Gaucher's disease.
b. Cooley's anemia.
c. Sickle cell anemia.

Does the size of the spleen determine the need for surgery?

No. Some of the best cures are obtained in cases in which the spleen is only slightly enlarged or not enlarged at all.

When does removal of the spleen become an emergency procedure?

When it has ruptured, surgery must be performed immediately as a lifesaving measure.

Is removal of the spleen a dangerous operation?

No. The mortality rate from this procedure is very low, except when performed upon patients who are moribund or those who are in the terminal stages of their illness.

When is it harmful to remove the spleen?

There are very few instances in which removal of the spleen is actually harmful to the patient. However, as stated previously, there are several conditions in which no benefit ensues.

Can people lead a normal life after removal of the spleen?

Yes, provided that the condition for which the spleen has been removed is alleviated.

Will other structures within the body take over the functions of the spleen after it has been removed?

Yes. The bone marrow and certain cells, called reticulo-endothelial cells, will perform the spleen's function.

Do diseases of the spleen often clear up by themselves, without treatment?

No. There is no medical treatment or medication which will bring about a cure of any of the major diseases of the spleen.

What kind of anesthesia is used for operations to remove the spleen?

General inhalation anesthesia.

What special preoperative preparations are necessary?

In certain cases, blood transfusions and vitamins will be given beforehand to fortify the patient. In other cases, it may be necessary to fortify the patient by giving him cortisone or similar substances before, during, and for some time following surgery.

How long does splenectomy (removal of the spleen) take to perform?

From three-quarters of an hour to two hours, depending upon the size of the organ and its adhesions to adjacent structures.

Where is the incision made for removal of the spleen?

An incision five to eight inches long is made in the left upper portion of the abdomen.

What special postoperative measures are necessary?

Blood studies must be carried out frequently to determine the progress of the patient. These studies may indicate what medications should be given. Blood transfusions, vitamins, and steroid medications such as cortisone are often administered postoperatively.

How soon after splenectomy do bleeding tendencies disappear, if the operation is successful?

This may take place immediately postoperatively, or within a few days.

Are special nurses needed after operations upon the spleen?

Yes, for a few days.

How soon after surgery can the patient get out of bed?

Within a day or two.

Does the spleen ever grow back once it has been removed?

In performing a splenectomy, it is essential to determine the presence or absence of accessory spleens. The original spleen, once removed, will not grow back again, but accessory spleens may grow to a large size if not removed at the original operation.

What are accessory spleens?

These are small structures, usually no larger than a nickel or a dime, which are identical in structure to the spleen and are located in the vicinity of the spleen. They are found in a small percentage of all normal people.

Are there any permanent after-effects of removal of the spleen?

No. The patient usually lives a normal life, or at least returns to his preoperative state.

Is it safe to become pregnant after removal of the spleen?

Yes, unless the spleen has been removed in the hope of improving some condition such as leukemia or a malignant tumor of the spleen.

How soon after removal of the spleen can one do the following:

Leave the hospital	Twelve to sixteen days.
Bathe	Two weeks.
Walk out on the street	Twelve to fourteen days.
Walk up and down stairs	Twelve to fourteen days.
Perform household duties	Six to eight weeks.
Drive a car	Six to eight weeks.
Resume marital relations	Six weeks.
Return to work	Eight weeks.
Resume all physical activities	Eight to ten weeks.

Should a patient be rechecked periodically after removal of the spleen?

Yes. It is especially important to have the blood examined every few weeks after the spleen has been removed. Such studies will reveal whether blood-clotting tendencies have returned to normal, whether the anemia has been alleviated, and whether normal blood production and destruction have been resumed. Bone marrow studies will also be carried out to obtain further information on blood cell production.

What is a splenic puncture?

It is a diagnostic procedure performed to make a specific diagnosis of a disease within the spleen.

How is a splenic puncture carried out?

A long needle is inserted, under local anesthesia, through the left lower chest wall directly into the spleen. The needle is attached to a syringe and the plunger is pulled out, thus causing some of the splenic cells to pass up through the needle into the syringe. These cells are then sent to the pathology laboratory for microscopic examination.

Is splenic puncture a dangerous procedure?

Not when carried out by one familiar with the technique.

What is the special value of a diagnostic splenic puncture?

There are many cases of splenic disease in which blood examination and examination of the bone marrow will not reveal the exact diagnosis. In certain of these cases, a final conclusion can be determined only through examination of spleen tissue itself.

CHAPTER 64

Sterility and Fertility

(See also Chapter 24 on Female Organs; Chapter 39 on Male Organs; Chapter 54 on Pregnancy and Childbirth; Chapter 60 on Sex)

What is sterility?

Sterility is the inability to reproduce. Since this definition connotes an absolute and irreversible state, it is more appropriate to use the term *infertility*. Infertility indicates a more temporary state which may, under certain circumstances, be reversed.

First-degree sterility relates to those couples who have failed to conceive after at least one year of effort. Second-degree sterility refers to those couples who have had one or more children and have then failed to conceive after repeated attempts over a prolonged period of time.

Couples who have had pregnancies which have failed to culminate in living children should also be included in the general classification of infertility, since the ultimate aim of reproduction is living, healthy children.

How often does sterility occur among married couples?

Although there are no absolutely accurate statistics, it is estimated that approximately one out of every five marriages fails to produce a living offspring.

How long does it take the average married couple to conceive for the first time?

Pregnancy will usually take place within a year, providing the couple

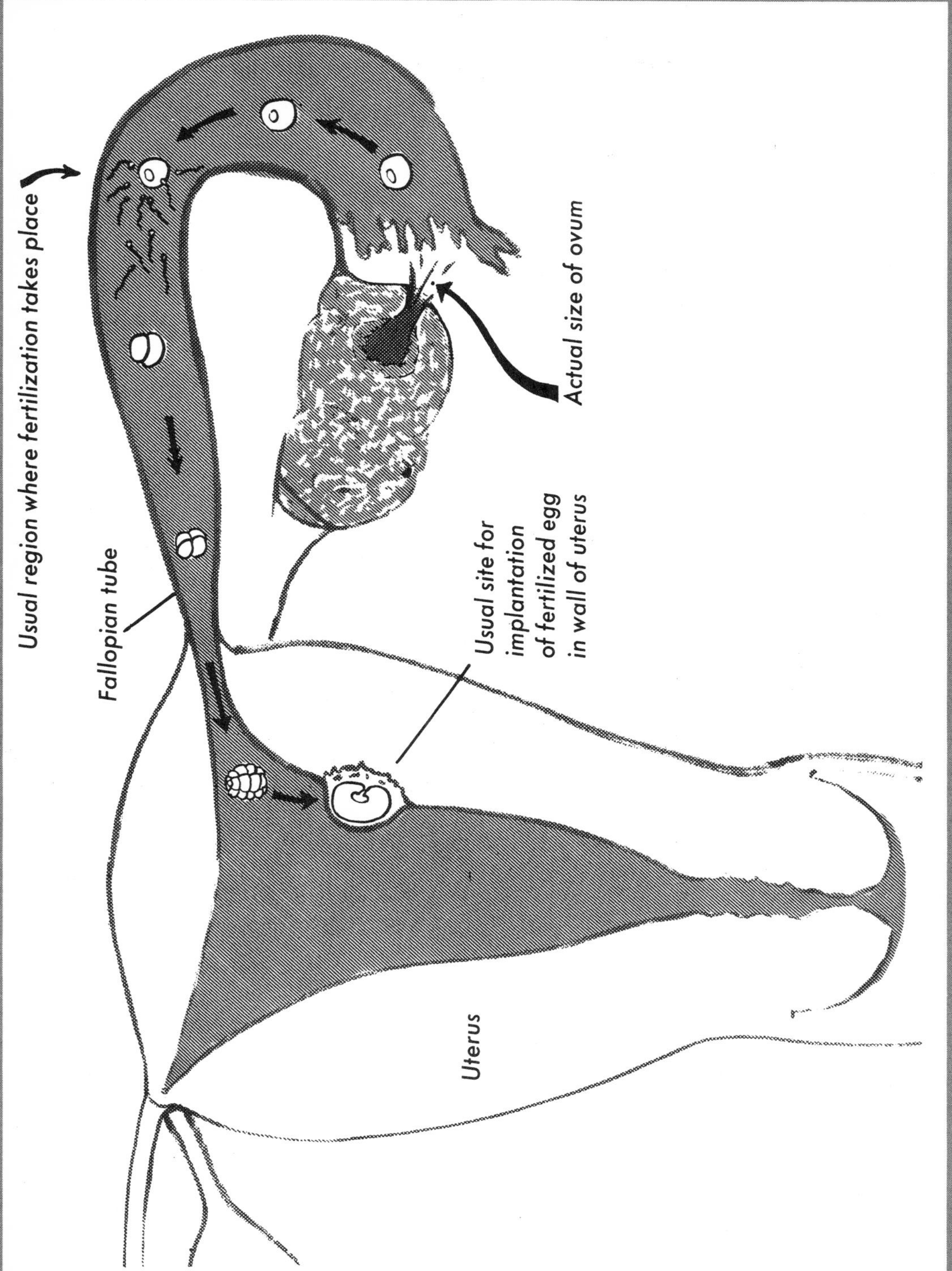

Fertilization of an Egg by a Sperm. This diagram demonstrates the route that sperm travel in order to reach the egg in the fallopian tube. After fertilization has taken place in the tube, the egg descends to the uterus, where it implants in the uterine wall.

has intercourse two to three times weekly and refrains from using contraceptive devices. The wife who conceives within the first month or two after trying is *not* the average woman. It is not at all unusual for normal young people to try for eight to ten months before being successful.

Must the wife have an orgasm for conception to take place?

No! Climax plays no role whatsoever in conception.

What factors are necessary for pregnancy to take place?

The woman must produce an egg from her ovaries; the Fallopian tubes must be open; healthy sperm must reach the egg while it is in the Fallopian tubes; there must be a place within the lining of the uterus for implantation of the fertilized egg; the woman must produce the proper hormones to nourish the fertilized, implanted egg.

FEMALE STERILITY

What are some of the common causes of sterility (infertility) in women?

a. Failure to ovulate or produce an egg. This can be the result of a congenital defect in the chromosomes, such as is seen in Turner's syndrome, or it can be due to an acquired abnormality in a female who is structurally normal.
b. Blocked Fallopian tubes, either due to infection or to a birth deformity in which the tubes are obstructed.
c. Glandular imbalance, particularly involving the pituitary gland, the thyroid, the adrenal glands, or the ovaries.
d. Failure of the sperm to pass through the cervix and up into the uterus. This may be caused by obstruction or infection at the cervix, the entrance to the womb.
e. Psychological factors, often elusive, vague, and difficult to evaluate. It has been known, however, that some sterile women will be able to conceive after a period of psychotherapy.
f. There is a large group of women who fail to conceive without

any discernible cause. In view of the fact that scientists are learning more all the time about the nature of chromosomes, genes, and cellular structure, it is quite likely that this group will be understood more fully and many additional reasons for sterility will be found.

Must all of these factors be present to prevent conception?

Obviously, no. These factors may exist singularly or in combination. It must be understood that infertility is a relative term and that minimal degrees of a number of factors can be as effective in causing sterility as one major factor.

What is the "fertile period" of the month?

The middle of the menstrual cycle, when ovulation takes place. In a twenty-eight-day cycle, this is usually about twelve to sixteen days after the onset of the menstrual period.

When is the "barren period" of the month?

Seven to nine days before the menstrual period, during the menstrual period, and the three to five days immediately following the menstrual period, depending upon the cycle and length of menstruation.

During how many days of the month is conception possible?

Since healthy sperm must be deposited in the vagina within two days before ovulation and not longer than two days after ovulation, it is obvious that out of the entire cycle of twenty-eight days, fertilization of an egg can occur on only three to four of those days.

Can one determine the "fertile period" and the "barren period" accurately?

In a woman who menstruates regularly, these periods can be determined with some accuracy by studying the basal body temperature charts from day to day.

If a woman fails to ovulate, how is this fact recognized?

a. By taking a careful menstrual history and noting any irregularities.

b. By recording basal temperatures over a period of several months.

a definite curve will be developed which will show whether or not the patient is ovulating.

c. By taking a biopsy (endometrial biopsy) of the lining membrane of the uterus just before the expected date of menstruation, the gynecologist can tell whether ovulation is present or absent.
d. Vaginal smears can be studied microscopically to reveal whether ovulation has taken place.

Can a woman be successfully treated if she fails to ovulate?

Yes. In the majority of cases, a glandular study will reveal the cause for failure to ovulate and will point the way toward the proper hormonal treatment. This will involve a careful study of the activity of the pituitary gland, the thyroid gland, the adrenal glands, and the ovaries.

How is a biopsy of the lining of the uterus (endometrial biopsy) performed?

This is an office procedure performed on an examining table. A speculum is inserted into the vagina and the cervix is grasped with a clamp. A small metal instrument is then inserted through the cervix into the uterus and the lining is scraped.

Is the taking of an endometrial biopsy a painful procedure?

There is slight discomfort, but it takes only a few minutes to perform and has no unpleasant after-effects.

What precautions should be taken before doing an endometrial biopsy?

It is important to determine that the patient is not pregnant at the time the biopsy is taken. For this reason, abstinence is advised from the time of the previous menstrual period until the time the biopsy is taken. This is necessary because an early pregnancy would be disturbed by an endometrial biopsy.

Will the patient bleed for two or three days after the taking of an endometrial biopsy?

Yes.

What are the common causes of blocked Fallopian tubes?

a. Previous inflammation of the pelvic organs, most frequently caused by gonorrhea, tuberculosis, or some other germ.

b. Peritonitis, most often secondary to a ruptured appendix.

c. Spasm of the Fallopian tubes due to tension and emotional factors.

d. A fibroid in the upper portion of the uterus which shuts off the entrance of the Fallopian tubes.

e. Endometriosis.

How are blocked tubes diagnosed?

a. By performing the Rubin test. This involves the pumping of a gas (carbon dioxide) through the cervix into the uterine cavity and noting that the gas has entered the abdominal cavity.

Hysterogram. This x-ray shows the outline of a normal uterine cavity and demonstrates that the right fallopian tube is open and the left fallopian tube closed. This is an extremely valuable test, as it demonstrates whether the passageway is open to allow pregnancy to take place. Conditions such as polyps or fibroids within the cavity of the uterus can also be diagnosed by performing a hysterogram.

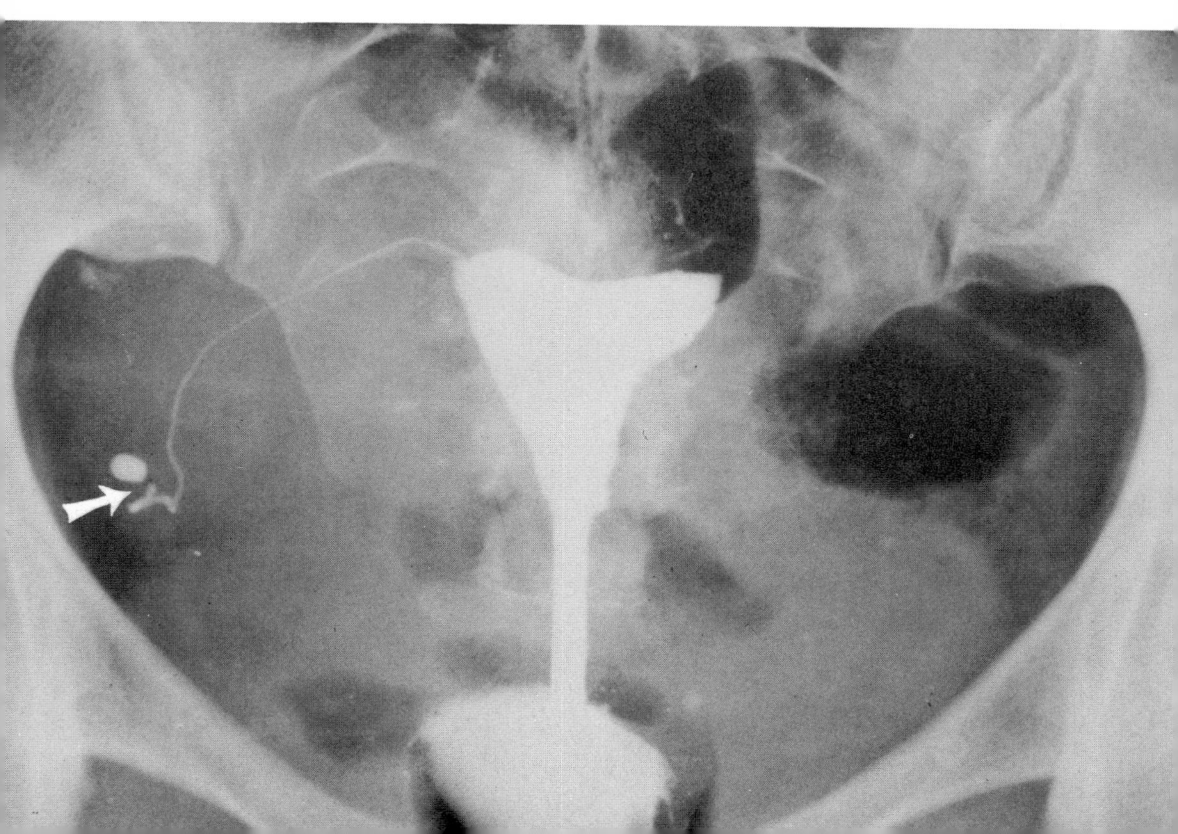

b. By an x-ray examination involving the insertion of a radio-opaque dye into the cervix to outline the uterine cavity and tubes (hysterogram).

How is the Rubin test performed?

As an office procedure, the patient is instructed to report about five to seven days after a menstrual period. On the examining table, the cervix is exposed and grasped with a clamp. A thin tubular instrument is inserted into the cervical canal. One end of this tubular instrument is attached to a container of carbon dioxide and to a recording machine. By the proper use of the valves, carbon dioxide is administered and passed up into the uterus at known pressures. The only outlet for this gas is through the Fallopian tubes into the abdominal cavity. If the tubes are open, the gas escapes into the abdominal cavity and the pressure recorded on the machine falls. If the gas does not go into the abdominal cavity, the pressure on the machine is maintained or is elevated. By listening through the abdominal wall with a stethoscope, the escape of gas through the tubes can actually be heard.

If the tubes are open, will the patient experience pain from the Rubin test?

Yes. The gas entering the abdominal cavity often produces pain in the shoulder region within five to ten minutes. This pain will subside in a short time and is not serious.

Is there any danger to the Rubin test?

If proper precautions are taken, there is little chance of anything going wrong with this test. In occasional cases, an inflammatory disease within the Fallopian tubes may be aggravated by this procedure.

Can patients resume marital relations following a Rubin test?

Not until two days after the test has been performed.

How is a hysterogram performed?

This test is performed in essentially the same manner as the Rubin test, except that the radio-opaque dye is inserted through the cervix and the results are obtained by taking an x-ray picture.

What precautions should be taken before a hysterogram is performed?

It must be ascertained that no infection exists within the vagina, uterus, or tubes.

Can blocked tubes ever be opened?

Yes. In occasional cases, performance of the Rubin test itself, by expanding the tubes with gas, will overcome the blockage. This test may be repeated at monthly intervals if it is not at first successful in reopening the tubes.

Are operations to overcome blocked tubes successful?

Yes, in approximately 20 per cent of cases.

What can be done if the blocked tubes are due to spasm or emotional factors?

The giving of antispasmodic medications and the treatment of the patient's emotional problems will often result in the release of spasm and in the opening of the tubes.

How does glandular or hormonal imbalance cause infertility?

By preventing ovulation or by failing to produce a proper atmosphere for the implantation of the fertilized egg in the wall of the uterus.

Are there any specific tests to note the presence or absence of glandular imbalance?

Yes. Hormone studies can be carried out by specific tests upon the urine and blood. Also, the basal metabolic rate and chemical analyses may give a clue as to the existence of glandular disturbance.

Can glandular imbalance be overcome?

Yes, in some cases, by appropriate treatment with hormones. An endocrinologist can best handle this type of case.

Does the cervix often block the passage of healthy sperm into the uterus?

Yes. This occurs frequently when the cervix is infected or blocked by the presence of thick mucus.

Are there any tests to determine the ability of the sperm to penetrate the cervix?

Yes. The Huhner test is performed by examining the sperm after they have been deposited in the vagina. The patient comes to the office about two hours after intercourse, and samples from the vaginal canal and from the cervix are taken and are examined under a microscope. Where a normal sperm analysis exists, a comparison of the sperm in the vagina and in the cervix will give a clue as to the ability of the sperm to penetrate into the uterus.

Do healthy sperm ever fail to reach the cervix because of a tipped womb or because of improper positions in intercourse?

Yes. Such situations do occur and may interfere with eventual conception.

If this situation does exist, can it be corrected?

Yes, by changing the position of intercourse or by taking the sperm and artificially depositing them in the cervix.

If failure of the sperm to pass through the cervix is due to an infection of the cervix, can this situation be corrected?

Yes, by cauterizing the cervix and by using antibiotics to get rid of the infection.

Is conception ever interfered with by a vagina that is too acid?

Yes. This is overcome by taking an alkaline douche with bicarbonate of soda before intercourse.

Do fibroids of the uterus ever cause sterility?

Yes, when the fibroids are located just beneath the lining of the uterus (submucous). Also, if the fibroids block the entrance to the Fallopian tubes, the sperm may not be able to reach the egg.

Do cysts of the ovaries ever cause infertility?

Yes, when the cyst is the type which results from or causes an upset in hormone production and balance. Pregnancy will often occur when such cysts are removed surgically.

If infertility is thought to be due to emotional factors, how can it be treated?

In many cases of this kind, psychotherapy has proved of great value and is often followed by conception.

Is sterility in a woman often caused by the prolonged use of contraceptive jellies?

No. It has never been proved that the use of these substances will interfere with conception, once they have been discontinued.

Will the prolonged use of contraceptive pills interfere with subsequent ability to conceive?

On the contrary, it has been shown that women who have been taking contraceptive pills for a long period of time are more prone to conceive during the months immediately after their use.

Can sterility result from "overindulgence" in intercourse?

No. This has no influence whatever on fertility.

What is meant by artificial insemination?

It is the introduction of live sperm, either the husband's or a donor's, in the vicinity of the cervix.

When is artificial insemination employed?

a. In cases where the Huhner test reveals that the husband's sperm (even though healthy) are not being deposited into the cervix, the sperm are collected and are deposited into the cervix by the gynecologist.
b. In cases in which the husband is sterile—that is, he possesses no live healthy sperm—and husband and wife consent, a sperm donor is employed.

How is artificial insemination carried out?

The patient reports to the office at an appointed time. She is placed on an examining table and a speculum is inserted into the vagina. Live sperm, taken either from the husband or from a donor, are injected with a syringe into the opening of the cervix. A small rubber cap which fits the cervix is then placed over the cervix to keep the sperm in contact with the cervix for a period of approximately a half-hour.

At what time of the month is artificial insemination carried out?

When it has been determined by investigation that the patient is ovulating.

How often is artificial insemination attempted?

During one menstrual cycle, it should be done every day for three days. These days should be just before, during, and after the ovulation date. This procedure should be repeated every month for four to six months.

How often is artificial insemination successful?

In about 30 per cent of cases.

How is a sperm donor selected?

The donor must be a healthy male who has been examined and found free of disease. A thorough history should be obtained to make sure that the donor's family is free from inherited physical or mental disease. (Such donors are usually recruited from college students, medical students, or internes.) The donor must remain anonymous to the couple! The couple must also remain anonymous to the donor! Complete accord must be reached and consent must be given by husband, wife, and donor in writing, preferably in the presence of an attorney.

What are the dangers involved in artificial insemination?

There are no physical dangers, but there may be some emotional injury to the husband when a donor is used. There may also be legal or religious entanglements, and these should be considered very carefully before artificial insemination is embarked upon.

MALE STERILITY

Is the male an important factor in sterility?

Yes. Any attempt to overcome infertility which does not have the complete cooperation of the male is worthless and should not be undertaken. *About 30 to 40 per cent of all infertile marriages are due to failure of the male, not the female!* Complete studies of the husband must be carried out by the urologist in all cases of infertile marriages.

What constitutes sterility in the male?

A sterile man is one who either has no sperm or has an insufficient number of normal, active sperm to make conception possible.

What is the difference between sterility and infertility in the male?

Sterility implies an absolute impossibility of conception or fertilization. In the male, this would be a situation in which there are no sperm to ejaculate. On the other hand, infertility suggests that conception and fertilization are possible but not likely because of a low sperm count.

What is a sperm count?

The ejaculate, which usually amounts to about one teaspoonful, normally contains upward of sixty million sperm per cubic centimeter. This count is obtained by microscopic examination of the ejaculate.

Are there any other features of the ejaculate which are important to examine?

Yes. The motility of the sperm, as well as their anatomical appearance and characteristics, is important to note.

What are the common causes of absence of sperm?

a. There are some developmental abnormalities in males that may cause them to be born without the ability to produce sperm. Such conditions have just recently been discovered through study of chromosomes and genes.

b. Old age is often accompanied by the loss of the ability of the testicle to produce sperm. This varies widely among individual men and may not have its onset in some until the eighth or ninth decades of life.

c. Orchitis, an inflammation of the testicle, may result in loss of sperm production. This is not uncommon following an attack of mumps in an adult. Other infections can also cause this form of male sterility.

d. Sperm may be absent because there is an interference with their migration from the testicle to the ejaculate. A previous infection, such as gonorrhea, may cause blockage of the passageway (the vas deferens) from the testicle to the seminal vesicle.

e. Of course, when the testicles are absent or are undescended (see Undescended Testicles), no sperm will be produced.

How can one tell whether the testicles are capable of producing sperm?

By a simple operative procedure known as testicular biopsy, a sample of testicular tissue is removed and submitted to the laboratory for microscopic examination. In most cases, this will demonstrate the capability of the testicle to produce sperm.

How is a biopsy of the testicles carried out?

It is done in an operating room of a hospital under light general anesthesia. A small incision is made in the skin of the scrotum and through this a small piece of testicle is snipped away.

What causes a low or reduced sperm count?

A natural reduction in the sperm content of the ejaculate follows frequent intercourse, a generalized debilitating disease, surgical operations, or any situation which temporarily weakens or depresses body activities. Low sperm counts of this type may be of a temporary nature. In other cases, however, men who are perfectly normal in all other respects may have low sperm counts.

What are the most common causes of a reduced sperm count?

a. Glandular or endocrine disorders.

b. Inflammation of the testicles secondary to mumps, gonorrhea, tuberculosis, or other diseases.

c. Diseases of the testicles which result in their shrinkage (atrophy), such as interference with their circulation, etc.

d. Old age.

Are potency and sterility related?

Yes, insofar as inadequate erections (poor potency) which do not permit proper vaginal penetration will naturally interfere with conception, since the sperm will not be properly deposited. This can take place even when the sperm count is perfectly normal.

Can a man be potent yet sterile?

Yes. Many men are able to effect intercourse in a normal manner but their ejaculate (semen) contains no live sperm. Such men are potent but sterile.

What are some of the common causes of impotence?

a. By far the most common cause is psychological disturbance.

b. Local disease of the genital organs.

c. Senility.

Is it important for men with low sperm counts to have adequate diet and vitamin intake?

Yes. Such men should take supplementary vitamins to make sure that their intake is at a satisfactory level.

Is treatment of sterility in the male ever successful?

Yes, in certain cases. Of course, if the testicles are absent or are markedly atrophied, nothing can be done about it. When the problem is one of a low sperm count, various types of hormone treatment are available which may result in an elevation of the sperm count.

Is treatment for male sterility always successful?

No, and the results are often unpredictable. However, treatment should always be carried out because, in a certain percentage of cases, pregnancy will result.

Are there methods, other than the glandular approach, for treating male sterility?

Yes. Any local disease should be eradicated. If there is an infection or a constriction of the urethra, this should be attended to. If there is an inflammation of the prostate gland, this must be corrected. If there is any disease within the scrotum, such as a hydrocele or varicocele, this should be treated surgically. If impotence exists, it should receive treatment from a psychiatrist.

How is it that parties to an infertile union, with no apparent abnormality on examination, will sometimes become divorced, remarried, and become fertile?

In some matings, despite the fact that each partner is found to be physically sound, there is a psychological or chemical barrier to conception. When such people remarry, subsequent circumstances may be such that these barriers no longer exist, and pregnancy results.

What is the "rebound phenomenon" in male sterility?

In some instances, it has been noted that if a man with a low sperm count is given medication to reduce his count to zero, and the medication is then withdrawn, his sperm count will rebound to a point higher than it was before treatment was begun. This form of treatment has been successful in producing pregnancies in some cases but not in the majority of instances.

At what age do most men become infertile?

This varies markedly. Some men remain fertile throughout their entire lives, even into the eighth and ninth decades of life.

Is there such a thing as a male menopause?

It is commonly believed that there is a period in a man's life during which he has menopausal changes, but this is not medically true. The age at which men become impotent, or at which they become infertile, varies widely. Some men lose their potency and become infertile in their forties or fifties; others remain both potent and fertile until the eighth or even ninth decade of life.

Will the giving of hormones cure impotence?

In the vast majority of cases, the giving of hormones has nothing more than psychological value. Most impotence in men is due either to a psychological maladjustment or to senility.

Will overindulgence in sex lead to premature impotence?

No. There is no proof that the sexual activity of the male will have any organic effect upon the age at which he becomes either impotent or infertile.

Is it advisable to continue male hormone injections over a long period of time in order to overcome male sterility?

No. If intensive treatment over a period of several weeks does not result in sperm production, it is perhaps best to discontinue this form of treatment. It is thought that the administration of male hormones over a period of several months or years may induce a dormant tumor of the prostate gland to become active.

Testicular Biopsy. Through a small opening in the scrotum, a snip of testicular tissue is removed for biopsy in order to determine whether infertility has resulted from damage to the testicle. The incision in the scrotum is then sutured as shown on the right.

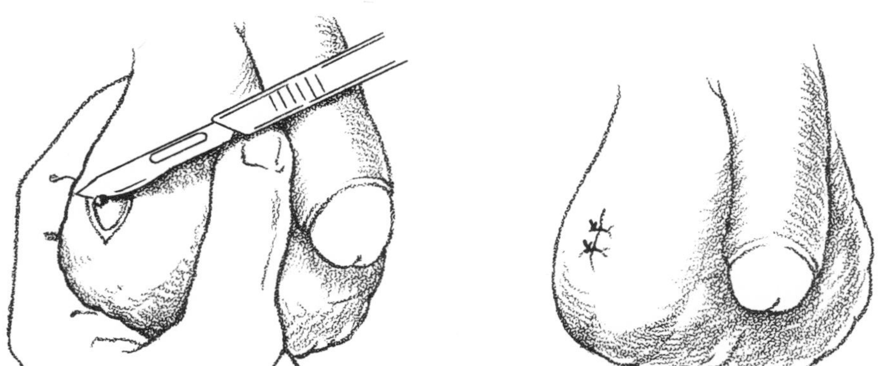

CHAPTER 65

The Stomach and Duodenum

(See also Chapter 22 on Esophagus; Chapter 26 on Gall Bladder and Bile Ducts; Chapter 37 on Liver; Chapter 46 on Pancreas; Chapter 62 on Small and Large Intestines; Chapter 75 on X-ray)

What is the stomach?

The stomach is a hollow pouchlike structure lying beneath the diaphragm under the ribs on the left side of the abdomen. The empty stomach is a sac measuring about six to eight inches in length by three to four inches in width.

What is the function of the stomach?

It is a common misconception that the stomach digests most of our foods. Its main function is to churn the food we have swallowed and to break it down into smaller particles. Its acid juice merely initiates digestion; the more important phases of digestion take place in the small intestine. Very little is absorbed directly through the stomach wall, except certain minerals, water, and alcohol.

What are the most common conditions affecting the stomach?

a. Chronic dyspepsia (indigestion).
b. Hyperacidity (too much acid).
c. Acute gastritis.
d. Chronic gastritis.
e. Ulcer.
f. Pyloric stenosis (obstruction of the stomach outlet).
g. "Upside-down stomach" (diaphragmatic hernia).
h. Benign tumors.
i. Cancer.

Where is the duodenum?

The duodenum is that segment of the small intestine extending for several inches immediately beyond the stomach. It is considered along with the stomach because conditions affecting the stomach so often affect the duodenum, too.

What is the function of the duodenum?

The wall of the duodenum manufactures juices (enzymes) which help digest foods. It is also the portion of small intestine into which the bile is deposited and the segment where the pancreatic juices empty.

What are the most common diseases of the duodenum?

a. Inflammation of the duodenum (duodenitis).
b. Duodenal ulcer.

Do diseases of the stomach or duodenum tend to run in families or to be inherited?

No.

What kind of person is most likely to develop trouble in the stomach or duodenum?

The energetic, nervous, neurotic type in the twenties, thirties, or forties. Men more commonly have stomach or duodenal trouble than women.

Is there any method to minimize stomach trouble?

Yes. To lead a well-ordered, sensible, adjusted life and to eat a moderate, bland diet at regular meal times. Excessive smoking and drinking, too, react badly on the stomach in certain people.

How does the physician make a precise diagnosis of stomach or duodenal disease?

a. By taking a careful history of the exact symptoms.
b. By fluoroscopic and x-ray examination, with the swallowing of barium to visualize the lining of the stomach and duodenum.
c. By passing a tube and analyzing stomach and duodenal contents.

What are the most common symptoms of trouble in the stomach or duodenum?

a. Heartburn.
b. Belching.
c. Nausea.
d. Vomiting.
e. Pain high in the abdomen.

Can the eating of improper foods and poor dietary habits lead to stomach and duodenal disease?

Yes, if continued over a prolonged period of time.

Is it true that certain combinations of foods, such as ice cream and pickles, will cause stomach upsets?

Not necessarily. It all depends upon individual tolerance to certain foods.

Is it true that certain combinations of foods will cause "food poisoning"?

No. Food must be spoiled or infected to cause food poisoning.

Can one live a normal life if part of the stomach has been removed?

Yes. This occurs frequently when one has had a gastrectomy (removal of part of stomach) for ulcer. (See the section on Peptic Ulcer in this chapter.)

Can one eat normally when part of the stomach has been removed?

Yes, but the amount of food should be reduced somewhat and the frequency of feedings increased.

X-ray of a Normal Stomach and Duodenum. People beyond the age of forty or forty-five should have an x-ray series taken of the stomach and duodenum every year or two. By such x-rays, ulcers, inflammatory conditions of the stomach or duodenum, and the presence of tumors can be diagnosed.

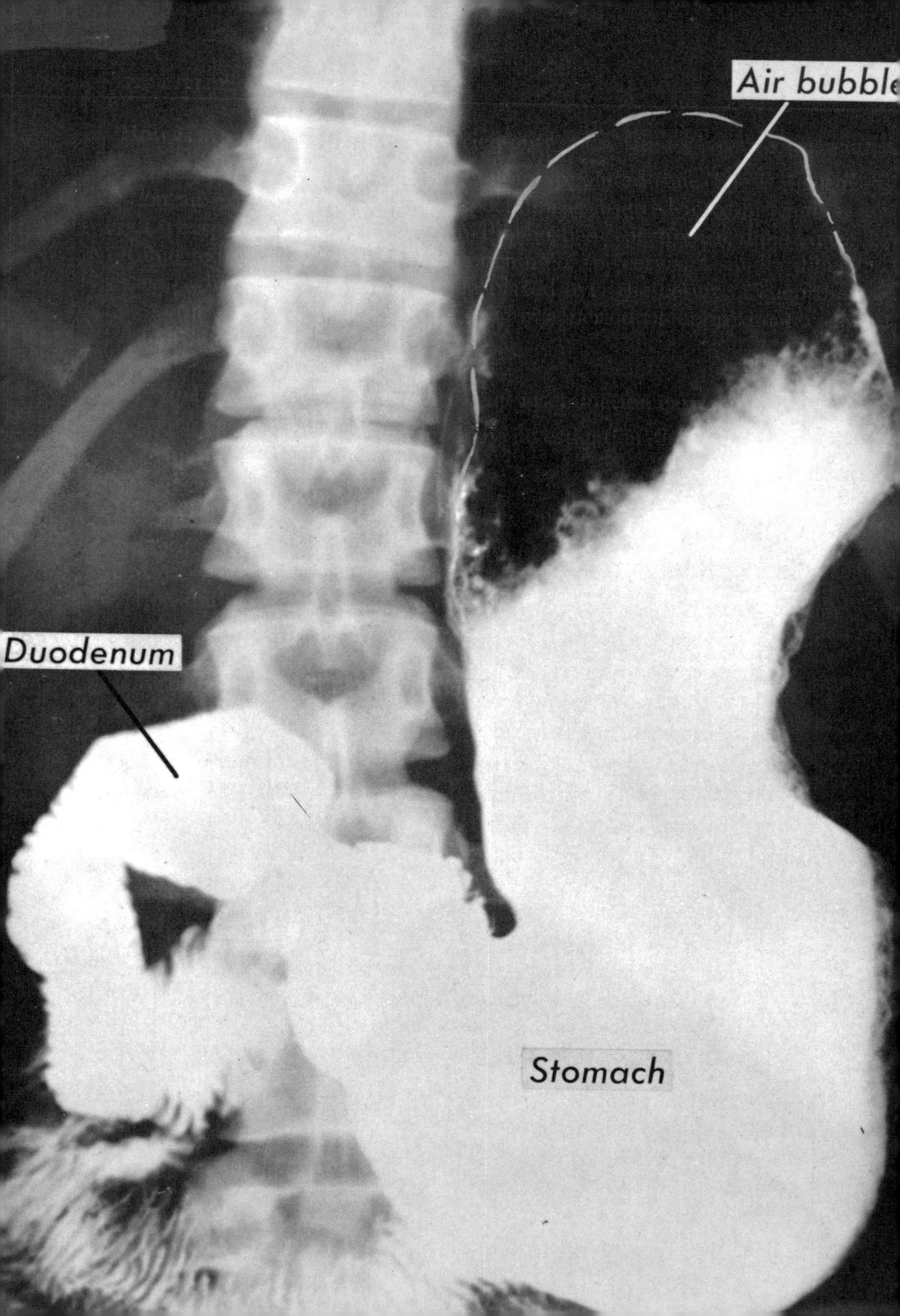
Air bubble
Duodenum
Stomach

Is it true that emotional instability, overwork, or worry can cause stomach trouble?

Definitely, yes. There is a marked psychic factor in conditions of the stomach and duodenum.

INDIGESTION
(*Dyspepsia*)

What are the common symptoms of indigestion?

A sense of fullness in the upper abdomen, heartburn, acid regurgitation of food, nausea, and vomiting.

What is heartburn?

A sensation of burning in the upper abdomen which ascends to the chest. Also, there is the taste of sour food in the back of the throat.

What causes indigestion?

a. Excess secretion of stomach juices and acid.
b. Eating too much.
c. Eating too rapidly.
d. Eating improperly prepared foods.
e. Eating too highly seasoned foods.
f. Eating the wrong foods, such as those containing too much fat, grease, etc.
g. Eating infected or spoiled foods.

What is the treatment for indigestion?

a. Fasting for several hours, or even for an entire day.
b. Eating a light bland diet.
c. Taking one of the innumerable medications which will neutralize excess secretion of stomach juices and acidity.
d. The administration of one of the antispasmodic medications to cut down on excess contractions of the stomach and duodenum.

Is it true that certain people are immune to the symptoms of indigestion and upset stomach?

Certain people do tend to have "stronger stomachs" than others.

Nevertheless, if improper food intake occurs or if infected material is eaten, even the strongest stomach can react violently!

Is it good practice for someone to make himself vomit when his stomach feels upset?

If this can be done without too much distress, it is often good treatment to empty the stomach when it is upset.

Are the terms "acute gastritis," "upset stomach," and "acute indigestion" really used to describe the same condition?

Yes, although some people erroneously associate the term "acute indigestion" with a heart attack.

What are the symptoms of an "upset stomach"?

Nausea, vomiting, cramps in the upper abdomen, loss of appetite. These occur usually within an hour or two after eating something that disagrees with the patient.

How can one differentiate between an upset stomach and a more serious condition such as appendicitis, a gall bladder attack, or a heart attack?

This is frequently difficult, and all people who have severe upper abdominal pain should contact their physician. Self-treatment is unwise if one has these symptoms.

Is it safe to take a laxative for an upset stomach or acute indigestion?

No, unless advised by your doctor.

When should one call a doctor for abdominal pain?

a. Whenever the pain is severe and the patient feels unable to tolerate it.

b. Whenever the pain persists for more than a few hours.

Are there any particular foods which are more apt to cause indigestion than others?

Yes; spoiled foods or foods which have been allowed to stand out in an open kitchen for several hours in hot weather (such as salads). Also, highly seasoned and greasy foods.

Is it true that certain foods cannot be eaten with other foods because they are incompatible?

No. This is a common misconception.

Is the drinking of liquids at meal time a bad habit?

On the contrary, it aids digestion.

Should one eat more lightly in hot weather than in cold weather?

Yes.

Should one avoid heavy meals before going to sleep at night?

Yes. It is best to permit all the organs of the body to rest during sleep.

Is it dangerous to eat a heavy meal immediately before swimming?

Yes, because the blood flow is diverted to the digestive tract instead of serving the muscular system, where it is most needed at such times. However, it has not been proved that eating before swimming will cause cramps and thus endanger the life of the swimmer.

How great a part do the emotions play in indigestion?

A very strong part. Every conceivable abdominal or intestinal symptom can be caused by emotional upset.

Is it true that a person tends to have more stomach trouble as he grows older?

Yes.

Are there certain foods which must be avoided when drinking alcoholic beverages?

No. It is a common misconception that certain foods will cause violent upset if taken along with an alcoholic beverage. Of course, an upset stomach may follow drinking excessive quantities of alcohol no matter what food is taken along with it.

Is it harmful to take iced drinks when one is overheated?

No, except when large amounts are taken rapidly.

STOMACH ACIDITY

Does the normal stomach contain acid?

Yes. Hydrochloric acid is secreted by the cells of the stomach in order to aid digestion.

Will excess stomach acids cause symptoms?

Yes. It is thought that excess acid is an important factor in the formation of an ulcer of the stomach or duodenum. Excess acid may also be associated with heartburn, inflammation of the stomach lining (gastritis), or inflammation of the duodenum (duodenitis).

Will lack of acid in the stomach cause symptoms?

Usually not, as the acid is not essential to normal digestion. On the other hand, in later life, a lack of acid is thought to make one slightly more prone to the development of a stomach tumor.

Can one live normally without stomach acid?

Yes. Approximately 10 per cent of all people have low acid or absence of acid in the stomach.

What causes lack of stomach acid?

a. Most people with lack of acid (achlorhydria) are born with it.
b. As people grow older and get into the sixth and seventh decades of life, they tend to manufacture less acid.

What are the symptoms of lack of acid?

Usually, there are none. Occasionally, a patient with low acid experiences some difficulty in digesting large quantities of meats.

What causes excess stomach acidity?

The exact cause is unknown. It is known that the emotionally disturbed, energetic, dynamic types tend to secrete more acid.

Also, certain highly seasoned foods, tobacco, and alcohol will cause the stomach lining to secrete large quantities of hydrochloric acid.

How does the physician test for acid in the stomach?

a. By passing a rubber tube through the nose or mouth into the stomach and analyzing the material which is withdrawn. This is called "gastric analysis."

b. There is a urine test which gives a fairly accurate picture of stomach acidity.

If a person has high stomach acidity, does this mean he will always have high acid?

Not necessarily. The factors producing excess acidity, such as periods of emotional strain, may subside and the acid content of the stomach may then return to normal.

How effective are the commonly advertised antacid medications?

Very effective to counteract excess acidity for a short period of time. However, they do not cure the condition; relief is only temporary.

Is there any harm in taking antacid medications over a long period of time?

No, but it is much wiser to seek medical aid to relieve the underlying cause of the excess acidity (hyperacidity).

What is the best treatment for excess stomach acidity?

a. Frequent bland feedings, every two to three hours.

b. Abstinence from smoking, alcohol, and highly seasoned foods.

c. Taking of antacid medications and certain gastric inhibitory medicines in the banthine group.

d. Attempting to live a more well-ordered, controlled emotional life.

What is the best treatment for lack of acid in the stomach?

Usually, no treatment is required. However, if symptoms do occur, appropriate amounts of acid can be taken orally.

What role does excess stomach acidity play in the cause of ulcers of the stomach or duodenum?

It is thought that the greatest single contributory factor toward ulcer formation is chronic hyperacidity.

ACUTE GASTRITIS AND GASTROENTERITIS

What is acute gastritis?

It is an inflammation of the lining of the stomach caused by bacteria, viruses, chemical irritants, or by eating spoiled foods.

What are the symptoms of acute gastritis?

Nausea, vomiting, upper abdominal cramps, fever.

Is gastritis usually associated with a similar inflammation of the small intestine?

Yes, and the condition is therefore referred to as gastroenteritis.

Is "ptomaine poisoning" another name for acute gastritis or gastroenteritis?

Yes, but this is no longer a term used by physicians.

What is the treatment for acute gastritis or gastroenteritis?

a. Bed rest.
b. Abstinence from food.
c. Moderate fluid intake when nausea subsides.
d. Antispasmodic and antacid drugs.
e. Drugs to quiet excess intestinal activity and to halt the diarrhea.

How soon do people with acute gastritis or gastroenteritis get well?

The condition usually subsides within one to three days. If it does not, examinations should be carried out to determine whether some more serious underlying disease exists.

How does one distinguish between acute gastritis and acute gastroenteritis?

The latter condition is accompanied by violent midabdominal and lower abdominal cramps, with episodes of diarrhea. When only the stomach is involved, diarrhea is not present.

Is it necessary to operate for acute gastritis?

No. This is a medical condition which will clear up with medical management.

CHRONIC GASTRITIS

What is chronic gastritis?

An inflammation of the lining of the stomach which persists over a long period of time.

What causes chronic gastritis?

The cause is not definitely known, but it is thought that prolonged and excessive use of spices, alcohol, and other irritants may eventually lead to a chronic inflammation of the stomach lining.

What are the symptoms of chronic gastritis?

Upper abdominal discomfort and pain, heartburn, and a sense of fullness in the region. Also, loss of appetite, loss of weight, nausea, and vomiting. With certain types, there may be hemorrhage, with the vomiting of blood or the passage of a black stool.

How does the physician make a diagnosis of chronic gastritis?

From the history of symptoms plus characteristic x-ray findings.

What is the best way to prevent getting chronic gastritis?

Avoid those substances which are thought to be predisposing toward the disease.

What is the treatment for chronic gastritis?

a. Stop smoking.
b. Refrain from alcoholic beverages.
c. Eat frequent, small, bland meals, with plenty of milk.
d. Refrain from eating spicy foods.

e. If the chronic gastritis is associated with excess stomach acidity, take appropriate antacid medications.

f. If there is an absence of acid, then medications will be given along with liver extracts and vitamins.

Does chronic gastritis ever clear up?

Yes, some cases will, after adequate treatment for several months. Others do not clear up but can be kept under control.

Is it ever necessary to operate for chronic gastritis?

Only if there is repeated hemorrhage.

Does chronic gastritis ever terminate in other diseases?

Yes. It has been found that certain types of chronic gastritis (hypertrophic gastritis) seem to predispose toward ulcer formation, while other types (atrophic gastritis) predispose toward cancer of the stomach.

How can one tell the progress of chronic gastritis?

a. By noting the activity of the symptoms.

b. By a medical checkup every few months, with x-rays of the stomach.

What is the difference between chronic hypertrophic gastritis and chronic atrophic gastritis?

Hypertrophic gastritis gives many of the symptoms of ulcer, is associated with excess acid secretion, and may be accompanied by hemorrhage.

Atrophic gastritis may be associated with loss of appetite, low or absent acid secretion, and anemia.

INFLAMMATION OF THE DUODENUM

(Duodenitis)

What is duodenitis?

An inflammation and irritability of the duodenum.

What causes duodenitis?

It is usually associated with excess acidity and with all the other factors that lead to the development of an ulcer.

What are the symptoms of duodenitis?

Very similar to those of ulcer. (See the section on Peptic Ulcer in this chapter.)

How does the physician make a diagnosis of duodenitis?

By noting the symptoms and by observing the characteristic findings of an irritable and spastic duodenum on x-ray examination.

What is the treatment for duodenitis?

The same as for peptic ulcer.

Is it ever necessary to operate for duodenitis?

No. This is strictly a medical condition.

Will duodenitis clear up by itself, if untreated?

It may, but it has a tendency to become chronic if not treated.

How effective are present-day measures in relieving duodenitis?

An ulcer regime will cause most cases to subside after a period of several weeks or months.

Do people who have had duodenitis at one time tend to develop it again?

Yes, if they are careless with their diet, drink to excess, and fail to observe medical instructions.

PEPTIC ULCER

(Ulcers of the Stomach or Duodenum)

What is meant by the term "peptic" ulcer?

It is a general term used to describe an ulcer in the stomach, duodenum, or the lower end of the esophagus.

What causes peptic ulcer?

The exact cause is not known, but the common underlying factor in almost all cases is hyperacidity, or the secretion of excess acid by the stomach.

What types of peptic ulcer are there?

a. Duodenal ulcer is the most common form.

b. Stomach (gastric) ulcer is next in frequency.

c. Esophageal ulcer is the least frequently encountered ulcer.

How common is an ulcer of the stomach or duodenum?

About one in every ten adults is thought to have a duodenal ulcer at some time or other. About one in every hundred adults will have a gastric ulcer at some time or other.

What type of person is most likely to develop peptic ulcer?

The energetic, dynamic, highly emotional person who is beset by many frustrations but who works at a fast pace in a highly civilized society. Men get ulcers more often than women.

Do ulcers of the stomach or duodenum tend to run in families or to be inherited?

Not really, except that there is a tendency for children to develop along the same lines as their parents. Thus, neurotic parents with ulcers may have offspring who develop the same tendencies.

What actually takes place when an ulcer of the stomach or duodenum is present?

The lining mucous membrane is eaten away and eroded, leaving a raw, uncovered area in the wall of the stomach or duodenum. Ulcers may vary in size from that of a pinhead to that of a half dollar.

Is there any way to lessen the chances of getting an ulcer?

a. Don't smoke.

b. Drink alcohol only in moderate amounts.

c. Eat bland, non-spicy foods.

d. Attempt to live within the bounds of one's ability and capacity.

Is the size of an ulcer significant?

Not necessarily. Small ulcers may bleed or rupture almost as easily as large ulcers. As a general rule, however, the larger and deeper the ulcer, the more difficult and the longer it will take to heal.

How can one tell if he has an ulcer?

The most characteristic symptoms are gnawing hunger pains in the upper abdomen occurring between meals. The pains are usually relieved for several hours by eating. Other symptoms include sour taste in the mouth, belching, and heartburn, relieved by the taking of antacid medications.

What tests are performed to make a positive diagnosis of peptic ulcer?

Most cases can be demonstrated by x-ray studies of the stomach and duodenum.

What are the harmful effects of peptic ulcer?

In addition to the pain and continued discomfort which ulcer patients suffer, there are the following possible complications:

a. A gastric (stomach) ulcer, if untreated, may develop into cancer. This happens in about one in fifteen cases.
b. As ulcers become chronic, they may form scar tissue which will obstruct the outlet of the stomach.
c. Ulcers may rupture and cause peritonitis.
d. Ulcers tend to cause severe hemorrhage. Death from loss of blood can occur during a bleeding episode.

What is the treatment for peptic ulcer?

More than 90 per cent of all ulcers will respond to medical treatment and will require no surgery.

Standard medical treatment for a patient suffering from a peptic ulcer will consist of:

a. Special ulcer diet, with frequent feedings of milk and cream.
b. Abstinence from all irritants, spicy foods, alcohol, etc.
c. Antacid medications.
d. Special medications which act through the nervous system so as

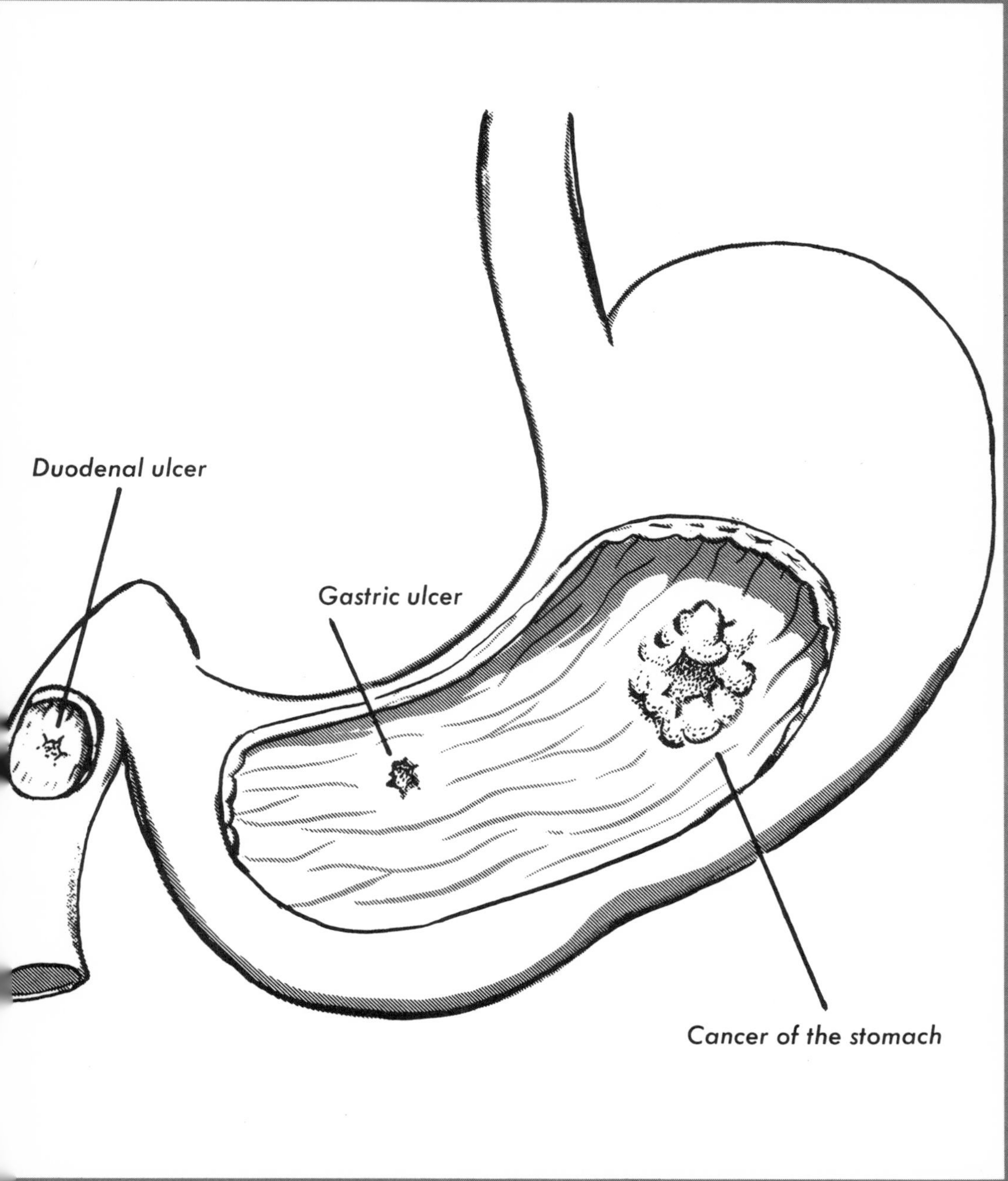

Cancer of the Stomach, Ulcers of the Stomach, and Duodenal Ulcer. This is a composite drawing showing three separate conditions which sometimes affect the stomach or duodenum.

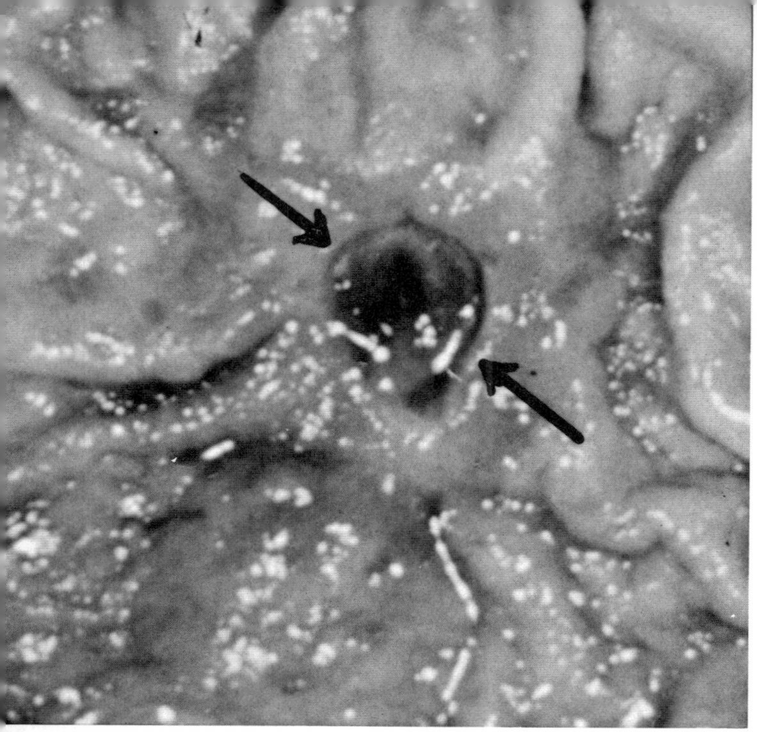

Ulcer of the Stomach. This is an actual photograph of a stomach ulcer which has been removed surgically. Note how the lining membrane of the stomach has been eaten away by the ulcer.

to cut down on the secretion of gastric juice and acid. These drugs are in the banthine group.

e. Stop smoking.

The remainder who do not respond to medical treatment should be operated upon if:

a. It is a gastric ulcer which shows no healing within a few weeks, as these ulcers have a tendency to become cancerous.
b. When pain and discomfort continue over the years despite conscientious attempts to bring about a cure through medical management.
c. When there is obstruction to the stomach outlet.
d. When the ulcer ruptures or threatens to rupture.
e. When there are repeated episodes of severe hemorrhage.

Do ulcers, once healed through medical management, have a tendency to recur?

Yes. As long as the stomach pours out an excess of acid there is danger of a new break occurring in its lining, with a resultant ulcer.

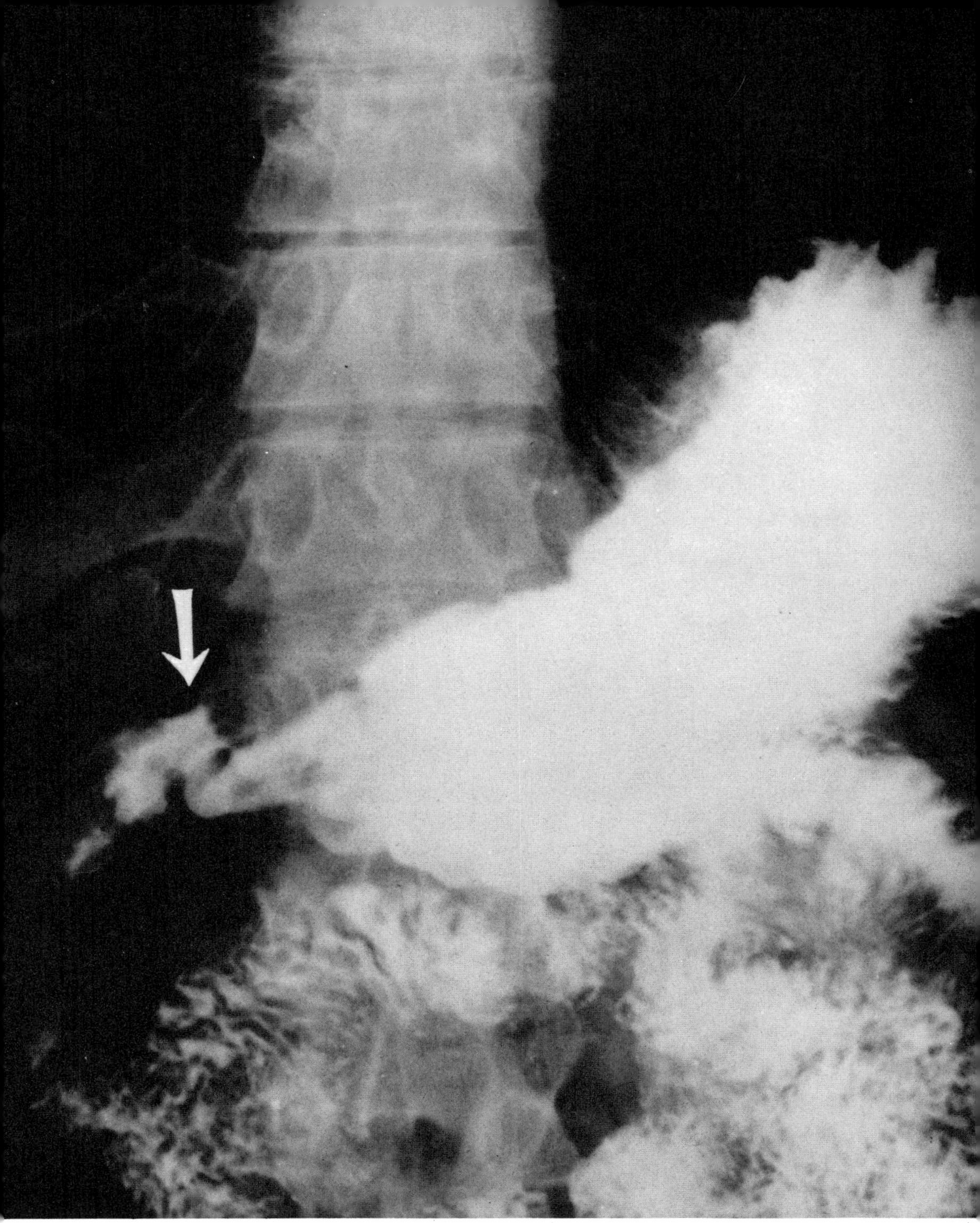

X-ray Showing Duodenal Ulcer. Compare the irregular outline of the duodenum in this x-ray with that of the normal duodenal outline seen in the x-ray of the normal stomach on page 1365

What are the causes for recurrence of healed ulcers?

Failure to maintain an ulcer dietary regime; continuation of smoking and drinking alcoholic beverages; the persistence of those situations in life which lead to emotional instability and stress.

What actually takes place in the lining of the stomach when an ulcer heals?

The lining membrane (mucosa) grows back over the raw, ulcerated surface.

Why is it more important to remove an ulcer of the stomach than an ulcer of the duodenum?

Stomach ulcers may form cancer; duodenal ulcers do not.

Are operations for peptic ulcer serious?

Yes, but approximately ninety-nine out of a hundred will recover from the surgery.

What operations are performed to cure peptic ulcer?

There are several procedures, each of which has special indications and each will result in cure in well over 90 per cent of cases.

1. For an ulcer located in the stomach (gastric ulcer), a subtotal gastrectomy is done. This involves the removal of approximately 3/4s of the stomach and the remainder is joined to the small intestine. (See accompanying diagrams.)
2. For an ulcer in the duodenum (the most common form of peptic ulcer) one of the following operations is performed:
   a. A subtotal gastrectomy, as described above.
   b. A vagotomy, in which the vagus nerves (which stimulate the stomach to secrete acid) are cut and approximately 50 per cent of the stomach is removed.
   c. A vagotomy is performed and the outlet of the stomach is altered so as to permit the regurgitation of bile from the alkaline duodenum into the stomach. This procedure is known as pyloroplasty.
   d. A vagotomy is performed and a short-circuiting opening is

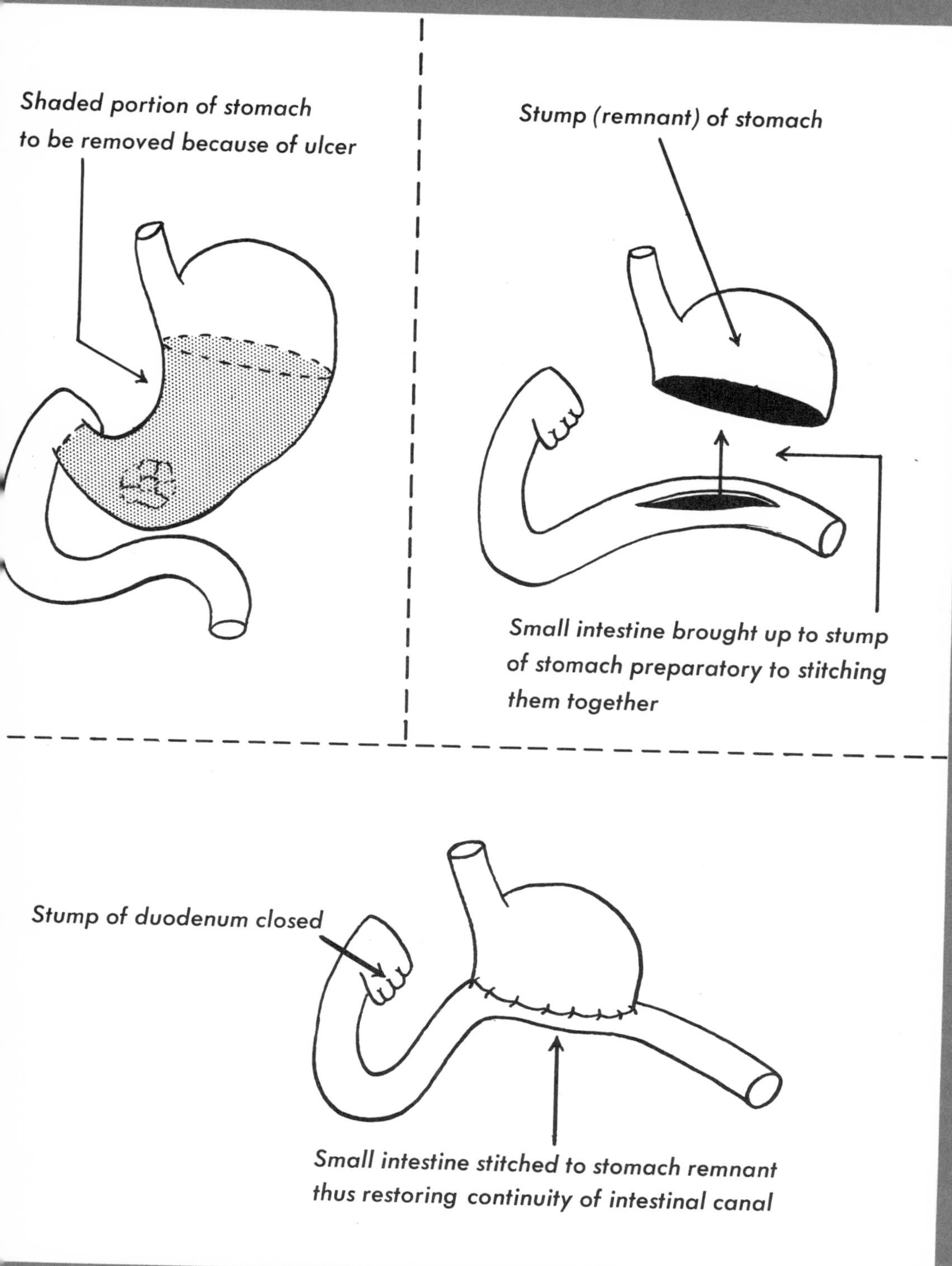

Subtotal Gastrectomy for Ulcer. These diagrams demonstrate the operative procedure most frequently used for cure of a stomach or duodenal ulcer. The results from this operation are good, with cure of the ulcer resulting in more than 90 per cent of cases.

made between the stomach and small intestine. This latter procedure is known as a gastro-jejunostomy.

Are all of the above operations equally successful in treating peptic ulcer?

Although all of the above operations give satisfactory results, recent statistical studies seem to show that the operations associated with vagotomy will give a somewhat higher cure rate than plain gastrectomy. This holds true for ulcers in the duodenum, but not for those located in the stomach.

How long a period of hospitalization is usually required for operations for ulcer?

Ten to fifteen days.

Will special preoperative preparations be necessary?

Yes. Patients are often admitted to the hospital a few days prior to surgery so that they can be prepared by liquid diet, washings of the stomach, intravenous medications, vitamins, and—if they have lost much blood—transfusions.

Will special nurses be required after an operation for peptic ulcer?

Yes, for several days.

How long does it take to perform an ulcer operation?

From two to five hours, depending upon the severity of the case and the type of operation performed. (Speed in surgery is not important.)

What anesthesia is usually employed in ulcer operations?

General inhalation anesthesia.

What special postoperative treatments are necessary after ulcer operations?

a. Liquid by mouth is withheld for two to three days, and food is not given for four to five days.

b. The patient is fed intravenously with glucose, proteins, minerals, and vitamins.

c. Stomach tubes are employed to keep the stomach or stomach remnant empty.

d. Antibiotics are sometimes given to prevent postoperative infection.

What takes over the function of the stomach or duodenum when part of it is removed because of an ulcer?

The remnant of the stomach dilates over a period of several months and, along with the small intestine to which it has been joined, a pouch is formed which serves as an excellent receptacle for food.

Do ulcers tend to recur after an operation has been carried out?

They recur rarely—in less than 3 per cent of cases.

What postoperative precautions must be followed after operations for ulcer?

a. Do not eat too large quantities of food at one time.

b. Highly seasoned foods and alcoholic beverages should be kept at a minimum for several months postoperatively, until one is sure that all ulcer symptoms have disappeared completely.

Can one *ever* return to completely normal eating after an ulcer operation?

Yes, within a few months.

What limitations on one's activities must be imposed after an ulcer operation?

None, after the patient has convalesced completely. (This may require three to four months.)

Does stomach removal for ulcer affect the span of life?

No.

Does stomach removal tend toward the development of anemia?

Yes, in some cases. However, this can be treated successfully with medications to build up the blood.

Is pregnancy permissible after an operation for peptic ulcer?

Yes.

How soon after an ulcer operation can one do the following:

Bathe	Ten to fifteen days.
Walk out on the street	Ten to fifteen days.
Walk up and down stairs	Ten to fifteen days.
Perform household duties	Five to six weeks.
Drive a car	Six to eight weeks.
Resume marital relations	Five to six weeks.
Return to work	Eight weeks.

How often should one return for a periodic examination after an ulcer operation?

Every four to six months.

If a patient has had gastrectomy for duodenal ulcer, is the ulcer itself always removed?

Not if it is technically too difficult to remove. Cure, in ulcer cases, is brought about by removing the acid-producing portion of the stomach, by cutting the vagus nerve which stimulates the production of acid, and by short-circuiting the flow of food so that it completely bypasses the duodenum. If this is done, the ulcer which has been left behind will heal very rapidly and will cause no symptoms.

Can digestion be normal even without stomach acids and without part of the stomach?

Yes. Approximately 10 per cent of all people have little or no acid in their stomach. Also, it should be remembered that the major phase of digestion of foods takes place in the small intestine, not in the stomach.

PYLORIC STENOSIS

(Obstruction of the Outlet of the Stomach in the Newborn)

What is pyloric stenosis?

An obstruction to the outlet of the stomach in infants during their first few weeks of life.

What causes pyloric stenosis?

An overgrowth of the muscle surrounding the pylorus.

Are male infants affected more often than female infants?

Yes. It is three times more common in males.

How common is pyloric stenosis?

It occurs in approximately one in one thousand births.

What are the symptoms of pyloric stenosis?

a. Forceful vomiting which sometimes shoots out of the mouth.
b. A lump, the size of a walnut, can usually be felt in the right upper portion of the abdomen.
c. Weight loss due to repeated vomiting.
d. X-ray findings demonstrating an obstruction to the passage of food from the stomach into the small intestine.

What is the treatment for pyloric stenosis?

The great majority of cases will require surgery. A small number can be treated successfully with antispasmodic drugs.

How long should one wait before deciding to operate, if symptoms persist?

No longer than one to two weeks.

What operative procedure is carried out?

A small incision, two inches long, is made in the right upper portion

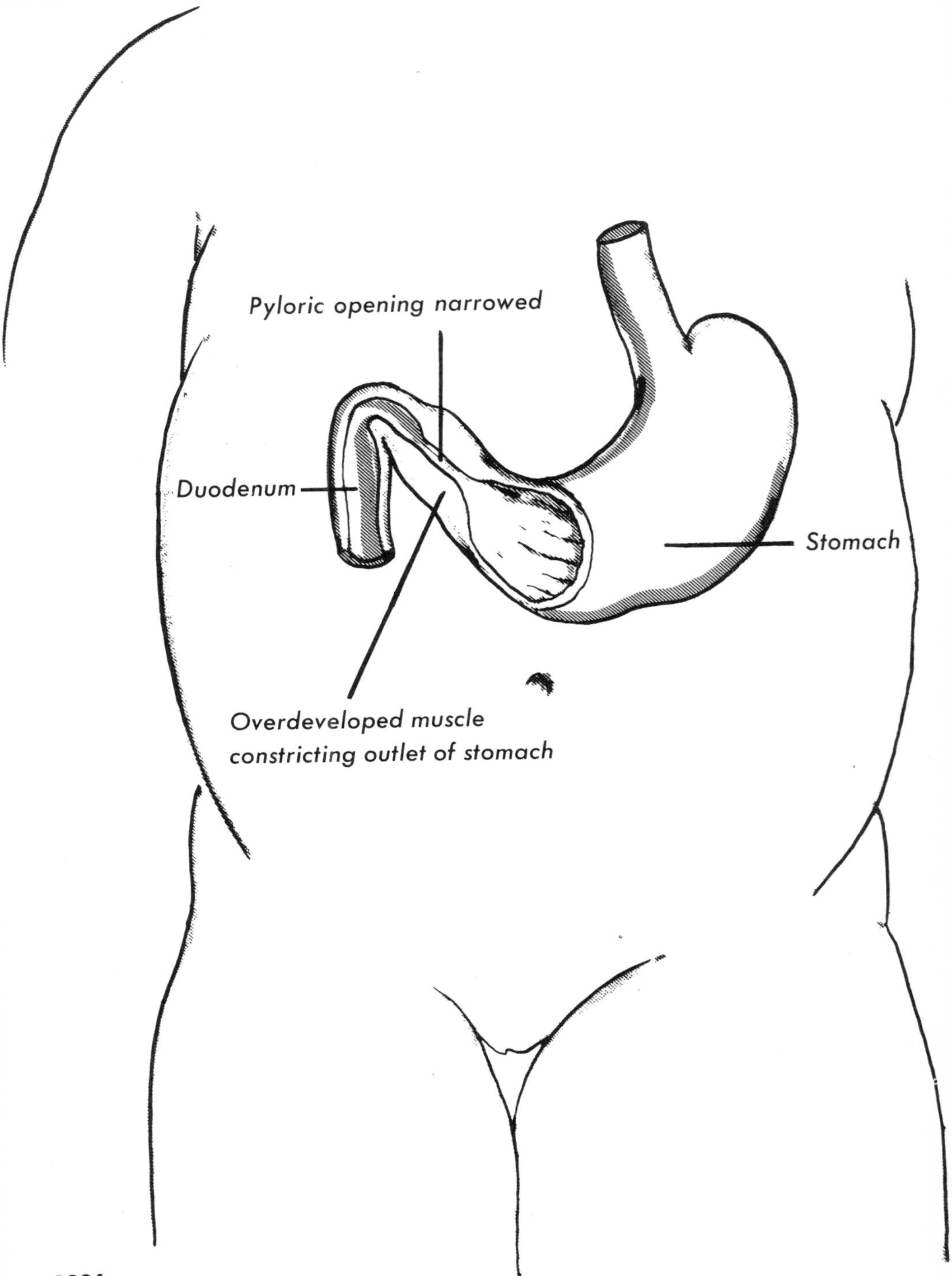

Pyloric Stenosis. This diagram shows how the outlet of the stomach is obstructed by excess muscle development. When these muscles are severed surgically, the condition is relieved.

of the abdomen. The pyloric portion of the stomach is grasped and the muscle fibers are cut. The mucous membrane lining is permitted to remain intact.

How effective is surgery in the cure of pyloric stenosis?

Practically all cases are cured by the operation described above.

Is this operation dangerous?

No. Recovery will take place in all cases, barring the exceptional complication which may accompany any surgical procedure.

What type of anesthesia is used in operating upon pyloric stenosis?

Ether inhalation anesthesia.

How long a period of hospitalization is usually necessary?

Five to seven days.

Are special nurses required for the infant?

No.

How long does it take the wound to heal after an operation for pyloric stenosis?

Seven to ten days.

How soon after surgery are feedings begun?

Within twenty-four to forty-eight hours.

Does pyloric stenosis, once operated upon, have a tendency to recur?

No.

How soon after an operation can the child be bathed?

As soon as the wound has healed.

Will the child live a completely normal life after pyloric stenosis?

Yes. Development will not be impaired once surgical cure has been obtained.

"UPSIDE-DOWN" STOMACH

(Hernia of the Diaphragm)

(See Chapter 28, on Hernia.)

CANCER OF THE STOMACH

What causes cancer of the stomach?

In most instances, the cause is unknown. Some cancers are thought to have their origin in ulcers of the stomach.

Are all tumors of the stomach cancerous?

No. There may be tumors of the mucous membrane lining or of the muscle wall which are nonmalignant. The most common nonmalignant tumors are polyps of the mucous membrane, lipomas (fatty tumors), and myomas (tumors containing muscle tissue).

Are nonmalignant tumors of the stomach curable?

Yes. They can be removed surgically, either by local excision or by removing that portion of the stomach in which they grow.

How common is cancer of the stomach?

It accounts for approximately one-third of all cancers in men, and one-fifth of all cancers in women.

Do statistics show that cancer of the stomach in this country is on the increase?

No. Peculiarly, recent statistical data would seem to indicate that cancer of the stomach is one of the few types of malignancy that is not increasing.

What age groups are most affected by cancer of the stomach?

This is a disease most often found in middle age and in the later years of life.

Does cancer of the stomach tend to run in families or to be inherited?

No.

Is there any way to prevent cancer of the stomach?

The prompt removal of an ulcer in the stomach may prevent it from becoming cancerous. Also, cancer might be apprehended in its early stages if more people would visit their physician for a regular physical examination and if more people who have gastro-intestinal symptoms would submit to thorough x-ray examinations.

How is the diagnosis of cancer of the stomach made?

By x-ray examination. The diagnosis can also be made in certain cases by passing a specially designed instrument known as a gastroscope through the mouth into the stomach. This may allow the gastroscopist to view the tumor directly through the instrument.

What are the symptoms of cancer of the stomach?

There are very few early symptoms. However, chronic indigestion, loss of appetite, slight weight loss, or pallor should stimulate one to seek an x-ray of his entire gastro-intestinal tract.

What is the treatment for cancer of the stomach?

Prompt surgery with gastrectomy (the removal of all but a small remnant of the stomach).

What special preoperative measures are necessary for cancer of the stomach?

The same as for peptic ulcer.

Are operations for cancer of the stomach very serious?

Yes, but with modern advances in surgery, well over 90 per cent will recover from their operation.

How long a hospital stay is necessary for cancer of the stomach?

Approximately two weeks.

What type of anesthesia is used?

Either general inhalation anesthesia or, in selected cases, a high spinal anesthesia.

How long does it take to perform an operation for cancer of the stomach?

Two to five hours, depending upon whether the entire stomach is removed or only a portion of it is removed. Also, a great deal will depend upon the extent of spread and the technical problems which are encountered.

Do ulcers of the stomach ever become malignant?

Yes. Large ulcers of the stomach (not the duodenum) have a tendency to become malignant.

Will a surgeon know whether a stomach ulcer has become malignant when he views it at operation?

Not always, but he will perform a gastrectomy, nevertheless. The tissue will be submitted for microscopic examination and this will tell the story within a few days.

Are blood transfusions given during operations upon the stomach?

Yes, in most cases.

What is the usual postoperative course and what are the postoperative routines employed in cases of cancer of the stomach?

Practically the same as those used after gastrectomy for ulcer, except that the patient is a good deal sicker after gastrectomy for cancer. (See the section on Peptic Ulcer in this chapter.)

For how long a period are special nurses necessary after this kind of operation?

For several days.

CHAPTER 66

Stress

(See also Chapter 41 on Mental Health and Disease)

What is the concept of stress?

The human body has within it certain innate mechanisms which allow it to protect itself from outside stresses. These stresses may be physical, such as excess heat or cold; or emotional, such as impending danger. The reaction of the body to the stress is called "adaptation." Adaptation is a complex mechanism involving the nervous system and the glandular (endocrine) system. These adaptation patterns vary, depending upon the nature of the stress and the basic character of the individual. In general, adaptational response to physical stress is physical; the adaptational response to an emotional stress is both psychological and physical. These latter responses may be expressed as an emotional pattern—anger, fear, disgust, etc.

What are some physical stress reactions?

One of the most important is the reaction to a sudden or severe injury. The body may react to such an injury by a generalized response known as shock, a state in which the blood content of the body is redistributed to those organs which need it the most. However, like many adaptational mechanisms, if the shock is permitted to persist too long, it may lose its ability to act as a protective mechanism and may lead to death.

Another common physical adaptational reaction to a physical stress is allergy. The allergic response, whether in the form of hay fever, asthma or hives, is the body's defense against a foreign substance (i.e., a pollen). However, when the protective reaction is too extreme (as in bronchial asthma), the reaction may be more serious than the stress which originally produced it.

What are some emotional stress reactions?

Just as a physical stress (pollen) can provoke a physical reaction (asthma), so can a psychological stress (impending danger) provoke a psychological reaction (fear). The adaptational reaction of fear is biologically designed to better prepare the person for the danger. Thus, when confronted with danger, the adrenal glands pour forth certain secretions which better enable the body to withstand the stress. However, the psychological elements of fear may become so overwhelming as to completely incapacitate the individual, while the physical elements, if they persist long enough, may actually cause physical illness. Some physicians call these physical illnesses, which result from psychological stresses, psychosomatic diseases.

What role does the stress mechanism play in health?

Certain of the stress reactions are essential for health. For example, the allergic reaction which is so troublesome to hay fever sufferers is the same mechanism as the one by which we develop immunity to certain diseases, either through actual exposure (you can have measles only once) or by inoculation (polio vaccine). Similarly, in any physical illness, the production of certain hormones by the adrenal gland is the means the body uses to fight disease, just as the doctor may fight disease when he prescribes drugs or medications.

What part does the stress mechanism play in physical disease?

It is thought that impaired adaptational responses, whether overactive or underactive, may result in actual physical disease. Allergy, as mentioned above, may be an example of a physical adaptational response which has gone askew. High blood pressure, on the other hand, is considered by many to be the result of emotional adaptational response becoming overactive. When a person becomes excited, his pressure rises and he becomes more affected. However, if excitement persists too long, his high blood pressure becomes fixed and he becomes physically ill.

On the other hand, in certain illnesses, the adaptational organs react as though they were exhausted. For example, the adrenal glands may excrete an insufficient amount of hormone (cortisone). Under such circumstances, the body may react defectively, and diseases such as arthritis or colitis may result. The administration of the adrenal hormone (cortisone) will help the patient to return to normal.

Is the stress reaction a helpful or harmful one in maintaining health?

This will depend upon the severity of the stress and the intensity of the adaptational reaction. Basically, the stress reaction is beneficial, since it is the biological system of self-protection. However, if the adaptational system becomes either overactive or exhaustive, it may produce actual physical or mental disease.

What are the so-called "adaptation diseases"?

They are those brought about through constant exposure to chronic stress.

What is the relation of the stress mechanisms to the so-called "psychosomatic disorders"?

Psychosomatic disorders are considered by many physicians to be the physical results of prolonged emotional tension. Such diseases as high blood pressure, peptic ulcer, and overactivity of the thyroid gland fall into this category. Other diseases, such as arthritis, colitis, and allergies, are considered to be the effect of underactivity of the adaptational system through exhaustion.

What role is stress supposed to play in the aging process?

It is thought by many investigators that aging is in some measure the result of frequent and continued insult which the body suffers over a prolonged period of time. Hardening of the arteries, for example, may result from prolonged high blood pressure and diabetes, both of which may be adaptational responses. The endocrine glands, especially, tend to become exhausted by frequent stresses and strains of life, and their underactivity tends to accelerate the aging process. It would appear that to prolong life, one should avoid excessive stresses of any type.

CHAPTER 67

The Throat

(See also Chapter 36 on Lips, Jaws, Mouth, Teeth, and Tongue; Chapter 45 on Nose and Sinuses; Chapter 59 on Salivary Glands; Chapter 68 on Thyroid Gland)

THE TONSILS AND ADENOIDS

What are the tonsils, and where are they located?

The tonsils are two ovoid, glandlike structures, measuring about one and one-half inches long by three-quarters of an inch wide, imbedded in the sides of the throat just behind and above the level of the tongue.

What is the normal appearance of the tonsils?

When normal, the tonsils are barely visible.

What is the appearance of the tonsils when infected?

They may occupy a major portion of the pharynx and may actually meet in the midline. They can be seen as large reddened masses and, when acutely inflamed, yellow spots of pus can often be seen on their surface.

What are the adenoids, and where are they located?

They consist of the same type of tissue as the tonsils and are located high up in the throat above the level of the soft palate. They cannot be easily seen on ordinary inspection of the throat. Normally, the adenoids are about half the size of the tonsils.

What is the function of the tonsils and adenoids?

They are composed of lymphoid tissue and are thought to serve as

Adenoids. Enlargement of the adenoids may lead to ear infections and often prevents breathing through the nose. In children, adenoids are removed at the same time as tonsils.

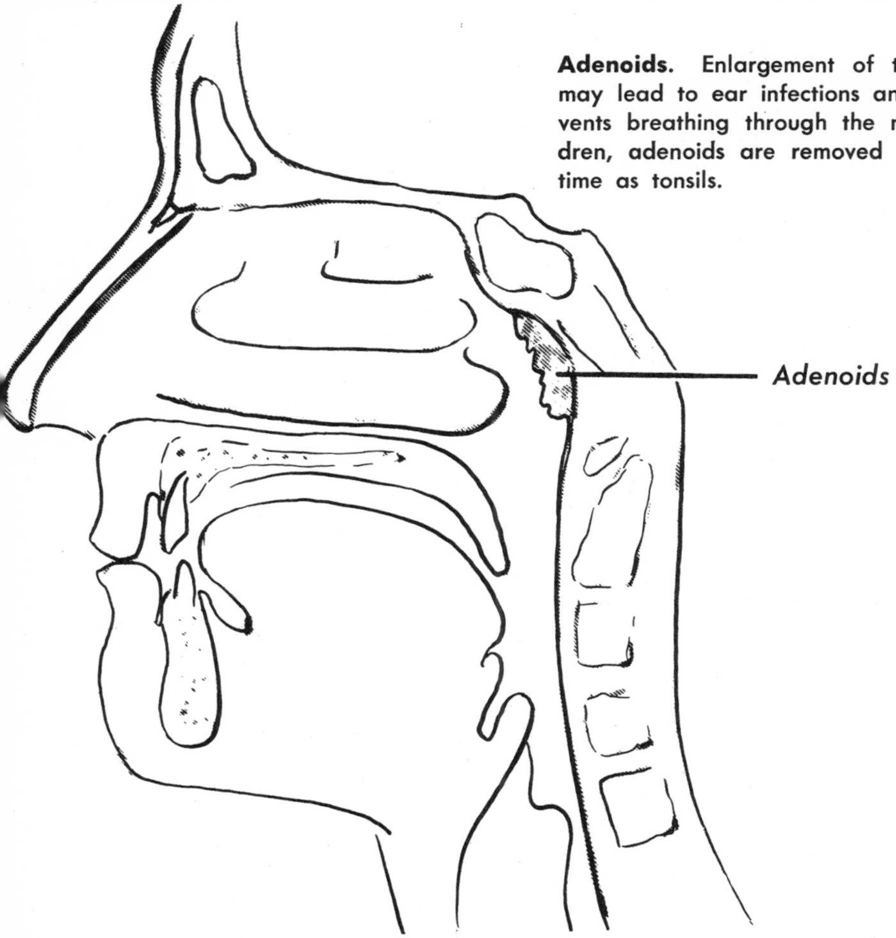

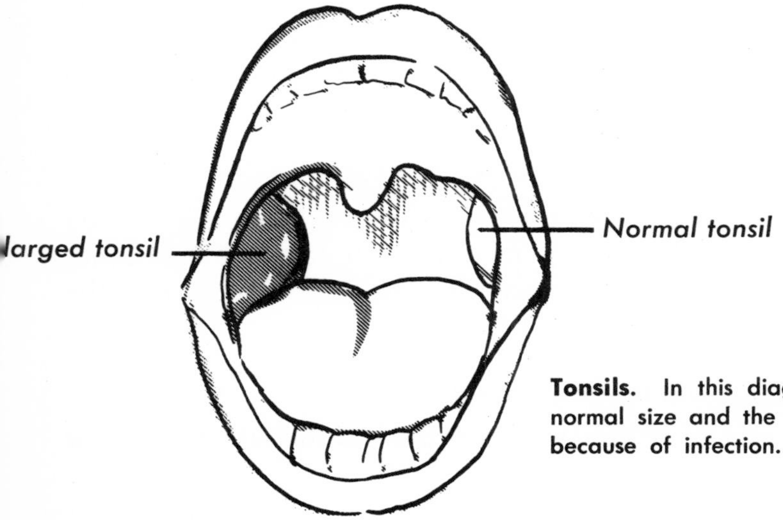

Tonsils. In this diagram, one tonsil is of normal size and the other one is enlarged because of infection.

a barrier which localizes and gives immunity to infections which enter the body through the mouth or nose.

Since tonsils and adenoids are supposed to perform a useful function, why are they so frequently removed?

Because their function is lost when they become chronically infected. Under such circumstances, they act as a focus of infection and may lead to disease of other organs, such as the eyes, joints, muscles, kidneys, or even the heart.

What are the symptoms of acute inflammation of the tonsils and adenoids?

Pain in the throat, high fever, and swelling of the glands of the neck. Infected adenoids may also cause infection of the sinuses, with obstruction of the air passages to the middle ear. This may eventually lead to ear infection and possible loss of hearing. With enlarged adenoids, the patient may develop into a mouth-breather. If this condition is permitted to go uncorrected for a long period of time, facial changes may occur, with the upper lip being pulled upward and the face taking on a stupid, languid expression.

When are tonsillectomy and adenoidectomy indicated?

Until recently, it was routine practice to recommend these operations for all children when they reached the age of three to five years. Now, it is advised only when the tonsils have become chronically infected or when diseased adenoids give rise to nose or ear complications.

What are the common causes of enlarged glands in the neck?

Acute infections of the tonsils, acute pharyngitis, infection of the adenoids, or infection of the sinuses.

Are tonsils and adenoids always removed at the same time?

In children, it is customary to remove both the tonsils and the adenoids at the same time. However, in infants and young children with ear infection, it is occasionally advisable to remove adenoids without removing the tonsils. Since adenoid tissue tends to shrink after the tenth year of life, tonsillectomy is usually performed without removing the adenoids in adults.

Are tonsillectomy and adenoidectomy dangerous operations?

These procedures are considered to be among the safest of all operations.

What kind of anesthesia is used for these operations?

General anesthesia for children and local or general anesthesia for adults.

What is the most favorable time of the year to remove the tonsils and adenoids?

Any time of the year is satisfactory.

Should allergic children, or those from an allergic family, undergo tonsillectomy or adenoidectomy?

Yes. However, the procedure should not be done in the hope of curing the allergy.

Should children of allergic parents have tonsillectomy or adenoidectomy performed between April first and October fifteenth?

No. It has been shown that tonsillectomy will increase their chances of developing into active hay fever patients during the following allergy season.

Will the routine be changed now that polio vaccine has been so widely given?

Many physicians now feel that it does not matter when tonsils are removed since infantile paralysis has been practically eliminated. However, since there is a very small number of cases still extant, it is perhaps better to advise continuation of the practice of removing the tonsils at some time other than the period from June to October.

What is the relationship of deafness to diseases of the tonsils and adenoids?

Enlarged and infected adenoids may cause recurrent middle ear infection and thus cause impairment of hearing. Also, adenoid tissue near the opening of the Eustachian tube, by mechanically obstructing the tube, may cause a faulty replacement of the air in the middle ear, thus interfering with hearing.

Will removal of chronically infected adenoids and tonsils improve hearing in children?

Yes, if the deafness has been caused by the infected adenoid.

How soon after an acute upper respiratory infection or an acute tonsillitis can tonsillectomy be performed?

At least two to three weeks should elapse. Usually, antibiotics are prescribed before and after such operations to minimize the chances of infection.

If a child has been exposed to a contagious disease, should tonsillectomy be postponed?

Yes, until all chance of catching the disease has passed.

Do abscesses ever form within the tonsil or near the tonsil?

Yes. Abscesses just behind or to the side of the tonsils are quite common. This is called a peritonsillar abscess or quinsy sore throat.

What is the treatment for quinsy sore throat?

Incision and drainage of the abscess. This can often be done with a little local anesthesia in the surgeon's office. On the other hand, if the abscess is very large it may perhaps be best to incise it in the hospital.

How is the diagnosis of peritonsillar abscess made?

The child will develop high fever, and on inspection it is noticed that there is a tremendous swelling and tenderness around the tonsil. There is also a characteristic voice change and an inability to open the mouth widely.

Do adults ever develop peritonsillar abscess?

Yes, but it is not nearly as common among them as it is among children.

Does quinsy sore throat ever produce suffocation?

Yes. If untreated, the entire back of the throat may become involved and may make it very difficult for air to reach the lungs.

Do acute infections of the tonsils require treatment?

Most definitely, yes. They should be strenuously treated with antibiotics. Failure to do this may result in bacteria getting into the bloodstream and affecting other parts of the body.

What other diseases can result from a poorly treated case of acute tonsillitis?

Rheumatic fever sometimes follows a streptococcal infection of the tonsils. Also, certain types of nephritis (kidney inflammation) can follow acute tonsillitis. In the rare case, the valves of the heart may become infected secondary to tonsillitis (endocarditis).

Will most acute infections of the tonsils and adenoids clear up by themselves?

Yes, but the chronic infections do not tend to clear up by themselves.

What is the best method to prevent recurring attacks of tonsillitis?

Remove the tonsils.

Do tonsils and adenoids ever grow back once they have been removed?

Yes, but only when they have not been removed completely.

What are the definite indications for tonsillectomy and adenoidectomy?

a. Obstruction to breathing.

b. Recurrent ear infections.

c. Recurrent sore throat.

d. When the tonsils are suspected of acting as a focus of infection for diseases in other organs.
e. Chronically infected tonsils or adenoids that no longer serve a useful function and are subject to recurrent acute infections.

Are special preoperative measures necessary before removing the tonsils and adenoids?

Some physicians will give antibiotics before this procedure in order to cut down on the possibility of infection. Other surgeons will prescribe vitamin K in order to minimize the chances of bleeding postoperatively.

Is it important to study a child's blood prior to removing his tonsils and adenoids?

Yes. The child must be examined thoroughly to make sure that he has no bleeding tendencies. This can be done on the day prior to, or the day of, the operation. Hemoglobin evaluation is also necessary, for if the child is very anemic, tonsillectomy will be postponed.

Should children be told that they are going to have their tonsils removed?

Yes. It is important that they be told the truth. If possible, children should see the recovery room several days prior to surgery. They should be told that the surgery is painless and that they will sleep through it. If it is to be performed in the surgeon's office, then the child should be told that his parents will be at his side when he awakens from the operation.

Why is it that some surgeons perform tonsillectomy in their offices, while others insist upon hospitalizing their patients?

If the surgeon has complete facilities, including beds for after-care and the proper anesthetic equipment, he will often advocate that the operation be performed in his office. If the facilities in the surgeon's office are not equal to those in the hospital, the surgeon will probably advocate hospitalization. Office surgery is done only rarely today.

What is the technique used in removing the tonsils and adenoids?

The tonsillar tissue is separated from its bed and is snared off close to the tongue. Adenoids are removed with a knife attached to a basket. The entire procedure usually takes about one-half hour to perform.

Do stitches have to be removed after tonsillectomy and adenoidectomy?

No.

What are the usual after-effects of these operations?

Pain in the throat or ears, or both, may persist for a week or ten days after surgery. This pain is often aggravated by eating, drinking, or merely swallowing. This pain can be minimized and kept under reasonable control by the liberal use of pain-relieving medications.

Do some children normally have a peculiar tone to their speech after removal of tonsils and adenoids?

Yes. This should occasion no alarm as it will last for only a few weeks or, at the most, for a few months.

How soon after surgery can a patient begin to talk?

Even though it is painful, the sooner the patient begins to talk the better, as this will return the muscles of the throat to normal working condition.

How long must the patient remain in bed after tonsillectomy and adenoidectomy?

One to two days.

Do children require special nurses after these operations?

The child should be watched for several hours after surgery to make sure that he is breathing properly and that no excessive bleeding is taking place.

How long a hospital stay is necessary after tonsillectomy?

One day.

How soon after operation can a child bathe?

Five to seven days.

How often does postoperative hemorrhage occur after tonsillectomy and adenoidectomy?

This occurs in only one in twenty-five cases. The routine use of the antibiotic drugs following surgery has cut down on the number of cases that bleed postoperatively.

What types of postoperative hemorrhages might be encountered?

a. Immediate bleeding, which may occur shortly after the surgery and can be controlled quite readily before the child leaves the operating room or the surgeon's office.
b. The delayed type of postoperative bleeding occurs on the fifth to the eighth day after operation. This is due to the falling away or loosening of the scab which has formed at the operative site. A small vessel or capillary may be exposed, which forms a blood clot and keeps the vessel open and produces the bleeding.

Is hemorrhage after tonsillectomy dangerous?

No. However, certain rare cases will bleed excessively and must demand the attention of the surgeon. The surgeon can control the bleeding readily by removal of the clot and the application of pressure.

How can hemorrhage after tonsillectomy be recognized?

Most children normally vomit blood mixed with stomach juices several hours after operation. Thereafter, there should be no further blood seen either in the nostrils, in the mouth, or in the throat. If a child vomits after being taken home, and if the vomit contains blood, the doctor should be notified at once.

Is any special postoperative diet required after these operations?

No, except to avoid highly spiced or highly seasoned foods. It is suggested that on the first day the patient be given water, milk, ice cream, etc., in small quantities. On the second day, in addition, he may have cereal, malted milk, Jello, junket, puddings, custard, broths, etc. On the third and fourth days; potatoes, eggs, toast, etc., may be added. On the fifth day, a normal diet may be resumed.

When is it necessary to use antibiotics before or after tonsillectomy?

When a child has had recurrent sore throats and colds without a free interval of two to three weeks, they should be given. In addition, it is now routine practice to give antibiotics for one week after surgery.

Should an ice collar be used for the sore throat following tonsillectomy?

No. It is of no value.

When can the patient be taken out of doors after operation?

About the fifth day, weather permitting.

How soon can the child return to school after tonsillectomy?

One week, if the temperature is normal.

When should an adult return to full activity after tonsillectomy?

Ten to fourteen days.

PHARYNGITIS

(Sore Throat)

What is pharyngitis?

An inflammation of the lining of the back wall of the throat, due either to an irritant or to a bacterial infection.

What are the symptoms of pharyngitis?

Pain in the back of the throat, difficulty on swallowing, and fever, often accompanied by a feeling of malaise.

Is sore throat always a disease entity in itself?

No. It often is the beginning of an upper respiratory infection, such as a cold or the grippe.

Does pharyngitis often herald the onset of some other infection?

Yes. There are innumerable diseases that begin with a sore throat.

What is the meaning of the term streptococcus sore throat?

While it is true that many cases of pharyngitis are caused by the streptococcus germ, many other bacteria and viruses can produce sore throats. The true streptococcus sore throat is an epidemic-like disease in the community, usually stemming from a common focus of infection, such as infected milk, etc.

What are the symptoms of a true streptococcus infection of the pharynx?

There is usually sudden onset, chills and fever, general weakness, headache and severe prostration. The throat appears very red and swollen and has gray patches upon it. A culture of the germs infecting the pharynx will show the hemolytic streptococcus.

What is the treatment of pharyngitis?

This will depend upon the cause. If it is bacterial in origin, antibiotics along with hot gargles and irrigations are prescribed.

Is local treatment of much value in treating pharyngitis?

No. However, in an isolated case, painting the back of the throat with silver nitrate may limit the spread of infection.

Are the antihistaminic drugs of much value in the treatment of pharyngitis?

No, since the symptoms of infection will continue as soon as the drugs are discontinued.

Are local medications, such as lozenges, medicated chewing gum, and gargling, of much value in the treatment of pharyngitis?

Although they may bring about temporary relief, they have no more than slight value. Most of their value is in the fact that they contain a local anesthetic agent.

Should antibiotics be given for all cases of pharyngitis?

Definitely not. The giving of excess antibiotics may sensitize the patient to their use, so that they will not have nearly as much value when they are truly needed for a serious condition. It must be remembered that most cases of pharyngitis will clear up by themselves within a few days.

What is the most soothing local medication for pharyngitis?

Warm gargles or irrigations containing salt and aspirin.

What is chronic pharyngitis?

This is a thickening in the lining membrane of the pharynx associated with repeated attacks of acute pharyngitis or secondary to chronic irritating factors.

What are some of the causes of chronic pharyngitis?

a. Repeated attacks of acute pharyngitis.
b. Excess tobacco smoking.
c. Excess use of alcohol.
d. Sinus infections.
e. Inhalation of irritating substances over a prolonged period of time.
f. Constitutional or generalized disease.

What are the symptoms of chronic pharyngitis?

Dry and sore throat, with a tickling sensation requiring repeated hawking and coughing.

Can a diagnosis of chronic pharyngitis be made on observation?

Yes. There is usually a thickening of the mucous membranes and an overgrowth of the lymphoid tissue.

What is the treatment for chronic pharyngitis?

The primary aim is to remove the cause to prevent further harm. Local treatment with stimulating medications is given along with other measures to improve the local oral hygiene.

THE LARYNX

What is the larynx?

A semi-rigid framework of cartilages held together by ligaments. It is lined with mucous membrane which is continuous with the throat above and the trachea (windpipe) below.

Where is the larynx located?

It forms a prominence in the neck commonly known as the Adam's apple.

What are the chief functions of the larynx?

The chief functions are speech, respiration, and action of the epiglottis which shunts food into the esophagus.

How is speech created?

By the passage of air through the larynx while the position of the vocal cords is varied so as to change the size of the opening and the degree of tension of the cords themselves.

How is the larynx concerned with respiration?

Air is permitted to enter the trachea and lungs by action of the laryngeal muscles which keep the vocal cords apart.

How does the larynx serve as a valve?

It has a valvular action which closes the entrance to the trachea to food or any foreign particles. This same action prevents the escape of air from the lungs when it is found necessary to hold one's breath.

Can the larynx be studied and examined by a physician on direct inspection?

Yes. This is done by mirror visualization and is called indirect laryngoscopy. It can also be seen by direct laryngoscopy, wherein a lighted hollow metal tube is inserted into the mouth and behind the tongue down toward the larynx.

What conditions can be noted by the physician when he views the larynx?

He can determine the presence or absence of infection; he can observe the action of the vocal cords to note whether they are functioning properly; he can detect the presence of growths within the larynx.

What are the symptoms of acute laryngitis?

Acute laryngitis is due to an inflammation of the mucous membrane of the larynx and is characterized by a hoarse voice, and pain and swelling in the region of the larynx. There may be rapid onset or it may be in a less acute form.

What causes acute infections of the larynx?

Any of the bacteria which can cause an infection elsewhere in the body.

Can inflammation of the larynx be caused by irritating substances, such as smoke, gas, fumes, scalding steam, dust, etc.?

Yes.

Is acute laryngitis usually a dangerous condition?

No. It usually appears as part of an upper respiratory infection and will run its course within a week to ten days.

What are the dangers of laryngitis?

The ordinary case of laryngitis is not dangerous. However, since the larynx is the bottleneck of the airway (it being the narrowest passage space to the lungs), any decrease in the area caused by swelling or any compression may produce a serious obstruction to breathing.

What is croup?

(See Chapter 30, on Infant and Childhood Diseases.) It is an acute inflammation of the larynx and may produce serious impairment of breathing in children.

What is the treatment for acute laryngitis?

a. Rest the voice and do not attempt to speak.
b. Humidify the air, usually by steam inhalations.
c. Take heavy doses of the antibiotic drugs, under the supervision of the physician.

d. If there is great difficulty in breathing, an oxygen tent may be necessary.
e. In emergency cases only, it may be necessary to do a tracheotomy to save life.

What are the usual causes of hoarseness?

Any factor which prevents the normal meeting of the two vocal cords in the midline will cause a change in the voice. This may be a slight swelling of the mucous membrane, a foreign body, a tumor, or a paralysis of one of the vocal cords.

What is the significance of prolonged or chronic hoarseness?

It indicates a disease of one or both of the vocal cords.

How soon should one consult his physician for hoarseness?

Any hoarseness that does not clear up within one to two weeks should be investigated by a physician.

What are the chief causes of chronic hoarseness?

a. A chronic inflammation of the larynx.
b. A paralysis of one of the vocal cords.
c. A tumor of one of the vocal cords.
d. Pressure from a growth, such as a goiter, upon the larynx.
e. A tumor of the wall of the larynx.

TUMORS OF THE LARYNX

Are tumors of the larynx very common?

Yes. This is a very commonly encountered condition. Fortunately, most of these growths are benign.

How is the diagnosis of laryngeal tumor made?

The larynx is inspected by direct or indirect laryngoscopy. The surgeon can usually tell, from the appearance and location of the tumor, whether or not it is benign.

How is a definite diagnosis of the type of laryngeal tumor made?

A small piece of the tumor tissue is removed through the laryngoscope and is examined under the microscope in the laboratory. This biopsy will tell whether the tumor is benign or cancerous.

What are the common symptoms of a laryngeal tumor?

Hoarseness is the chief symptom and may be the only one. If the tumor becomes very large, which is unusual, it may obstruct the airway and result in difficult breathing. Less common complaints are coughing, pain, difficulty in swallowing, and a blood-tinged sputum.

What is the treatment for benign laryngeal tumors?

They must be removed surgically. This can frequently be done in an office under local anesthesia through the laryngoscope. Occasionally, hospitalization is required and the tumor is removed under local or general anesthesia. Although the procedure may be unpleasant, it is not painful or serious.

What are the results of surgery for benign laryngeal tumors?

Excellent. Most of these lesions are nodes or polyps. Some have a tendency, once removed, to recur. Thus, removal may have to be done again.

Is hoarseness cured by the removal of a benign laryngeal tumor?

Yes, but it is important to emphasize that the voice should not be used for two to three weeks following surgery.

How frequent is cancer of the larynx?

It is a relatively uncommon disease, seen mainly in men over fifty years of age.

What is the cause of cancer of the larynx?

The cause is unknown. However, the history of most patients with cancer of the larynx indicates that they have been heavy smokers or people who abuse their voice. Also, a history of drinking excessive quantities of straight alcohol is often obtained.

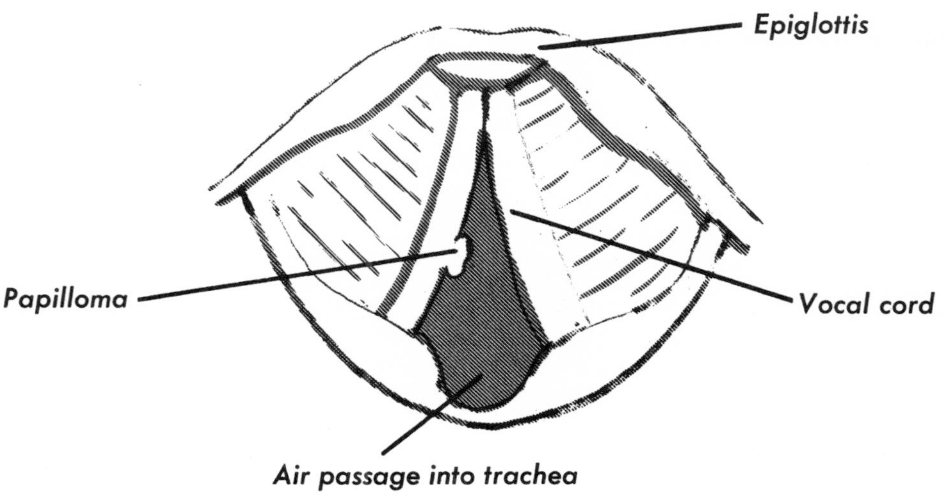

Papilloma of the Vocal Cord. This diagram shows a warty growth, known as a papilloma, on one of the vocal cords. Such a tumor will cause persistent hoarseness. This tumor lends itself to easy surgical removal and cure.

How is a definite diagnosis of cancer of the larynx made?

By taking a piece of the tissue and submitting it to microscopic examination.

What is the treatment for cancer of the larynx?

a. X-ray therapy.
b. Surgical removal of the larynx.
c. A combination of x-ray treatment and surgical removal of the larynx.

Is removal of the larynx (laryngectomy) a serious surgical procedure?

Yes. However, in expert hands, operative recovery takes place in the vast majority of cases.

Can a cure of cancer of the larynx be obtained?

Yes, provided the operation has been performed when the cancer is in a relatively early stage of development. Or, if x-ray therapy has been the treatment of choice, a cure can frequently be obtained if treatment is begun during the early stages of the tumor growth.

Are blood transfusions given during operations for removal of the larynx?

Yes. Also, special nursing care is an absolute necessity, as patients who have undergone such operations have a tracheotomy tube which must be carefully tended.

How long a hospital stay is necessary following laryngectomy?

Usually two weeks, but sometimes as long as three or four weeks.

Can people who have had their larynx removed talk again?

Yes, but the voice is markedly changed and speaking is accomplished only after they have received several weeks or months of special instruction.

If the entire larynx has been removed, will people breathe normally or will they have to use a tracheotomy tube?

When a total laryngectomy has been performed, the patient must breathe through a tracheotomy tube placed in the neck.

Can a useful voice be developed after a total laryngectomy?

Yes. This is accomplished by learning how to bring up air from the stomach. Also, there are electrical devices which act more or less in the same manner as a larynx.

THE TRACHEA

(*Windpipe*)

What is tracheitis?

It is an inflammation of the mucous membrane lining of the trachea, extending from below the Adam's apple down into the lungs.

What are the symptoms of an inflammation of the trachea?

a. A tightness and burning in the chest and under the breastbone.

b. A cough and wheezing.

c. The bringing up of sputum.

d. Fever, malaise.

What are the causes of tracheitis?

It is most often seen as an accompaniment of an acute upper respiratory infection and can be caused by the usual causes of these conditions.

Can tracheitis also be caused by irritants, such as smokes, vapors, chemicals, and fumes?

Yes.

What is the treatment for acute tracheitis?

The same as for the other upper respiratory infections which usually accompany it.

Does tracheitis often appear as a forerunner of bronchitis or pneumonia?

Yes. Tracheitis is usually seen as part of a general respiratory infection.

TRACHEOTOMY

What is a tracheotomy?

It is an operation in which an artificial opening is made into the trachea through an incision in the neck below the level of the larynx.

What conditions require tracheotomy?

a. Suffocation due to obstruction of the airway above or at the level of the larynx.
b. Postoperative conditions in which mucous secretions block the bronchial tubes, cause severe respiratory difficulties, and the patient is unable to expel the mucus voluntarily.

What are the main symptoms of obstruction of the larynx?

a. Difficulty in breathing.
b. Pallor and restlessness.
c. Bluish discoloration of the lips.
d. Rapid respiration and rapid pulse.

What are the most common causes of obstruction of the larynx?

a. Abscess formation.

b. Inflammation of the lining of the cartilages of the larynx.
c. Severe croup.
d. Acute inflammation involving the tissues surrounding the larynx. This may occur from neck infections extending from the floor of the mouth (Ludwig's angina).
e. Injuries or wounds of the larynx or nearby structures, with swelling of the tissues composing the larynx.
f. A foreign body which gets stuck in the larynx. This occurs in children who sometimes swallow coins or peanuts, etc.
g. Burns of the larynx from drinking scalding liquids or inhaling live steam.
h. Inhalation of severely irritating chemicals or vapors.

What first aid should be given to someone choking from a foreign body in the larynx or trachea?

a. Try to retrieve the foreign body by inserting a finger into the throat of the patient.
b. Turn the patient upside-down and hold him in that position.
c. Encourage coughing.
d. Transport the patient, in a sitting position, to the nearest emergency room of a hospital.

When should a tracheotomy be performed?

When the laryngeal obstruction has developed to such an extent that the patient is unable to breathe at all and life is obviously threatened.

How is an emergency tracheotomy performed?

If necessary, this operation can be done without anesthesia or any attempt at sterilization. In an emergency, to prevent total suffocation, a knife is inserted into the neck over the trachea in the midline just below the Adam's apple. Air is allowed to reach the lungs from a point below the obstruction.

When an elective tracheotomy is performed, how is the opening into the trachea kept open?

By insertion of a tracheotomy tube. This tube has a double lining

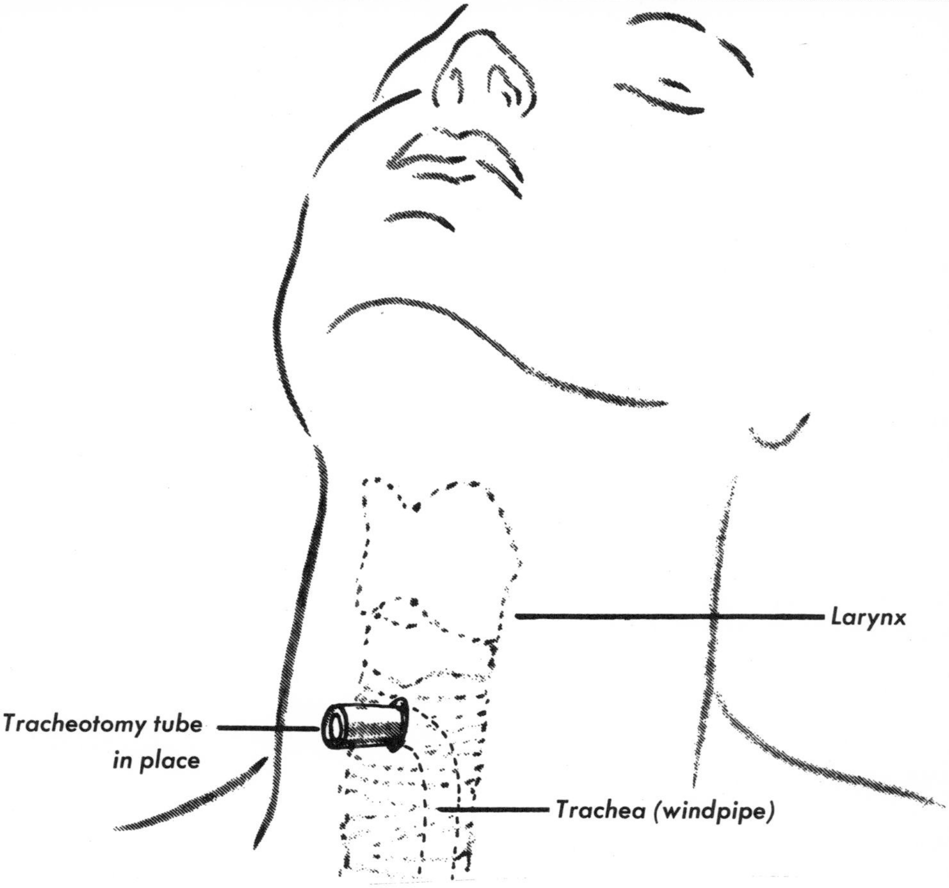

Tracheotomy. This diagram shows how the trachea has been opened and a tube inserted in order to restore a free airway. This procedure is performed whenever there is danger of suffocation due to obstruction in the throat or larynx. When the obstruction has been relieved, the tube is removed, the hole will heal, and the patient will resume normal breathing through the nose.

and the inner lining can be taken out as often as necessary to keep it clean and free of mucus collection.

When the tracheotomy tube is removed after the obstruction has disappeared, will the hole heal readily?

Yes. Once normal breathing has been resumed and the tube removed, the tracheotomy hole will close within a few days.

Does a tracheotomy interfere with normal eating?

No!

BRANCHIAL CYSTS

(*Gill Slits*)

What are branchial cysts?

They are pouches which persist as remnants from incompletely absorbed grooves seen in embryonic development.

Where are branchial cysts usually encountered?

They appear in the neck as remnants of improper and incomplete absorption of the gill slits during embryonic life.

When are branchial cysts usually noted?

During childhood or early adult life, an unusual opening may be seen on the side of the face or behind the ear or along the lateral aspect of the neck as far down as the collarbone.

What is the treatment for branchial cysts or openings?

If they show evidence of enlargement or if there is a discharge from an abnormal opening, they should be removed surgically.

Are operations for removal of branchial cysts dangerous?

No, but they may be complicated by the fact that the cyst may have to be traced far up into its opening in the throat.

Do branchial cysts have a tendency to recur once they have been removed?

If incompletely removed, they may recur and this will require a secondary operation.

Are branchial cysts common?

No.

CHAPTER 68

The Thyroid Gland

(See also Chapter 4 on Adrenal Glands; Chapter 48 on Parathyroid Glands; Chapter 52 on Pituitary Gland)

Where is the thyroid located?

It is around the windpipe (trachea), in the lower portion of the front of the neck. Normally, it is made up of three portions, one lobe on each side of the windpipe and a connecting portion called the isthmus. Each lobe measures about two by one inch in diameter, and there is a mid-portion measuring one-half to one inch in diameter which crosses over the front of the windpipe.

What is the function of the thyroid gland?

It is one of the most important organs in the body, as it regulates metabolism (the rate and manner in which we turn food into energy and expend that energy).

Is the thyroid one of the endocrine glands?

Yes. It secretes the hormone called thyroxin.

What is the function of the thyroid hormone?

It regulates the manner and rate at which the tissues utilize food and chemical substance for the production of energy. It is also concerned with the elaboration of body heat and muscular energy, body growth and development, and distribution and storage of body water and salt.

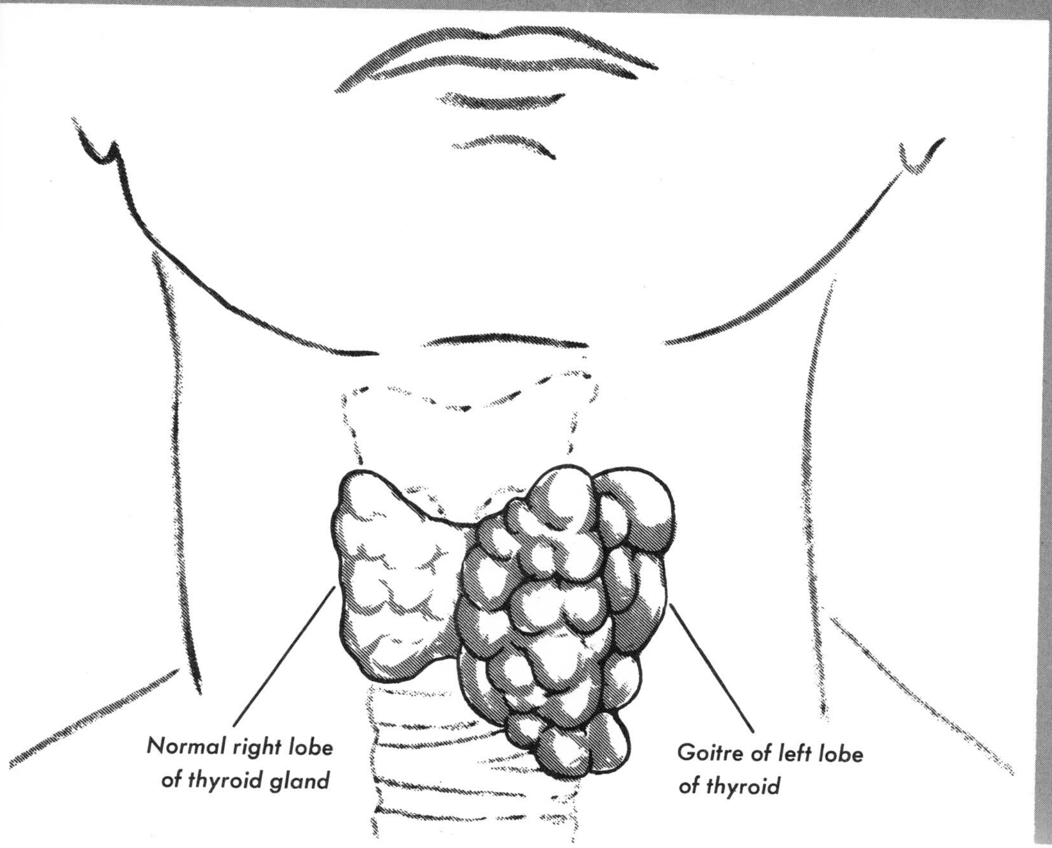

The Thyroid Gland. This diagram shows a thyroid gland with a right lobe of normal size and a left lobe involved in goiter formation.

What symptoms occur when there is an absence of the thyroid gland or when it functions underactively (hypothyroidism)?

a. Its incomplete development or absence at birth leads to a condition known as cretinism. This condition is characterized by markedly retarded mentality and a dwarfed body.

b. Milder inactivity and underfunction of the gland, either in adolescence or adult life, may lead to overweight, lack of energy, and a slowed mentality.

What happens when there is persistent overactivity of the gland (hyperthyroidism)?

This condition may lead to bulging of the eyes, marked weight loss, nervousness, irritability, and eventually serious heart damage.

Is the cause for malfunction of the thyroid gland known?

It is thought that the disturbances in the function of this gland are caused either by the effect of the pituitary gland upon the thyroid, or by disturbances within the thyroid gland itself.

How does one determine the activity of the thyroid gland?

a. By testing the basal metabolic rate (BMR).
b. By determining the protein-bound iodine (PBI).
c. By measuring the uptake of administered radioactive iodine by the thyroid gland.
d. Each year newer and more sophisticated laboratory tests are being evolved and used to assist the diagnosis when the aforementioned tests are either borderline or inconclusive.

What is the basal metabolic rate?

This is a breathing test which determines the relative rate of oxygen consumption by the body as a whole in the resting condition. A high BMR indicates excessive thyroid gland activity, as in hyperthyroidism. A low BMR may indicate underactivity of the gland, hypothyroidism.

How is a basal metabolism test performed?

The patient comes to the doctor's office early in the morning, before he has had breakfast. He is put at complete rest and then breathes pure oxygen through a tube placed over the nose and mouth.

Is a basal metabolism test unpleasant to take?

No.

Is it important to have the metabolism test taken when the patient is at rest, has an empty stomach, and is emotionally composed?

Yes. If the patient has recently eaten, undergone physical exercise, or is upset, the metabolism will be elevated and the test will be worthless.

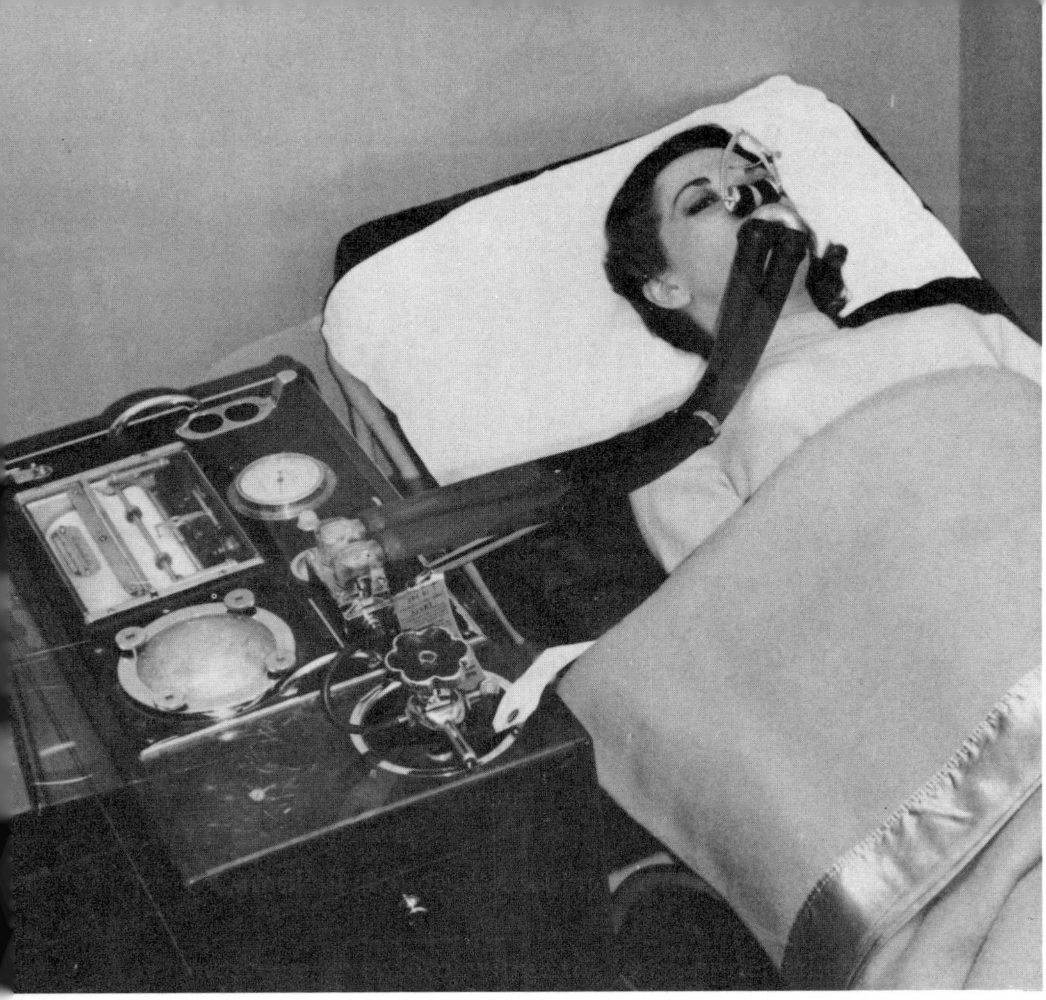

Basal Metabolism Test (BMR). This picture shows an actual basal metabolism test being given. In the performance of this test, the patient breathes oxygen through a tube. This is not an anesthesia machine; the patient remains awake throughout the test.

How is a protein-bound iodine determination made, and what is its significance?

This is a test performed by chemical analysis of blood, and is even more reliable as an indicator of thyroid function than the BMR test.

What is a goiter?

A goiter is a swelling or enlargement of the thyroid gland.

What are the most common causes for enlargement of the thyroid?

a. Colloid goiter. This is a diffuse, even swelling of the gland and is usually unaccompanied by symptoms or evidence of changes in metabolism or in the patient's state of well-being. It is seen most commonly in young adults in regions where the iodine content of drinking water is low.

b. Nodular goiter. This is characterized by a lumpy, irregular swelling either as a single area in the gland or as multiple irregularities within the gland.

   There are two types of nodular goiter:

   1. The non-toxic goiter which occurs in either sex at any time during adult life. These usually produce no symptoms but they are dangerous because some 7 to 10 per cent of them may, at some future time, turn into cancerous growths.
   2. Toxic goiter. These consist of small areas within the gland which cause overactivity of the entire gland and an increase in the basal metabolic rate.

c. Hyperthyroidism, or overactivity of the thyroid. This is often associated with a diffuse, smooth enlargement of the gland. This is the type of goiter most often seen with bulging eyes, tremor, extreme nervousness, loss of weight, irritability, profuse sweating, and heart palpitation.

Do goiters tend to run in families?

No. However, the colloid goiter may appear in several children in the same family, because they live in a vicinity where an iodine insufficiency exists.

What is the treatment for the simple colloid goiter?

In the early stages, a few drops of an iodine solution given by mouth may have curative results. Later on in the course of the disease, this form of treatment is of no value. In these instances, regulated doses of thyroid extract taken over a prolonged period of time may cause considerable shrinkage of the goiter.

Is there a satisfactory medical treatment for the toxic goiters which cause an elevation in the metabolic rate?

Yes. A great number of the cases of overactivity of the thyroid gland can be treated successfully by medical means. This will consist of the giving of iodine preparations in proper amounts and also the use of a group of medications which curtail the production of thyroid hormone. This latter group of medications is called the antithyroid drugs. A third method of treatment, the giving of radioactive iodine in certain selected cases, is also successful in halting overactivity of the thyroid gland. If these methods of treatment fail, then surgical excision is advisable.

THYROIDITIS

(*Inflammation of the Thyroid*)

What is thyroiditis?

An inflammatory reaction within the gland, caused by either bacteria or virus. Recent studies have shown that a considerable percentage of these cases are really caused by auto-immune mechanisms. In other words, for some unknown reason the individual starts to produce antibodies which attack his own thyroid gland.

Is thyroiditis a rare condition?

No, it is more common than previously suspected.

What are the symptoms of thyroiditis?

Fever, pain and tenderness in the neck over the region of the gland, hoarseness, and discomfort upon swallowing.

What is the treatment for thyroiditis?

This varies in different types of cases. The majority get well without treatment. In recent years cortisone has been used to alleviate the discomfort and limit the damage to the thyroid gland. Occasionally, antibiotics or x-ray therapy is used. Only occasionally is it necessary to perform surgery for complications of this condition.

SURGERY OF THE THYROID GLAND

When is it necessary to operate upon the thyroid gland?

a. When the goiter presses upon the windpipe or causes continued hoarseness.

b. When the hyperthyroidism (overactivity of the gland) continues despite thorough treatment with iodine and the antithyroid drugs.

c. When the thyroid has one or more isolated nodules (lumps) which can be felt by the physician. Surgery is advised in these cases to forestall the development of cancer or the development of toxicity within one of these nodules.

When is it possible to avoid surgery in thyroid disease?

a. When a simple colloid responds satisfactorily to the intake of iodine.

b. When diffuse hyperthyroidism responds satisfactorily to the taking of the antithyroid drugs.

c. When there is a recurrent hyperthyroidism after surgery and there is satisfactory response either to the antithyroid drugs or to radioactive iodine.

Is special preparation necessary before a thyroid operation?

Yes, if the gland is overactive because of a goiter. In this event, the giving of proper doses of iodine and the antithyroid drugs will precede surgery in order to bring the basal metabolic rate down to normal. No special preparation is necessary before an operation upon a simple colloid goiter or a non-toxic nodular goiter.

Is it possible to tell before operation whether a nodule in the thyroid is cancerous?

In the great majority of cases, the surgeon can make a correct diagnosis. However, the most accurate diagnosis can be made by the microscope after removal of the lump.

What harmful effects can there be if a diseased thyroid is not operated upon?

a. An enlarged simple goiter may cause dangerous compression of the windpipe and an inability to breathe properly.

b. The continuation of the toxic effects of an overactive gland will cause serious and irreparable damage to the heart.

c. As mentioned previously, 7 to 10 per cent of the small nodular goiters may become cancerous if not removed.

Do goiters often recur after surgery?

In occasional instances, a new nodule may form in the remnant of the gland left behind after surgery.

Can anything be done to prevent a goiter from recurring?

Yes. The incidence of recurrence is diminished greatly by giving the patient thyroid pills each day. In order to assure that no recurrence takes place, it is necessary for the patient to take these pills indefinitely.

Are thyroid operations dangerous?

No. They may be classified as simple major operative procedures with very little risk.

Is this a painful operation?

No, although there may be a certain amount of discomfort in the neck for a few days and some difficulty in swallowing for a few days after surgery.

Are thyroid operation scars very noticeable?

Usually not. In many cases it is impossible to find a scar a year or two after operation. The surgeon will always attempt to make his incision in one of the natural skin lines of the neck.

Does the surgeon usually remove the entire gland when performing a thyroid operation?

No, except when operating for a known cancer. It is customary to remove about 90 per cent of the gland and to allow the remainder to carry on with normal thyroid function.

Can the remnant of the thyroid, after surgery, carry out satisfactory thyroid function?

Yes. There is some regrowth of the remnant of gland which permits perfectly normal thyroid function.

How long does the operation take to perform?

Anywhere from three-quarters of an hour to two and a half hours,

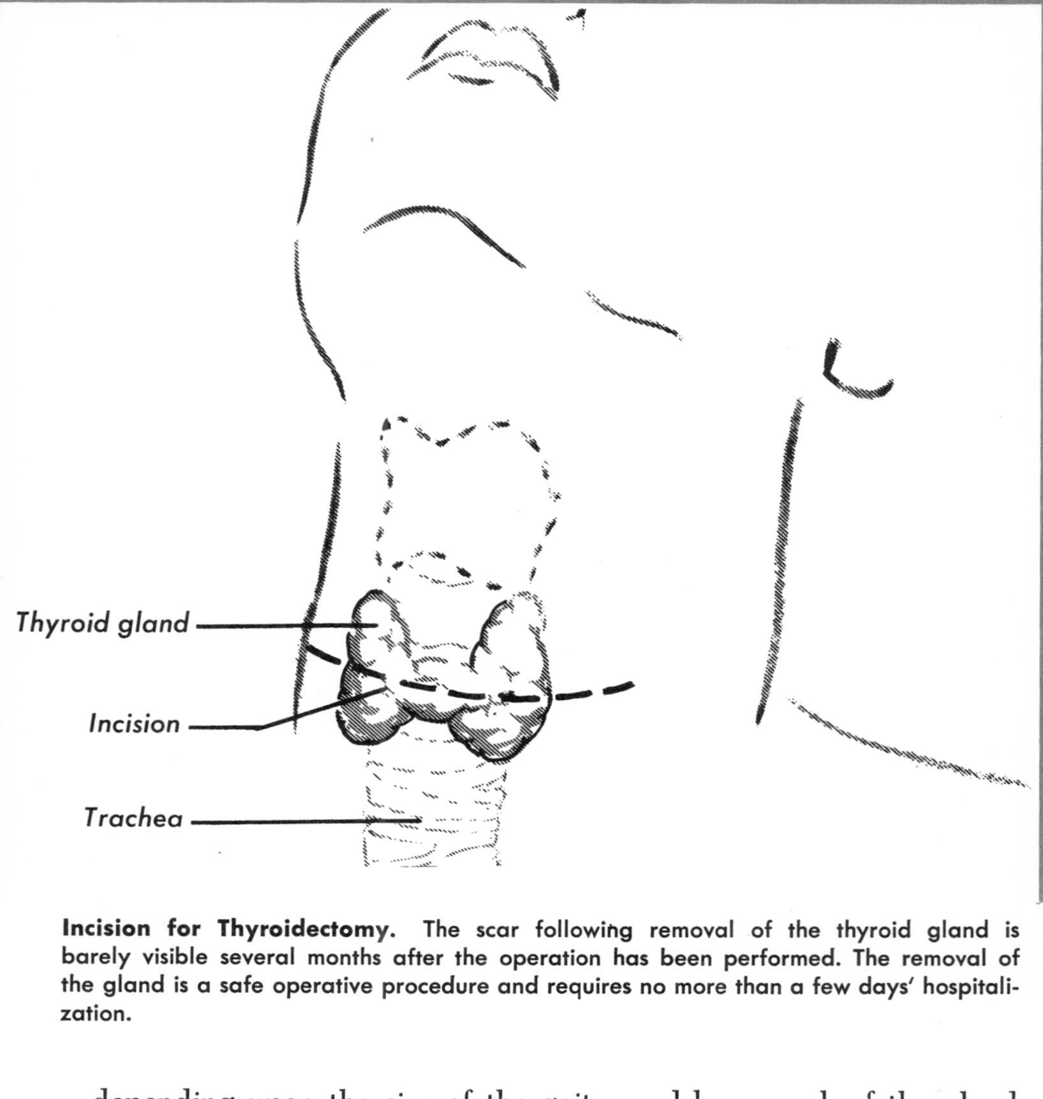

Incision for Thyroidectomy. The scar following removal of the thyroid gland is barely visible several months after the operation has been performed. The removal of the gland is a safe operative procedure and requires no more than a few days' hospitalization.

depending upon the size of the goiter and how much of the gland is to be removed.

What anesthesia is used for thyroid operations?

A general inhalation anesthesia is usually used, although the operation can be performed under local anesthesia.

Are the wounds drained after thyroid operations?

Yes, and there may be leakage of serum for a few days postoperatively.

Are special postoperative measures necessary?

Usually not, unless there was marked hyperthyroidism preoperatively. The patient is usually out of bed the day after surgery and special nurses can be dispensed with after a day or two.

What are the results of removing the thyroid gland?

In almost every type of thyroid operation, the results are excellent, with disappearance of the symptoms within a few days.

Does an overactive gland ever become underactive after surgery?

This does occur occasionally. In this event, the condition is controlled by the giving of thyroid pills.

Will the bulging of the eyes disappear after thyroid surgery?

It may recede somewhat, but if there has been marked bulging before surgery, a good measure of it will remain.

Will a patient with an overactive gland gain weight after surgery?

Yes.

Will all patients gain weight after removal of the thyroid?

Not if some of the gland has been left behind and not if thyroid pills are taken postoperatively.

Does removal of the thyroid gland affect one's sex life?

No.

How long a convalescent period is usually necessary after thyroidectomy?

Approximately three weeks.

Are there permanent voice changes after a thyroid operation?

No. Occasionally, however, it is necessary to disturb the nerve going to the larynx when removing a thyroid. If this has been necessary, hoarseness or voice changes may result for several weeks or even months.

Can one smoke immediately after thyroid surgery?

This is not advisable, since the throat may be sore after this operation.

Can cancer of the thyroid be cured by surgery?

Many cancers of the thyroid have been permanently cured by removing the gland.

How long a hospital stay is necessary for thyroid surgery?

Approximately four to seven days.

How long does it take for a thyroid wound to heal?

Approximately a week to ten days.

Can one return to a completely normal life after removal of the thyroid?

Yes.

Can a woman permit herself to become pregnant after cure of a thyroid condition?

Yes.

Should one return for periodic checkups after thyroid surgery?

Yes, about once every six months.

How soon after thyroid surgery can one do the following:

Bathe	Ten days.
Walk out on the street	Five to six days.
Walk up and down stairs	Five to six days.
Perform household duties	Three weeks.
Drive a car	Four weeks.
Resume marital relations	Three to four weeks.
Return to work	Four weeks.
Resume all physical activities	Four to six weeks.

CHAPTER 69

Transplantation of Organs

(See also Chapter 23 on Eyes; Chapter 27 on Heart; Chapter 34 on Kidneys and Ureters; Chapter 37 on Liver; Chapter 38 on Lungs)

Is it ever possible to transplant and replace worn-out organs or tissues?

Yes, in certain instances, tissues and organs can be grafted. Unfortunately most tissues transplanted from one individual to another, or to a human from an animal, will not survive more than a few days or weeks.

Is it possible to transplant an organ or a tissue from one part of a patient's body to another?

This can often be carried out with good chances for permanent success.

What are the most frequently transplanted tissues or organs?

By far the most commonly transplanted tissue is skin, but cartilage, bone, blood vessels, and occasionally a kidney or adrenal gland are transplanted from one part of the body to another. Hearts, livers, kidneys, corneas, and lungs have been transplanted successfully from one individual to another.

What is an autotransplant?

It is a graft of an organ or tissue from one part of the same body to another.

What is a homotransplant?

It is a graft of an organ or tissue from one human to another.

Is it technically possible to transplant an entire organ?

Yes, from the purely surgical point of view this is often feasible. There are now many cases on record in which an entire heart has been transplanted from one individual to another; there are also a considerable number of cases in which a kidney or liver has been transplanted from one patient to another.

Do transplants from one individual to another always survive?

Unfortunately, no. The reason for this is that all humans have antibodies and immune bodies circulating in their bloodstreams. It is the function of these substances to protect the individuals from the invasion of foreign bodies. Foreign bodies usually consist of bacteria, viruses, or inert particles that enter the body through infection or a break in the normal tissue barriers, or through an injury or wound. The body of the host reacts the same way toward transplanted organs or tissues as it does toward any other kind of foreign body and the protective cells within the host often bring about the ultimate destruction of the grafted tissue.

What is this reaction of the host to the transplant called?

There are two popular names for this phenomenon, namely, the *rejection reaction* and *transplantation immunity.*

Do all transplants from one individual to another die?

No. There are now many successful transplants of kidneys, livers, and hearts from one person to another. Also, segments of tissue, such as the cornea (the thin, clear membrane covering the pupil of the eye), have been successfully transplanted in innumerable cases from one individual to another.

Is it ever possible to have a successful graft of tissue from an animal to a human?

Yes. Animal cartilage has been frequently transplanted successfully in plastic surgery. Such cartilage is used to build up a receding chin or saddle nose. Recently, there are several reports in the medical literature of grafts of whole kidneys from chimpanzees or dogs that have survived for several months and up to two years.

Is it ever possible to overcome the rejection reaction or transplantation immunity?

Yes, a great deal of progress has been made within the past few years in this field. To overcome the rejection reaction it is necessary to temporarily immobilize or inhibit the antibodies of the recipient of the transplant. A substance known as *antilymphocytic globulin* has recently proved most effective in this connection.

What are some of the organs that technically can be transplanted from one human to another?

The heart, the lung, the liver, the kidney, the adrenal glands. Again it must be emphasized that the ability to perform a surgical procedure for transplantation does not guarantee that the transplanted organ will survive indefinitely.

Is it necessary to protect the patient during the period when his antibodies and fighting mechanisms are inactive?

Yes. Large doses of antibiotics and steroid drugs such as cortisone are given. If this were not done, the patient would succumb to overwhelming infection.

How does one attempt to overcome the rejection reaction to a transplanted organ?

a. Before grafting from one human to another, careful tissue matching is carried out. Tissues which match poorly are not grafted.
b. Chemicals are given, such as Imuran, which will temporarily suspend the ability of the recipient's antibodies to act against the organ.
c. It has been found that large doses of x-ray radiation to the area of the transplant or to the host's entire body will also temporarily inhibit the action of the antibodies and immune bodies.
d. In some cases, it has been discovered that the removal of the thymus gland beneath the breast bone, or of the spleen, will aid in the inhibition of the antibodies and thus allow a grafted organ to survive.

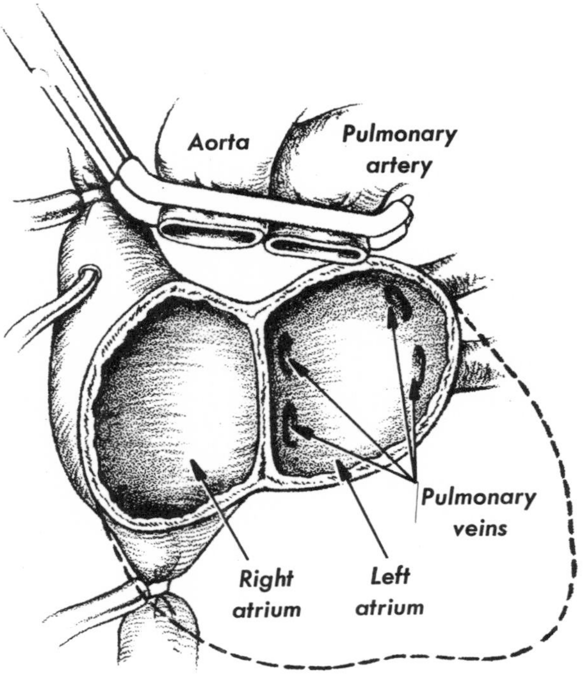

Heart Transplant. In the drawing above, the major part of a diseased heart, shown by the dotted lines, has been cut away. The upper chambers of the heart and the main vein and arteries are left. As shown in the bottom drawing, they are all sutured to the new, or donor's, heart to which blood circulation and function are restored.

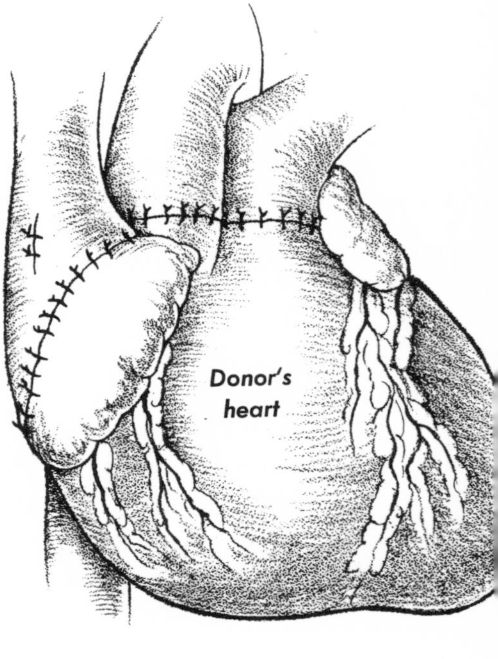

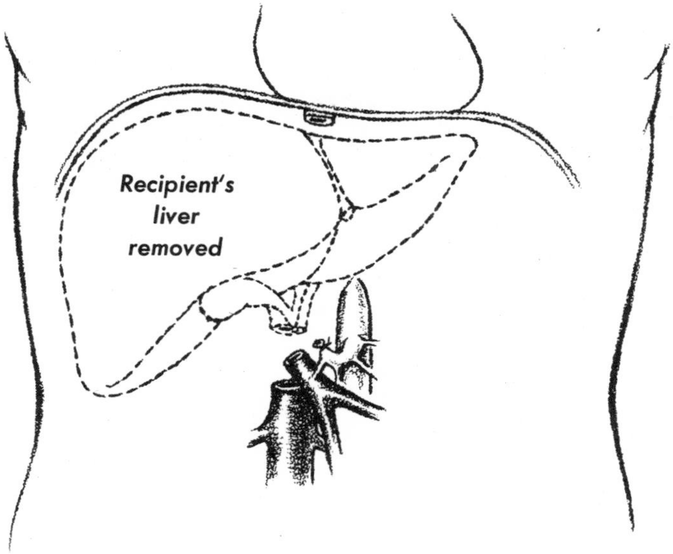

Liver Transplant. In the drawing at top, the dotted lines outline the patient's diseased liver, which is cut off from the main veins and arteries. In the bottom drawing, the donor liver has been placed in position and sutured to the large blood vessels, and function is restored.

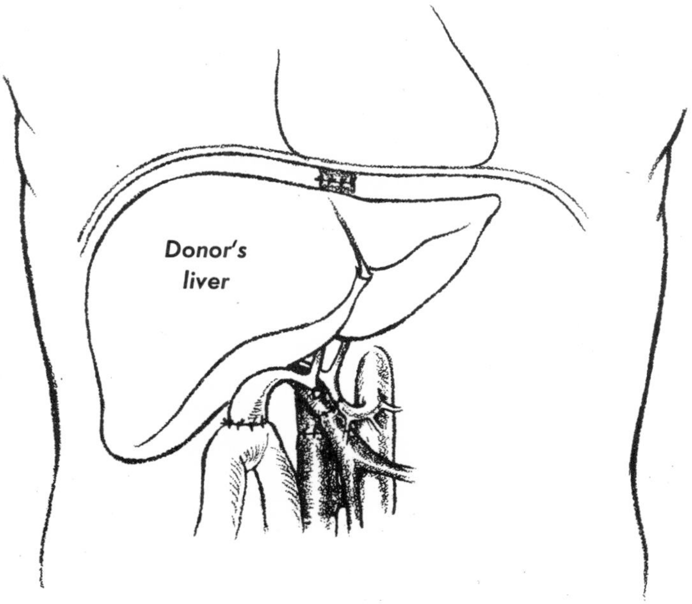

e. Antilymphocytic globulin is administered.
f. A combination of the above forms of treatment is usually employed to overcome the reaction phenomenon so as to permit the transplanted organ to survive.

Does a successfully transplanted organ always react normally in its new environment?

No. It has been discovered in animal experiments that sometimes healthy transplanted organs may develop the same disease as the structure it has replaced.

Can diseased arteries and blood vessels be replaced with a transplant?

Yes, this is one of the most successful areas for grafts and transplants. However, it has been learned that the transplantation of nonliving substances such as Dacron and Teflon are more satisfactory than the use of living tissue.

For what diseases of blood vessels are transplants advisable?

There are many conditions that are benefited by the use of Dacron or Teflon grafts. Some of these are:

a. In certain cases of stroke, it has been found that the cause lies in arteriosclerosis of the carotid artery in the neck. This can be helped in many cases by coring out the narrow passageway of the carotid artery in the neck (endarterectomy) and by supplying a patch graft of Dacron or Teflon.
b. There are many cases in which there is such marked arteriosclerosis of the aorta in the abdomen that insufficient blood supply reaches the legs. In these cases, the abdominal aorta may be replaced with a Dacron or Teflon tubular graft or its narrow passageway may be reamed out and a patch graft applied.
c. There are quite a large number of cases in which high blood pressure is due to arteriosclerosis and narrowing of the main artery to the kidney. In these cases, the renal artery can be cored out and a patch graft applied to it in order to broaden its passageway.
d. There are a large number of cases in which the circulation to the leg and foot is threatened by arteriosclerosis affecting the arteries in the pelvic region or in the thighs. In some of these

cases, it is possible to replace the narrowed blood vessels with Dacron or Teflon grafts. When bypassing the arteries at the knee, most surgeons prefer to use a vein graft rather than a nonliving Dacron or Teflon graft.

e. An aneurysm of the aorta in the chest or abdomen is one of the most common reasons for the employment of a graft. An aneurysm is a bulging and blistering out with a thinning of the wall of an artery. If this is allowed to persist, the vessel may burst and may cause the patient's death. To overcome this, a Dacron or Teflon tubular graft can be used to replace the diseased segment of aorta.

f. Within recent years, it has been found that certain of the arteries within the abdomen which supply large segments of the intestinal tract may undergo arteriosclerosis, and in these cases a replacement with a Dacron or Teflon graft is feasible.

Can one look forward to a day when there will be an extension of the life span as a result of organ transplantation?

There is no question but that within the next few decades the life span of many individuals will be prolonged by the successful transplantation and exchange of a healthy organ for a diseased one. Of course, in order for a patient to live extra years as a result of a transplant, other organs in his body must be in a relatively healthy state, for it is not possible to transplant all of the worn-out structures.

CHAPTER 70

Tuberculosis

(See also Chapter 38 on Lungs)

What is tuberculosis?

It is a communicable (contagious) disease caused by the tubercle bacillus, a germ, which is transmitted from one person to another by "droplet infection," that is, by sneezing, coughing, or spitting.

What progress has been made in the control of tuberculosis?

At the beginning of the 20th century, it was the most common cause of death in the U.S.A. with a mortality of about 200 per 100,000 persons per year. By 1961, it had fallen to 16th place among the causes of death with a mortality of only 5.4 per 100,000 persons per year.

Does tuberculosis always affect the lungs?

No. It usually does, but it may also involve the skin, bones, joints, intestinal tract, kidney, bladder, genital organs, lymph glands, or the brain and nervous system.

Are there different types of tubercle bacilli (germs)?

Yes. The human type, the bovine (cattle) type, and the avian (bird) type. This last type is very rare in human infections. The bovine (cattle) type is now practically insignificant in this country because it has been almost completely eradicated by the pasteurization of milk and the eradication of tuberculosis among cattle. It still causes a considerable amount of disease in some European countries where tuberculosis in cattle still exists. When this type of disease occurs in man, it usually is of the extra pulmonary (outside the lungs) variety, involving lymph glands, kidney, intestines, bones, and joints.

How do the tuberculosis germs enter the body?

Usually in three ways:

a. Inhalation of droplets or dust particles spread by coughing, sneezing, or spitting from tuberculous patients.
b. Swallowing of material from contaminated foods and eating utensils, and drinking milk from tuberculous cows.
c. Rarely, by direct inoculation of the skin with some contaminated object.

Is tuberculosis ever inherited?

No. Some population groups (American Negroes, American Indians, Mexicans, etc.) seem to be more prone to acquire a severe, rapidly fatal form of the disease, but this is probably due to greater exposure opportunities among them, occasioned by poor living conditions and overcrowding. This occurs most often when they move into large cities after having lived in the country.

Why is early recognition of a case of tuberculosis so important?

Because every new case of tuberculosis comes from an old case of tuberculosis! "Tuberculosis causes tuberculosis—every case comes from another."

Is anyone immune to tuberculosis?

No. Anybody, rich or poor, can contract the disease, but it is more apt to occur under poor living conditions and in people whose general health is bad. It can spread easily from one member of a family to another, from a teacher to her pupils, from one pupil to another, and even by less close contacts, such as coughing, sneezing, spitting in public places, etc. Children may become infected by being kissed by parents or relatives who are unaware that they have the disease, or by carrying the germs to their mouths from contaminated eating utensils or toys.

How can tuberculosis be prevented?

By following sensible rules of health: getting plenty of rest; eating nutritious foods; avoiding overcrowded living, playing, or traveling conditions; and by staying away from people who sneeze, cough, or spit. Also, by the examination of all contacts of a patient who has a positive tuberculin test, and by treating those who are found to have active tuberculosis.

Does age play any part in tuberculosis infection?

Yes. Infants up to the age of five years are more apt to get a severe, rapidly fatal type of the disease. Between the ages of five and fifteen, the incidence of fatal disease is at its lowest, and gradually increases from then on. Young girls from fourteen to twenty are particularly susceptible. The greatest number of "chronic" cases occur in middle life (thirty to fifty years of age). When tuberculosis first occurs in the elderly, it may be acute and severe.

Are there always early symptoms of tuberculosis?

No. Some people who are apparently perfectly well may have tuberculosis which can be detected only by x-ray examination, before any symptoms of the disease appear.

What are the symptoms of tuberculosis?

The early warnings may be few and they may progress and be disregarded unless they are properly evaluated and respected. They are:

a. Fatigue leading to exhaustion.
b. Loss of weight and energy.
c. Indigestion and loss of appetite.
d. Cough. This is often disregarded and passed off as a "cigarette cough."

Occasionally, the onset of the disease may be sudden and dramatic; it may start with a sudden hemorrhage from the lung or with acute pain in the chest due to pleurisy.

How is tuberculosis diagnosed?

The most positive methods are the x-ray examination and the sputum examination. Physical examination with the stethoscope and examination with the fluoroscope may help establish the diagnosis, but they are rarely sufficient to determine a positive diagnosis.

What is the tuberculin test?

It is a test used to see if there is a skin reaction to tuberculin, a product of the tubercle bacillus. A "positive" test means that the person has been infected at some time during his life but does *not* tell whether the disease is active. Only the x-ray examination and sputum examination can determine whether or not the disease is active.

Who should have tuberculin tests done routinely?

All children entering elementary school should be tested. Those found to react as "positive" should be x-rayed and all their contacts should be examined for the purpose of discovering active cases. All children of twelve to thirteen years of age should be tested again; those found to be "positive" should be x-rayed annually throughout their lives, and all their contacts should be examined, x-rayed and followed periodically.

Is it important for apparently healthy people to have periodic x-rays of the chest?

Yes. After the age of fifteen or sixteen it would be well to have x-rays made every few years. In that way, signs of disease in the lungs would be detected early.

Some people, such as student nurses and doctors and other employees working in hospitals where there are tuberculous patients, or anyone found to have a positive tuberculin test, should have a chest x-ray every six months to one year.

Is it important for young children to have periodic x-rays?

No. The incidence of active lung tuberculosis among children up to the age of sixteen is very small. However, those who have been found to have positive tuberculin tests should have such x-rays.

What factors aside from poor living conditions lower one's resistance to tuberculosis infection?

Prolonged fatigue, alcoholism, severe illnesses—especially diabetes. Also, industrial exposure to silicon dust, such as in sandblasting, etc.

What determines which of the positive tuberculin reactors will develop active disease?

The establishment of active infection depends upon the number and virulence of the invading germs, and the degree of immunity or resistance of the patient. A large number of "strong" germs may overcome the resistance of a relatively immune person, or a small number of "weak" germs may be enough to cause infection in a susceptible individual or in one whose resistance has been lowered by malnutrition, alcoholism, etc.

What is meant by a primary tuberculous infection?

It is the process which occurs following the first contact of the patient with the germ of tuberculosis. A small area of inflammation occurs (like a small patch of pneumonia), and the lymph glands in the region become inflamed too, but they wall off the spread of infection. Unless the infection is overwhelming, healing begins to take place, and scar tissue and, finally, calcium replace the inflamed portion of lung. The primary complex can then be recognized on the x-ray as a small area of calcification (chalky deposit) with some enlargement of the lymph glands.

As a result of the primary infection, the tuberculin skin test becomes positive. The positive skin test is really an allergic reaction to the tuberculin which has invaded the system.

What happens to people once they have had a primary infection?

Nothing more happens to about nine out of ten such people. A very small number, at some later date, develop active chronic pulmonary tuberculosis. This is the type usually seen in adults and may follow months or years after the primary infection.

How may the primary type of tuberculosis be recognized?

There are usually no signs or symptoms except for some unexplained fever and weight loss. The x-ray finding of the "primary complex" may not appear until years later, when calcium has been deposited within the infected area. The change from a "negative" to a "positive" tuberculin skin reaction indicates that a tuberculosis infection has taken place somewhere in the body.

Is the chronic form of lung tuberculosis due to fresh infection or to the breakdown of an old primary infection?

It may come about in either way.

What course does chronic tuberculosis take?

It can follow either one of two courses. It can heal by scarring, or it can destroy lung tissue and cause involvement of other portions of the lung or spread to other parts of the body.

Is the healing process ever complete in lung tuberculosis?

Probably not. Some bacteria deep in the diseased tissue may remain in a dormant state until such time as the patient's resistance is lowered, and then resume their active destructive processes. However, healing can take place in one area while the disease is still active in other areas.

How may other areas of the body become involved from lung tuberculosis?

The larynx, the throat, and the intestinal tract may become involved when the patient swallows sputum which has been coughed up from cavities through the bronchial tubes. On occasion, the disease may be spread by way of the bloodstream to other organs.

What are the early signs and symptoms of chronic lung tuberculosis?

There may be no early signs, the first evidence often being the x-ray appearance of the disease. Some cases start like acute pneumonia, others like grippe or influenza, with fever, weakness, and malaise which may persist for weeks. Most cases, however, begin very insidiously, with gradually increasing fatigue and weakness, loss of appetite, loss of weight, and low-grade fever. Cough and expectoration of sputum, sometimes bloody, may be early or late signs of the disease. Drenching night sweats may occur. Chest pain occurs usually only where the disease process is close to the pleural surface. Wheezing may occur if there is partial obstruction of the bronchial tubes with sputum.

Can the doctor always diagnose tuberculosis of the lungs by examination alone?

Usually not. In early cases, the area of lung involved may be too small to give signs that can be recognized by physical examination. It is therefore very important to have a chest x-ray in every case in which there is any suspicion of tuberculosis.

Is the x-ray examination alone sufficient for a positive diagnosis of lung tuberculosis?

No. Many other diseases can cause x-ray shadows that are indistinguishable from those of tuberculosis.

What procedure, aside from physical examination and x-ray examination, is most important for the positive diagnosis of pulmonary tuberculosis?

The sputum examination. When properly done, sputum examination is positive in over 90 per cent of active cases.

Suppose a patient does not expectorate any sputum. Can a positive diagnosis still be made?

Yes. If sputum is swallowed, it can be obtained by analysis of the stomach contents.

If sputum examinations by the usual "smear" method are negative, does that definitely prove the absence of tuberculosis?

No. The sputum should then be cultured so that any germs present will grow out and multiply.

Are guinea pigs ever used in the diagnosis of tuberculosis?

Yes. They were used before refined culture methods were available; and even now, when cultures are negative, sputum can be injected into a guinea pig and the animal examined (by autopsy) approximately six weeks later. If tuberculosis is found, this is proof positive that the sputum came from a tuberculous individual.

What constitutes an "active" case of tuberculosis?

One in which sputum or gastric contents show the presence of the tuberculosis germs. Also, one in which the x-rays reveal changes over a period of time.

When is the disease considered to be inactive or arrested?

When the patient seems well and when the sputum is negative and the x-rays are stable (show no change) over a prolonged period of time.

What are some of the diseases which must be differentiated from pulmonary tuberculosis?

All lung diseases with cough, fever, and x-ray changes; these include the pneumonias, bronchiectasis, lung abscess, tumors of the lung, the dust diseases, the diseases caused by yeasts and fungi, and sarcoidosis. Heart disease may cause secondary changes in the lungs, which may be confused with tuberculosis.

How may tuberculosis spread from the lungs to cause disease in other parts of the body?

a. By direct spread along the bronchial tubes to involve the pleura and the larynx, and by swallowing of sputum to involve the intestinal tract.
b. By way of the bloodstream to involve the entire body (generalized miliary tuberculosis)—the kidneys, liver, spleen, brain, testes, adrenal glands, and even the eyes.

How does tuberculosis affect pregnancy?

It has no effect on the ability of the woman to "carry to term" or to have a normal delivery. Most patients, even with active disease, can carry to term and tolerate labor and delivery. (This does not mean that pregnancy is desirable in a patient with tuberculosis.)

How does pregnancy affect tuberculosis?

Badly. If the disease has been inactive for over two years, pregnancy may be allowed fairly safely, but it should not be allowed if active disease is present or has been present within two years. Though the patient may tolerate pregnancy and delivery well, she must be watched very carefully after delivery, because that is when the disease is most likely to be reactivated.

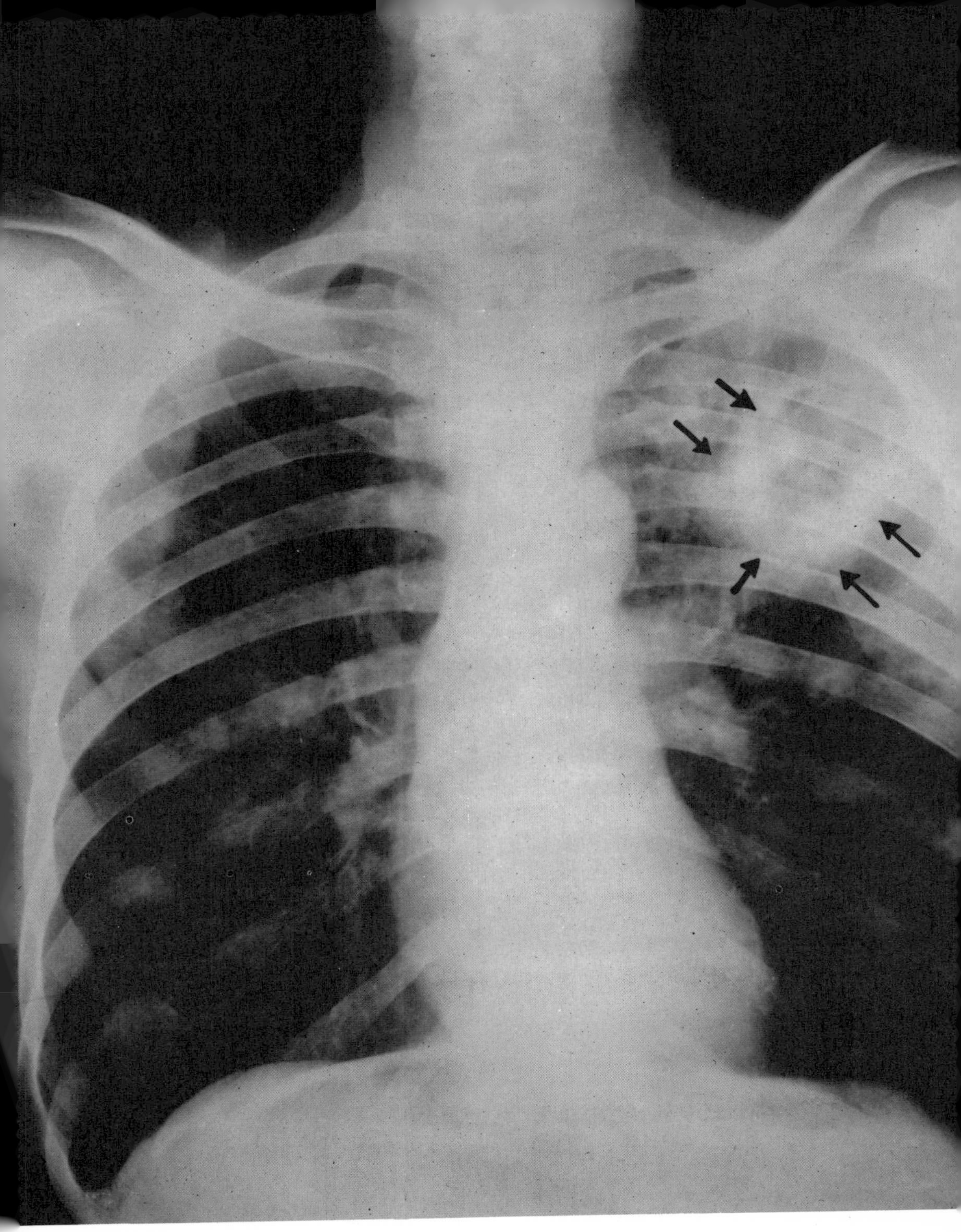

Tuberculosis. This x-ray shows tuberculous cavities in the upper portion of the left lung field.

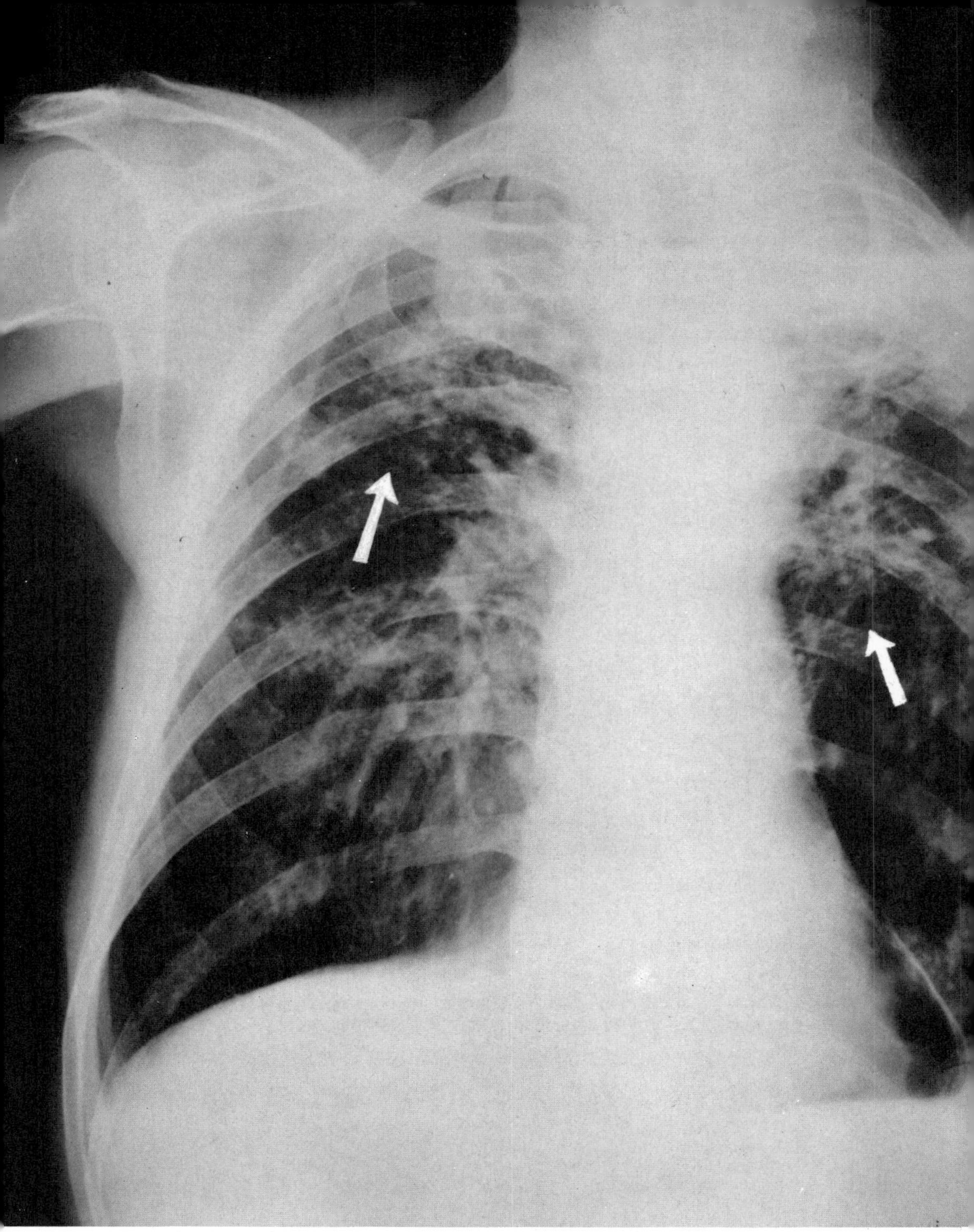

Active Spreading Tuberculosis. This x-ray shows infiltration of both lungs with tuberculosis. In former years there was a high mortality in patients with this type of infection. Today, with the newer drugs, the vast majority of tuberculosis patients can be saved.

What is the outlook (prognosis) in a case of pulmonary tuberculosis?

This depends upon several factors:

a. The general health and resistance of the patient.
b. The nature and extent of the lung involvement.

The better the general health of the patient, and the smaller the area of involvement, the better will be the outlook. The presence of cavities increases the seriousness of the disease. The larger the cavities, the more serious is the outlook.

The disease has a poorer prognosis in infancy and early childhood, and especially in adolescent girls.

With the newer drugs used in treatment, the outlook has improved tremendously in the past ten years.

What are the most important factors in preventing the spread of tuberculosis in the community?

a. Finding the active cases.
b. Isolation of active cases.
c. Treatment of active cases.

What is the best program for preventing the spread of tuberculosis in the community?

a. Mass x-ray surveys to pick up unknown cases.
b. Investigation of known contacts of active cases in the family or community.
c. Prevention of overcrowded living conditions and transportation.
d. Slum clearance.
e. Pasteurization of milk.
f. Control of tuberculosis in cattle.
g. Provision of adequate treatment facilities.

What is BCG?

The initials stand for bacillus Calmette-Guerin. It is a vaccine that was developed in France. It is made from a weakened tubercle bacillus, and is believed to have some value in producing immunity against tuberculosis in those with negative skin tests who are unavoidably exposed to the disease—doctors, medical students, nurses.

What does BCG vaccination accomplish?

It converts non-reactors (people with negative tuberculin tests) to reactors; it gives them positive skin tests. It is believed that this causes the body to react in such a way as to localize the disease and promote healing if exposure has occurred.

TREATMENT IN TUBERCULOSIS

Is complete bed rest necessary in the treatment of pulmonary tuberculosis?

No. Excellent results are now achieved without complete bed rest. Limited physical activity is desirable during the early stages of treatment with the antituberculous drugs, but many patients are treated on an ambulatory basis.

Is hospital or sanitarium care necessary for proper treatment, or can it be carried on just as well at home?

In the early active phases of treatment there is no question but that hospital treatment should be recommended. Not only can proper isolation of the sick person from his family be achieved to a much better degree than at home, but all the necessary aids to diagnosis, such as x-ray equipment, laboratory facilities, and expert consultation, are at hand in the hospital.

How long a period of rest is required?

There is no set time. Rest should be continued until the symptoms, such as cough and expectoration and weight loss, have been brought well under control and until the x-rays show stabilization and the sputum has become negative. In the case that does well, it usually takes about six to nine months of rest and drug treatment to achieve these ends. Under present circumstances, the first three months are best spent in a hospital and the remainder of the period of rest at home, if home conditions are suitable.

When is absolute bed rest necessary?

Critically ill patients and those with fever should be kept at complete bed rest, with meals in bed and bed baths. Bathroom privileges should be allowed as soon as the patient can tolerate a short walk.

Is it all right for the patient to move about in bed, or must he lie "stock still"?

Nowadays, we feel that there is no objection to sitting up in bed, moving about, shaving, washing, reading, etc.

How soon can the patient resume normal physical activity?

When sputum cultures have been converted to negative, and when such symptoms as fever, cough, expectoration and weight loss have subsided. However, drug treatment must be continued.

How long does a patient have to rest if he has had part of his lung removed surgically?

It is best to have such a patient rest for about six months after surgery, since some diseased tissue is undoubtedly left behind.

Is climate important in treatment of pulmonary tuberculosis?

No. Formerly, it was thought to be important, but now it is felt that as long as extremes of heat, cold, and altitude are avoided, it does not matter whether the patient is in the city or the country, or in the north or the south.

Is the tuberculous patient allowed to be out in the sun?

Yes, but undue exposure of the chest to direct sunlight, to the point of sunburn, is to be avoided because it increases the chances of hemoptysis (blood spitting) and reactivation of disease.

Is there any specific diet for tuberculosis?

No. A well-balanced diet with enough calories to allow for a moderate gain in weight, along with a vitamin supplement, is desirable.

What is the purpose of rehabilitation programs?

These are programs set up by states, cities, hospitals, and social service agencies with the idea of so directing and supervising the patient's convalescence that he will be able to resume his place in society, industry, and the community, to as "normal" an extent as possible. The programs involve training in activities of daily living, occupational training, and training in new and possibly less strenuous fields of activity.

For how long a time should the successfully treated patient take care of himself?

There is some danger of relapse for about five years after treatment is completed. Physical activity should be kept within bounds during this time. Rest periods during the day and adequate sleep at night (ten to twelve hours) are desirable.

Should the patient with tuberculosis be allowed to smoke?

Since tobacco smoke (no matter what its dangers are in relation to cancer of the lung) is an irritating substance, it should be avoided by the patient who has or has had tuberculosis.

How frequently should the patient who has recovered from the disease have x-ray examinations?

At least every six months, for several years. More frequent x-rays are indicated in cases where there is a suspicion of residual disease.

Is there any drug which *cures* tuberculosis?

No. However, there are several drugs which, when used properly, are highly effective against the disease. Most tuberculous infections are arrested promptly by the administration of these drugs, and healing is accelerated by their prolonged use.

Is any particular drug, combination of drugs, or set dosage of drugs, used routinely in treatment?

No. Each case must be evaluated individually by the physician. Over varying periods of time, one, two, or even three anti-tuberculous drugs may be used for any case.

Should every patient with active tuberculosis be treated with the anti-tuberculous drugs?

Yes. Whenever active disease is recognized it should be treated.

However, the particular drug or drugs, the problem of home or hospital care, and the duration of treatment must be individualized.

What is the usual length of time that treatment is continued?

It is now thought that drug treatment should be continued for at least two years after the last positive culture is obtained. Cases with open cavities and negative sputum are treated for more prolonged periods. There are some who feel that drug treatment should be continued for an indefinitely prolonged period.

What are the effective drugs in the treatment of tuberculosis?

The most commonly used, either separately or in combination, are Streptomycin, P.A.S. (para-amino-salicylic acid), and I.N.H. (isonicotinic acid hydrazide). Several others, such as cycloserine, ethionamide, pyrizinamine, and kanamycin, are still being evaluated.

Since the drugs have been shown to be effective, how are the previous forms of treatment to be regarded?

a. Bed rest can be modified and the length of time shortened.
b. Collapse therapy can be almost completely dispensed with. Pneumothorax and thoracoplasty are rarely used nowadays, and pneumoperitoneum is used as a temporary measure only occasionally.
c. It is still important to maintain adequate nutrition, to avoid respiratory irritants such as tobacco smoke, and to get adequate rest under the best possible living conditions.

How long should the treated patient be kept under observation?

At least several years, so that any relapse can be detected early.

How many cases relapse in tuberculosis?

Before the era of drug treatment, about 50 per cent of arrested cases suffered relapses. Now, with modern, adequate treatment, only about 10 per cent relapse.

What does "pulmonary resection" mean?

The surgical removal of a portion of lung so as to actually remove the diseased tissue.

In pulmonary resection, what portion of the lung is removed?

Anything from a small wedge-shaped segment of a lobe (segmentectomy) to a number of such segments, an entire lobe (lobectomy), or an entire lung (pneumonectomy) may be removed.

Which cases are suitable for resection therapy?

This decision must be based on mature medical and surgical judgment in each individual case. The cases considered are those with open cavities and positive sputum, which have failed to respond to adequate medical treatment. Some cases with open cavities and negative sputum have been resected on the theory of preventing subsequent breakdown of diseased tissue in cavity walls.

Is the surgical treatment of lung tuberculosis safe and effective?

Yes. When performed on suitable cases, the results are most encouraging.

Why aren't most people with pulmonary tuberculosis treated surgically?

Because most cases are unsuited to this form of treatment and will respond satisfactorily to medical management.

Lobectomy. The drawing on the left shows the two normal lungs with their bronchial tubes. At the right, the diseased upper lobe of the right lung has been removed and the bronchial tube has been left to maintain function in the lower lobe of the lung.

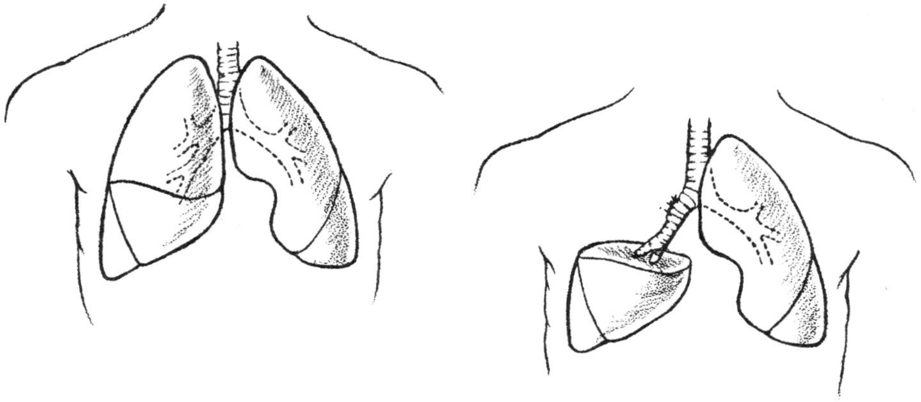

CHAPTER 71

Upper Respiratory Diseases

(See also Chapter 32 on Infectious and Virus Diseases; Chapter 38 on Lungs; Chapter 45 on Nose and Sinuses)

THE COMMON COLD

What is the common cold?

An acute inflammation and infection of the nose and the throat.

What causes the common cold?

A virus (a group of infecting agents which are much smaller than bacteria; they are so small that they cannot be seen under an ordinary microscope).

Is the common cold contagious?

Extremely contagious.

How is the common cold transmitted?

By coughing, sneezing, or close contact with another person.

What predisposes people toward catching a cold?

a. A general weakness or rundown condition.
b. Enlarged infected tonsils or adenoids, which reduce the ability to stave off infections of the nose and throat.
c. Any other disorder of the mucous membranes or the upper respiratory tract.
d. Allergies of the nose and throat which weaken local resistance.

Is a common cold the same as the "grippe"?

No, but grippe is also caused by one of a group of viruses, under some circumstances, the same as that which causes colds. Many different types of viruses can cause either the common cold or grippe, or even more severe infections.

What is the difference between the common cold and the grippe?

The grippe is a more severe infection, with higher temperature, and is associated with muscular aches and pains varying in degree.

Does grippe often start out as a common cold?

Yes.

What is the incidence of the common cold?

It is the most frequently encountered of all medical conditions. Statistics estimate that one in eight people in this country currently has a cold!

What other diseases have their onset as the common cold?

Such illnesses as grippe, influenza, measles, whooping cough, and several other diseases of the upper air passages frequently start as a common cold. Also, hay fever and other allergies may masquerade as colds for a short time.

What is the usual course of the common cold?

An uncomplicated cold lasts from four to seven days. Minor complications may persist for a few days longer.

How can one prevent the common cold?

There is no sure method of prevention. Vaccines and cold injections are not of proven value, but both inactivated and live vaccines are under investigation and combinations of viruses in vaccines are being studied as well. These may one day prove effective.

Do vitamins help in preventing colds?

Not specifically, although if the patient has a generally weakened condition, the taking of vitamins A, C, and D may build up resistance to all types of infection, including the common cold.

Are the antihistamine drugs of any value in preventing colds?

Actually, they are not. They do tend to dry the nasal secretions and probably are somewhat effective in those mild allergic conditions which are mistaken for the common cold. They may also postpone the full-blown appearance of a cold for a day or two.

Is the taking of large quantities of fresh fruit juice helpful in preventing colds?

No, except that this is a good practice to ensure adequate vitamin intake.

Are the antibiotic drugs of value in the treatment of the common cold?

No. As a matter of fact, they may do harm because they may sensitize patients to their use. Then at some future date, when the patient is ill and really needs these drugs, they may be ineffective or the patient may not be able to take them.

What is the best treatment for the common cold?

Adequate rest at the very onset of the cold is probably the best treatment. By resting and by isolating himself, the patient not only helps himself but prevents spread to others with whom he comes in contact. Simple remedies, such as aspirin, nose drops, and antihistamine drugs, make the patient more comfortable, but actually have no specific curative effects. Drinking large quantities of fluids is advisable, as in any acute upper respiratory infection. If fever or a distressing cough develops, it is best to have a medical examination to determine if a complication has set in.

What are some of the complications of a cold?

Most common colds do not develop complications. However, since the nose and throat are lined by a membrane which extends into the sinuses and the ears, down into the trachea (windpipe), bronchial tubes, and lungs, any one or all of these organs may become involved. If the virus infection extends beyond the nose and throat, this may be followed by sinusitis, middle ear infections, laryngitis, tracheitis, bronchitis, and even pneumonia, as complications of the common cold.

When are complications most likely to occur?

When the patient fails to take care of the common cold by adequate rest and treatment. Also, if the patient's resistance is low or he has had some other recent debilitating illness.

Is it important to take the temperature when one has a cold?

Yes. This should be done three times daily. An elevated temperature may herald the beginning of a complication.

How long should one wait after a cold to resume normal activities?

The patient should rest until he has had no symptoms and no fever for at least two full days.

Having recovered from a cold, does a person develop any resistance against getting another one?

For a period of several weeks, yes. However, unfortunately, no permanent resistance develops.

Is there any truth to the statement that one should "starve a cold" by not eating?

No. Normal light diet should be taken while one has a cold.

Is there any truth to the statement that one should "feed a cold"?

No.

Is the taking of a large quantity of whiskey helpful?

No.

THE LARYNX

(See also Chapter 67, on the Throat.)

What is the significance of hoarseness?

Hoarseness means that the larynx or voice box is involved by any one of a variety of conditions. Symptoms may vary from a slight huskiness of the voice to a complete loss of voice.

What conditions can cause hoarseness?

a. Inflammation, such as the common cold, influenza, tonsillitis, bronchitis, whooping cough, diphtheria, etc.
b. Inhalation of irritating dust, fumes, tobacco smoke, or chemicals.
c. Nerve involvement of the vocal cord, secondary to pressure upon it from an enlarging mass in the neck.
d. A goiter which presses upon the nerves supplying the larynx, or an injury to the nerve, secondary to an operation upon the thyroid.
e. Allergies which cause swelling of the larynx.
f. Benign tumors (fibromas) of the vocal cords.
g. Cancer of the vocal cords.

What is croup?

It is an acute inflammation of the larynx with swelling of the vocal cords, often accompanied by difficulty in breathing. (See Chapter 30, on Infant and Childhood Diseases.)

What is laryngitis?

An inflammation of the voice box or larynx, usually caused by a virus or bacterial infection.

Are there other causes for laryngitis?

Yes. Certain cases can be caused by a tuberculous infection, and others may be caused by a syphilitic infection of the larynx.

What are the usual symptoms of acute laryngitis?

a. Slight to moderate fever.
b. Hoarseness or complete temporary loss of the ability to speak.
c. Pain in the throat.
d. A dry, hacking cough.

What is the treatment for acute laryngitis?

a. Do not talk!

b. Drink large quantities of fluids, such as water, tea, and fruit juices.
c. If there is difficulty in breathing, take steam inhalations.
d. If the infection is severe, antibiotic drugs are sometimes prescribed.
e. Stay in bed until the temperature is normal for at least twenty-four to forty-eight hours.
f. Aspirin, or some similar drug, will often relieve accompanying aches and pains.

Does the voice always return after an attack of laryngitis?

Yes. The inability to speak will last for only a few days.

BRONCHIAL TUBES

What is acute bronchitis?

A self-limited acute infection, usually occurring as a complication of the common cold or the grippe.

What is the usual course of acute bronchitis?

It runs a parallel course to the underlying infection and will clear up soon after the cold or the grippe subsides.

When is bronchitis most prevalent?

During the winter months. It is often associated with exposure, chilling, and fatigue.

What is the most common complication of bronchitis?

Pneumonia.

Is there a tendency for some people to get recurrent attacks of acute bronchitis?

Yes. These people probably have a chronic source of infection, such as the sinuses or tonsils. Allergic individuals are also unusually susceptible to episodes of acute bronchitis.

What is the outstanding symptom of bronchitis?

A hacking, stubborn cough, with varying amounts of sputum being expectorated.

Should coughing be stopped by medication when one has bronchitis?

No. While coughing is a distressing symptom, it is also a beneficial one in that it gets rid of excessive mucous secretions which have accumulated in the bronchial tubes. Attempts should be made to keep the cough "loose" so that these secretions can be expectorated without difficulty.

When does acute bronchitis become chronic bronchitis?

Acute bronchitis should last no more than two to three weeks. If it has not been given the proper care and attention, it may persist longer and develop into a chronic infection.

If acute bronchitis does not subside, what diseases should be looked for as possible complications?

Pneumonia, tuberculosis, sinus infection, bronchiectasis (dilatation of the small bronchial tubes), asthma, a foreign body in the lung, or even a lung tumor.

Should one who has a persistent bronchitis or persistent cough be x-rayed?

Yes, by all means.

Should smoking be permitted during any one of the upper respiratory illnesses such as a common cold, grippe, influenza, bronchitis?

No. Tobacco smoke is particularly irritating to the lining membranes of the nose, throat, and bronchial tubes.

What is a "cigarette cough"?

This occurs commonly in the heavy smoker, but should not be interpreted as arising solely from the irritation of the tobacco smoke. Anybody, whether he is a heavy smoker or not, who coughs continuously should be investigated for an underlying lung or bronchial disease, as mentioned above.

Is the quantity and character of sputum raised by coughing of importance in determining the extent or character of the underlying condition?

Yes. In simple bronchitis the sputum is usually scant. In bronchiectasis, it is more profuse, thicker, and may be yellow or green in color. In lung abscess, it has a foul smell and may be bloody. In tuberculosis, it is usually blood-tinged. In lung cancer, it may also contain blood.

Does blood in the sputum always indicate tuberculosis or lung cancer?

No. It also occurs in rather minor conditions, including plain acute bronchitis, sinusitis, etc.

Does blood in the sputum always call for further careful investigation?

Yes. This is a definite indication to see your physician.

BRONCHIECTASIS

What is bronchography?

A procedure in which a liquid mixture is allowed to run down into the bronchial tubes so as to outline and fill them with an opaque substance. On x-ray, excellent outlines of the large and small bronchial tubes will be demonstrated.

What is bronchoscopy?

It is a procedure in which a rigid metal tube (bronchoscope) is inserted into the throat, past the vocal cords, into the trachea, and down into the bronchial tubes.

What can be seen on bronchoscopy?

Bronchoscopy is of inestimable value in lung conditions in which the x-ray and sputum examinations do not give a definite diagnosis. It may show the site of origin of bleeding; it may demonstrate foreign bodies that have been aspirated into the lungs; it may show a tumor in the bronchus, or the location of a cancer of the lung. It will also show the point of blockage of a bronchus.

What other value has bronchoscopy?

Since suction can be carried out through a bronchoscope, it is used to remove pus and mucus from areas which are wholly or partially blocked by these substances. Also, pieces of tissue may be removed through the bronchoscope (biopsy material) for various laboratory examinations to determine the exact nature of an existing disease process. Sometimes, an area of ulceration or bleeding may be cauterized through a bronchoscope, thus effecting a cure.

What is bronchiectasis?

It is a chronic disease in which the bronchial tubes are widened, either generally or in small localized areas.

What are the forms of bronchiectasis?

a. Congenital bronchiectasis (existing from time of birth).

b. Acquired bronchiectasis.

What are the symptoms and complications of bronchiectasis?

Chronic, long-standing cough, usually with profuse expectoration, asthma, thinning of the air sacs of the lungs (emphysema), hemorrhage from the bronchial tubes, lung abscess formation, or pneumonia.

Can bronchiectasis be diagnosed by an ordinary x-ray of the chest?

Not definitely. It may be necessary to pass a tube into the bronchial tubes (bronchoscopy) or to perform a bronchogram in order to clinch the diagnosis.

What are the principles of treatment for bronchiectasis?

a. Maintenance of adequate drainage of the mucous secretions from the bronchial tubes. To accomplish this, the secretions must be loosened, and certain expectorant medications are given toward that end.

b. The giving of antibiotic drugs to control the infection.

c. The use of inhalations of various drugs which may dilate and open the bronchial tubes.

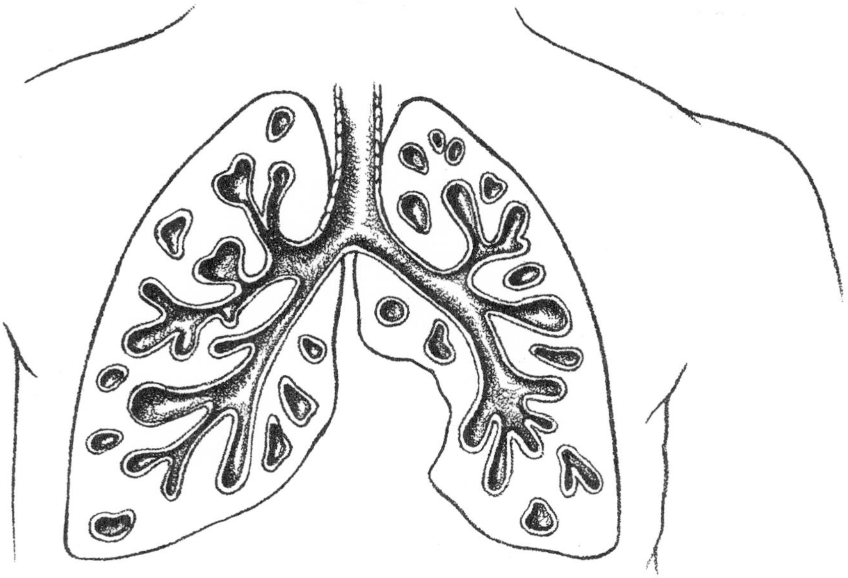

Bronchiectasis. The cutaway drawing of the lungs, above, shows the abnormal widening of the bronchial tubes that is typical of bronchiectasis.

Bronchoscopy. The drawing below shows a sideview of a bronchoscope in position. The metal tube allows a doctor to view the bronchi and make a definite diagnosis.

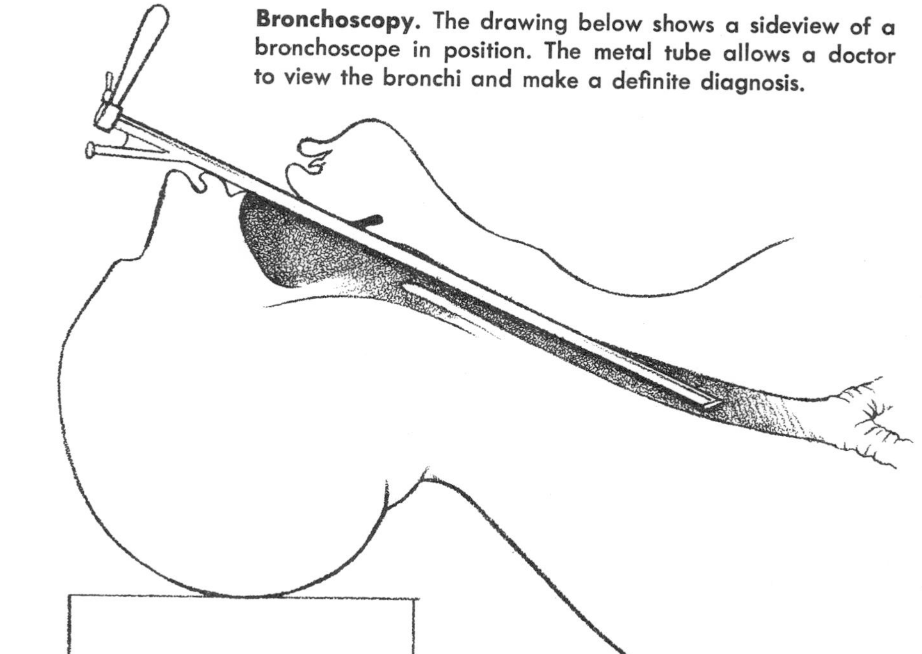

d. Postural drainage (coughing in various positions with the upper part of the body dependent or hanging down over a bed or table) may be very helpful in ridding the bronchial tubes of pus and mucus. This type of exercise should be done several times a day.

Is surgery ever indicated for bronchiectasis?

Yes, if the bronchiectasis is localized; that is, if there is widening in a small area of the lungs. In such an event, that portion of the lung can be removed successfully by surgery. Also, severe hemorrhage from bronchiectasis is an indication to remove that area of the lung.

Is surgery for bronchiectasis dangerous?

Today, operations for removal of part or all of the lung (lobectomy or pneumonectomy) can be carried out safely by chest surgeons.

What are the chances of recovery following surgery for bronchiectasis?

Well over 95 per cent will recover and be cured, provided all of the diseased portions of the lung is removed. The amount of lung tissue that can be removed safely can be determined by properly performed pulmonary function tests.

How long a period of hospitalization is necessary?

(See Chapter 38, on Lungs.)

LA GRIPPE AND INFLUENZA

What is "la grippe"?

It is a term used to denote a condition similar to influenza or "flu"; that is, a highly contagious virus disease with fever, muscular aches and pains, cough, running nose, sore throat, and inflammation of the respiratory passages.

Are the exact causes of grippe or influenza known?

The domestic type may be caused by at least two specific viruses, A and B, which have been isolated. There are undoubtedly many other virus strains which also produce these infections.

What are the distinguishing features between the common cold and grippe or influenza?

Patients with grippe or influenza have more severe symptoms, including headache, lack of appetite, weakness, and higher temperature ranges (up to 103° or 104°) than those suffering from the common cold.

How long does grippe usually last?

The acute phase, with fever, lasts from four or five days to a week or ten days, but is often followed by a period of weakness that may last for several weeks.

What is the significance if fever continues longer than four to five days?

It probably signifies that a *bacterial* infection has been superimposed upon the *virus* infection.

What are the main complications of grippe or influenza?

Bronchitis or pneumonia.

Is there a vaccine that will prevent grippe or flu?

There is an influenza A and B vaccine which is thought to be effective against these two types of infection but not against other types. However, many investigators feel that they have very limited value, if any. (See the section on Asiatic Influenza in this chapter.)

How often should these vaccines be repeated, if they are to be given at all?

About once a year.

Are the antibiotic drugs of value in the treatment of grippe or influenza?

Yes, but only to a certain extent. Their action is not to cure the grippe or virus infection, but rather to prevent secondary infections from taking hold. Thus, complications, such as sinusitis, bronchitis, pneumonia, are much less likely to take place while the antibiotics are being used.

Is there any specific method of diagnosing grippe or influenza?

Not really, except during an influenza epidemic, which occurs every few years.

What is the incubation period of grippe?

One to three days.

Does immunity result from an attack of grippe or influenza?

Yes, but it lasts no more than a few months.

How long should one remain in bed with grippe or influenza?

At least forty-eight hours after the fever has come down and all medications have been discontinued. Longer periods of rest may be necessary if cough is a prominent symptom.

How soon after an attack of grippe or influenza can one resume full activity?

Not until all the symptoms, including fatigue, weakness, and dizziness, have disappeared. Too early resumption of activity may lead to a relapse.

Aside from the antibiotic drugs, what other measures should be used routinely for the treatment of grippe or influenza?

The same measures as are advocated for the common cold. (See the section on the Common Cold in this chapter.)

Does the onset of cough during an attack of grippe or influenza necessarily indicate that pneumonia has set in?

No. Cough can occur when any part of the respiratory tract becomes irritated.

When should the patient decide to call a physician when a respiratory illness occurs?

Physicians should be called when an elevated temperature persists for more than twenty-four hours.

ASIATIC AND HONG KONG INFLUENZA

What is Asiatic flu?

It is a variety of influenza, usually seen in widespread epidemics throughout the world, caused by a variant of the Type A influenza virus as well as by several other virus strains.

What are the symptoms of Asiatic flu?

They are very similar to those of the more commonly known types of influenza and include weakness, chills, fever, headache, muscular pains, and, sometimes, intestinal symptoms.

What is the course of the disease?

It usually lasts five to ten days and then subsides, unless complications develop.

Can an accurate diagnosis of this type of influenza be made?

Since the symptoms are those of the common variety, it cannot always be diagnosed specifically but will probably be classed with the usual types of flu or grippe. Positive diagnosis depends upon complicated laboratory studies, which are not carried out in the ordinary case.

How is the disease spread?

By droplet infection from one patient to another, in the same way as in the ordinary type of flu.

What is the incubation period?

Twenty-four to seventy-two hours.

What are the complications of Asiatic flu?

Epidemics of influenza A seem to be associated with greater incidence of serious complications than those due to influenza B. The most common complications are viral pneumonias, bacterial pneumonias, tracheobronchitis, myocarditis (inflammation of the heart muscle), and certain neurologic complications, such as encephalitis and various forms of neuritis.

Is it a serious disease?

No. Although the attack rate is very high, the disease is usually mild and few people become seriously ill. Those most prone to its serious effects and complications are people with chronic heart, lung and kidney disease, the older age group (over fifty-five), and pregnant women. Vaccination is highly recommended for these people.

Is there any specific treatment?

There is no specific treatment for the disease itself, but antibiotics are of value in the prevention and treatment of complications.

Is there any way to prevent Asiatic flu?

Yes, by the use of influenza virus vaccine, polyvalent, Types A and B, containing several strains of domestic and Asian Type A virus and Type B virus.

How soon does immunity develop after vaccine is administered?

Usually within two weeks, although this may vary considerably.

For how long a period of time is the vaccine effective?

It appears that immunity following vaccination may persist for about four months and, in some instances, up to one year.

Is the vaccine effective in all cases in which it is given?

Vaccination has been found to be only 60 to 75 per cent effective in preventing the disease.

Is it safe for everyone to take the Asiatic Strain vaccine?

No. Those people who are allergic or sensitive to eggs, chickens, or chicken feathers should not be vaccinated, as the vaccine is prepared from chick eggs. Others can take it without serious ill effects.

Does Hong Kong flu differ markedly from Asiatic or other forms of influenza?

Only in degree. A recent epidemic was especially severe and was accompanied by a larger than usual number of complications. Also, the variety popularly called Hong Kong flu had a higher mortality rate than other recent forms of the disease.

CHAPTER 72

The Urinary Bladder and Urethra

(See also Chapter 24 on Female Organs; Chapter 34 on Kidneys and Ureters; Chapter 39 on Male Organs; Chapter 56 on Prostate Gland; Chapter 73 on Venereal Disease)

Where is the urinary bladder, and what is its function?

The bladder is a hollow, muscular organ situated at the bottom of the abdominal cavity behind the pubic bone. It is capable of changing in size, depending upon the amount of urine it contains or expels. The bladder receives urine from the kidneys via the ureters (which enter on either side) and expels the urine through the urethra, which connects with the outside. In the male, the neck of the bladder is in close proximity to, and is surrounded by, the prostate gland. The urethra in the male courses through the penis and is the same length as that structure. In the female, the urethra is short and terminates through a separate opening between the lips of the vulva.

BLADDER INFECTION
(*Cystitis*)

Is cystitis a common disease?

Yes. It is perhaps the most prevalent disorder of the urinary tract. It occurs in children as well as in adults.

What is the most frequent cause of cystitis?

A bacterial infection with such germs as the staphylococcus, streptococcus, colon bacillus, and bacillus proteus.

How do bacteria reach the bladder?

From the outside through the urethra, from infection in the female genital organs, from the kidneys, and from the intestinal tract.

What are different forms of cystitis?

a. Acute.
b. Chronic.
c. Interstitial.

What are the symptoms of acute cystitis?

The onset is usually sudden, characterized by frequent painful urination and not infrequently by the presence of pus and blood in the urine.

What is the treatment for acute cystitis?

a. The administration of the appropriate sulfa or antibiotic drug.
b. The liberal intake of fluids.
c. Bed rest.
d. A bland diet, with special care to avoid highly seasoned foods and alcoholic beverages.
e. Sedatives to relieve pain or spasm.

How long does an attack of acute cystitis usually last?

If treated promptly and adequately, the acute symptoms may subside within a few days. Some disability may persist for a week or two. The urine may take this amount of time to clear.

What are the symptoms of chronic cystitis?

Essentially the same as for acute cystitis, except that the symptoms may be less severe, more prolonged, and may tend to recur. Patients with this condition usually have associated disease in other parts of the urinary tract.

What is interstitial cystitis?

It is a form of chronic cystitis seen mainly in older women. This type of cystitis is characterized by marked thickening of the bladder wall and decreased bladder capacity.

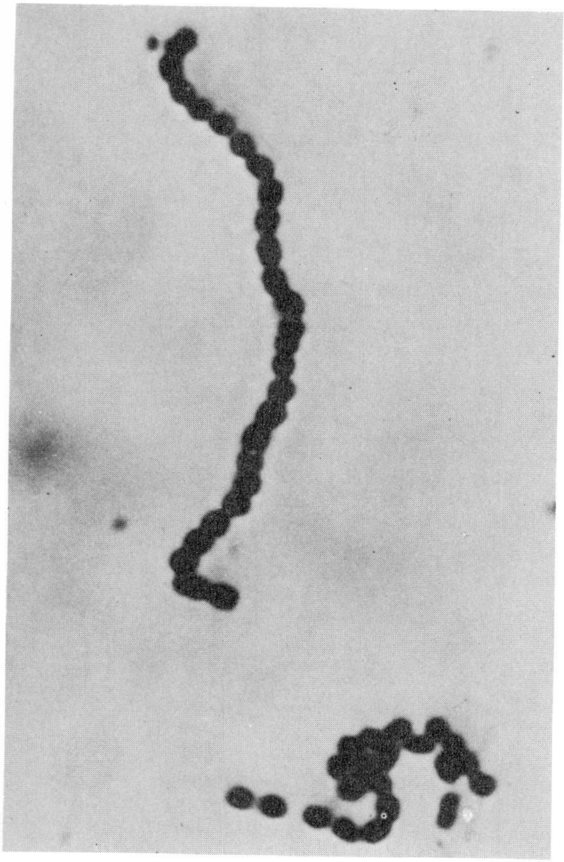

Infection-Causing Bacteria. Two germs which can cause infections of the bladder and other organs are shown in these photomicrographs. At the left is the easily identified chainlike formation of streptococcus bacteria. In the picture below are the characteristic grapelike clusters of staphylococcus bacteria.

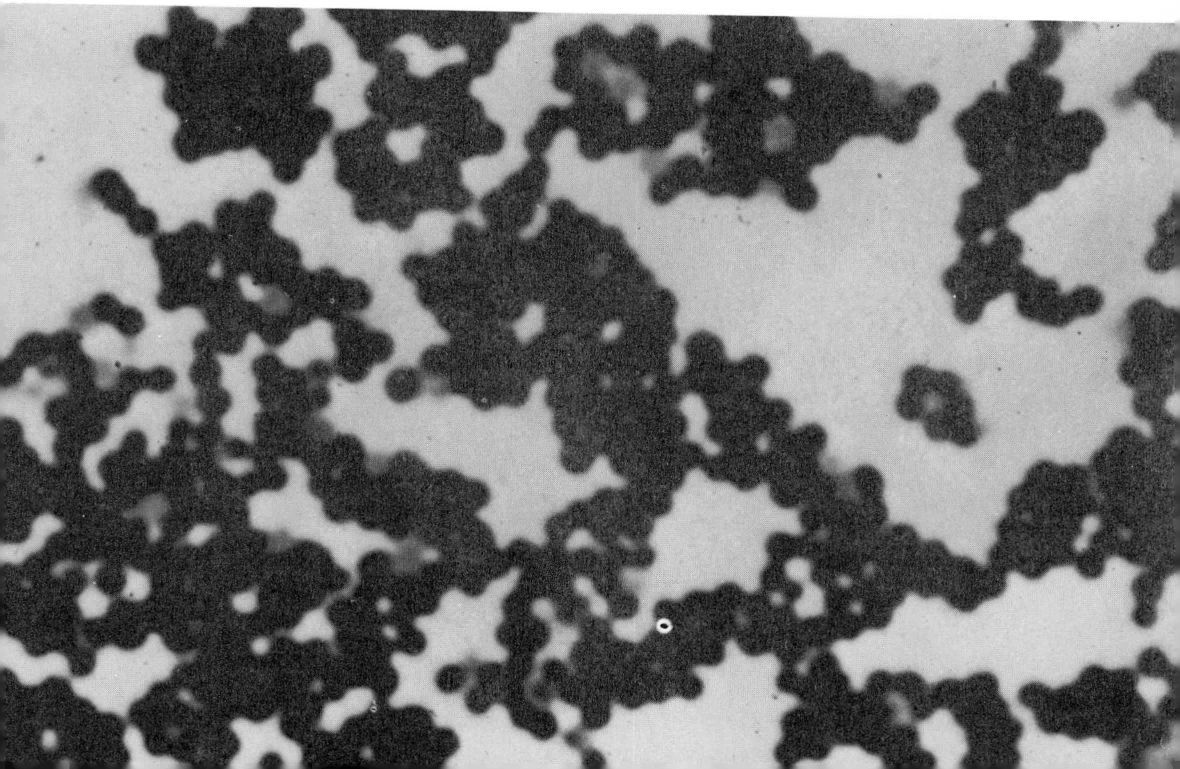

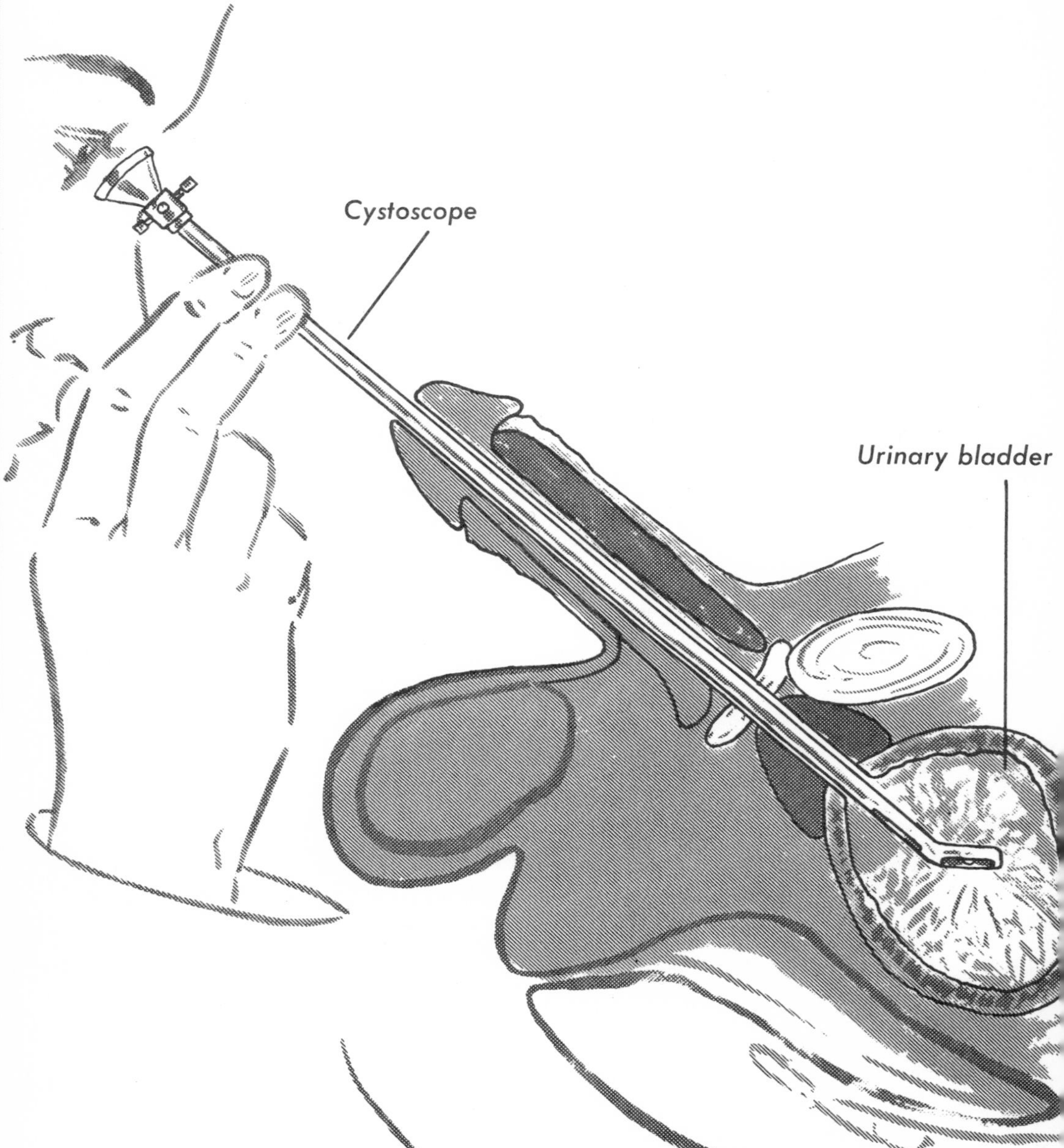

Cystoscopy. This diagram shows a cystoscope being passed into the urinary bladder. By peering through this instrument, the urologist can see disease within the bladder. Tumors, portions of enlarged prostate glands, and bladder stones can often be removed through the cystoscope.

How does one make the diagnosis of cystitis?

By finding pus cells, bacteria, and blood in the urine, and by noting the symptoms listed above.

Is it necessary to cystoscope all patients who have cystitis?

It is not necessary if the symptoms and infection subside quickly. However, if there have been recurring attacks or if the condition has become chronic, the entire urinary tract should be studied, by cystoscope as well as by other means. This is important in order to rule out disease more serious than cystitis. (See the section on Cystoscopy in this chapter.)

What conditions within the urinary tract may produce cystitis?

a. A stone in the kidney or ureter.
b. A tumor in the kidney or ureter.
c. A stone or tumor in the bladder.
d. Any obstructive condition within the urinary tract, such as an enlarged prostate, a cystocele in a female, etc.

CYSTOSCOPY

What is a cystoscopic examination?

One in which the interior of the bladder is viewed directly through a metal tubular instrument known as a cystoscope. Cystoscopes are equipped with lights and lenses which permit excellent visualization of the inside of the bladder. In addition, the outlets of the ureters from the kidneys may be studied through this instrument, as may the internal size and configuration of the prostate gland.

Is a cystoscopic examination painful?

In the female, it is virtually painless. In the male, there is some discomfort, but this can be minimized by using local anesthetic agents. In children, cystoscopy is performed under general anesthesia.

What are the after-effects of cystoscopy?

Some temporary urinary discomfort and possibly some blood in the urine. There also may be a rise in temperature for a day or two.

Is it necessary to be hospitalized for a cystoscopic examination?

Usually not. Most cystoscopic examinations can be done in the urologist's office. When catheters are to be placed through the cystoscope into the ureters and up toward the kidneys, hospitalization is often advised. When such catheters are to be left in place for a few days, hospitalization is mandatory.

BLADDER FISTULAS

What is a bladder fistula?

An abnormal communication between the bladder and some neighboring organ such as the vagina, the intestine, the uterus, etc.

What are the causes for the development of a bladder fistula?

They may result from a severe infection, a malignant growth, an injury secondary to a difficult labor, or as a complication of a surgical operation.

What is the most commonly encountered bladder fistula?

A connection between the bladder and the large bowel, secondary to an inflammation of the large bowel (diverticulitis). Another frequently encountered fistula is one between the bladder and bowel, secondary to a tumor of the bowel.

What are the symptoms of a bladder fistula?

If the fistula extends between the bladder and bowel, the patient will pass gas, feces, or food particles with the urine. If the fistula is between the bladder and vagina, the patient will leak urine from the vagina and will lose control over bladder emptying.

What is the treatment for bladder fistulas?

This will depend upon the cause. Small fistulas that are secondary to injury or infection may heal spontaneously, or they will close by diverting the urine with a rubber catheter. Most fistulas, however, will require surgical correction if a permanent cure is to be obtained.

If the underlying cause is malignant disease, the primary growth as well as the involved portions of the bladder wall must be removed. If diverticulitis (inflammation of the colon) has produced the fistula, the diseased segment of the colon must be removed as well as the involved portion of bladder wall.

Are operations for fistula serious?

Yes, but recovery is the general rule. In cases where malignant disease is the cause, extensive surgery may be indicated.

Are bladder fistulas always cured on the first attempt?

No. Recurrence does take place in a small proportion of cases and these must be reoperated to obtain a satisfactory result.

BLADDER STONES
(*Calculi*)

Are stones often encountered on examination of the urinary bladder?

Yes.

What causes bladder stones?

a. Those that form directly in the bladder usually are the result of poor emptying, with stagnation and pooling of urine.
b. Other stones may form as a result of a bladder disease such as chronic cystitis, a tumor, or diverticulum of the bladder wall.
c. Many bladder stones originate in the kidney and pass down into the bladder from above.

What symptoms do bladder stones produce?

Frequent, painful, bloody urination. Occasionally, stones may cause sudden blockage of the urinary outlet, with resultant inability to void.

How is a positive diagnosis of bladder stones made?

By x-ray examination or by direct visualization through a cystoscope.

What is the treatment for bladder stones?

If small, they often pass spontaneously, without treatment. More often, however, they must be removed. This is accomplished either by opening the bladder surgically or by crushing the stones with a specially designed instrument which is passed through a cystoscope. This latter procedure is called lithopaxy.

When is lithopaxy performed?

When the stones are not too large or firm, and when there are not too many of them. Also, since this procedure is carried out through instrumentation and not by open operation, it is more applicable to those people who are unable to withstand major surgery.

How are the stones removed from the bladder after they have been crushed?

By irrigation. In this manner, they are washed out of the bladder.

When is an open operation (cystotomy) for removal of stones indicated?

When the stones are very firm and therefore cannot be crushed. When they are very numerous, stones should be removed surgically. If there is an enlargement of the prostate along with bladder stones, the surgeon may elect to do an open operation so that he can remove the prostate at the same time.

TUMORS OF THE BLADDER

Do tumors often form within the bladder?

Yes.

Are most bladder tumors malignant?

It is thought that most are either malignant or potentially malignant.

What are the benign tumors of the bladder?

These are wartlike growths known as papillomas.

What are the symptoms of bladder tumors?

Painless bleeding on urination. Occasionally, there is frequency of urination or the passage of infected urine when cystitis supervenes.

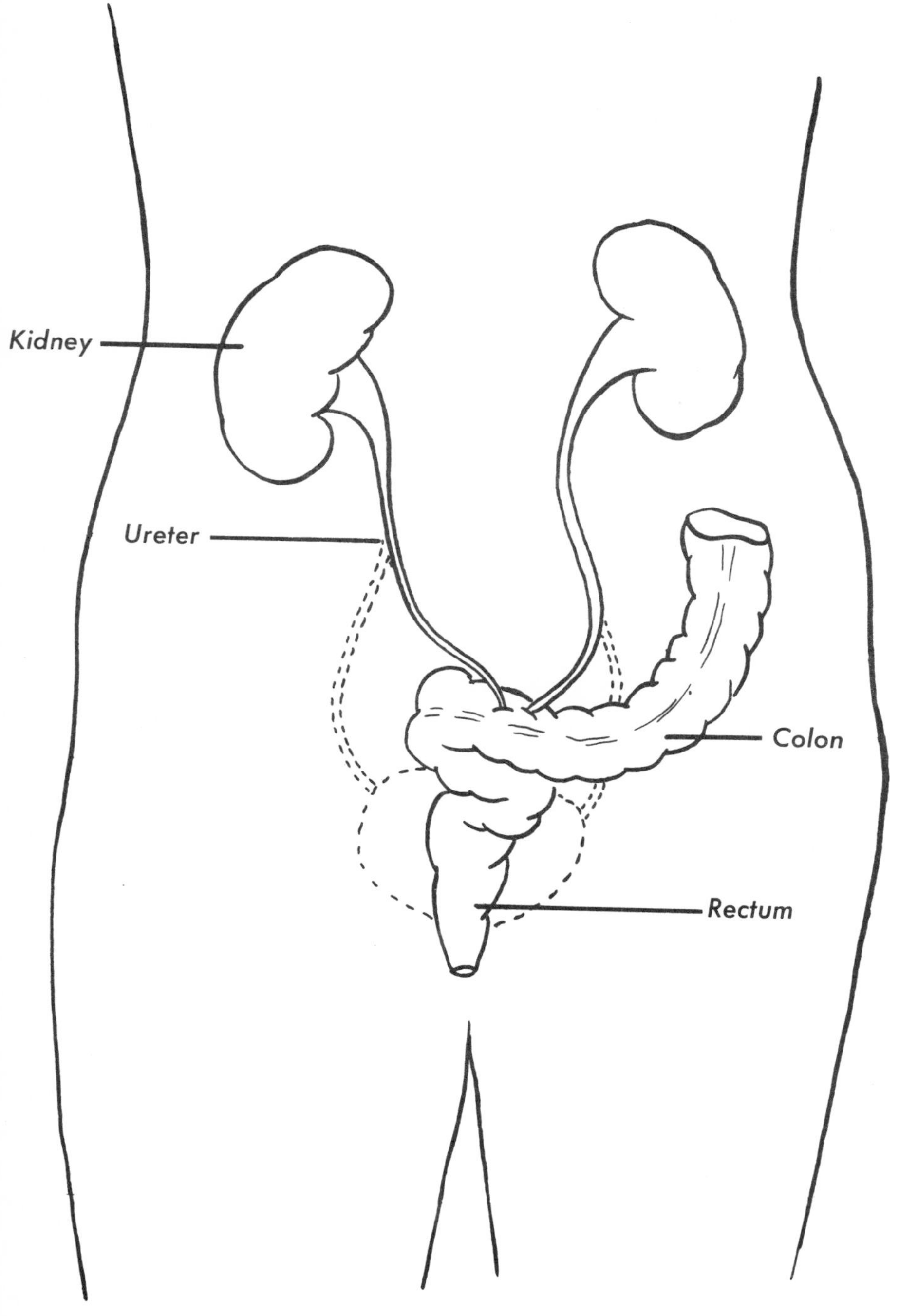

Ureteral Transplant Operation. This diagram shows the ureters being implanted into the large bowel after the urinary bladder has been removed for cancer. Operations more recently devised utilize a portion of small bowel for the implantation of the ureters (ileal bladder).

How is the diagnosis of a bladder tumor made?

By visualization through a cystoscope. A piece of the tumor is removed through the cystoscope and is submitted for microscopic examination.

What is the treatment for bladder tumors?

This will depend upon the size, location, and multiplicity of the tumor. Simple superficial tumors, which do not interfere with the flow of urine from either kidney and are readily accessible, are burned away by electrofulguration through a cystoscope. Large tumors, or ones that penetrate the wall of the bladder deeply, should be removed by cutting out that section of the bladder wall.

When the bladder is extensively involved by a highly malignant growth, it is necessary to remove the entire structure. This procedure is called a cystectomy. When this is done, some disposition must be made of the ureters to provide drainage of urine. Accordingly, the ureters are transplanted either to the skin (cutaneous ureterostomy) or they may be implanted into the large bowel (ureterocolostomy), or a pouch is constructed from a segment of small intestine and the ureters are attached to this pouch. This procedure is known as an ileal bladder operation.

How does one pass his urine when the ureters are transplanted into the large bowel?

Urine is passed through the rectum.

How does the urine drain when the ureters are transplanted into the small intestine?

This segment of small intestine (the ileum) is brought out to the skin and the opening is attached to a plastic or rubber bag which fits snugly to the skin.

Are operations for transplantation of the ureters and removal of the bladder serious?

Yes. They are of great magnitude, but it should be remembered that they are lifesaving procedures, performed in most instances to eradicate cancer.

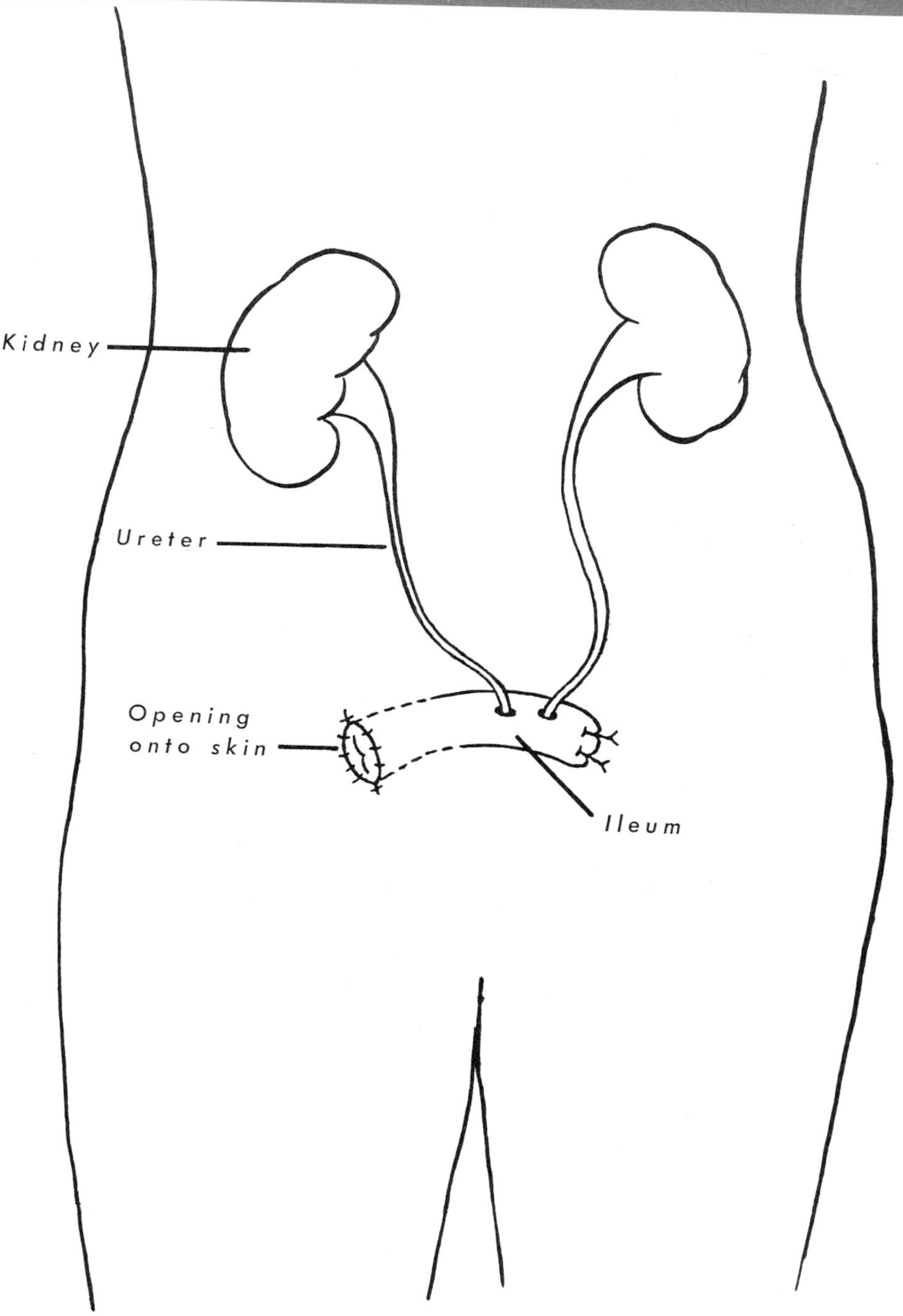

Ileal Bladder Operation. In this operation, a segment of small intestine (ileum) is isolated from the rest of the bowel. One end of the ileum is closed tightly and the other end is left open and is stitched to the skin. The ureters are implanted into this segment of bowel and the urine will drain into it and out onto the skin. A special apparatus is attached to the opening of the ileum which drains the urine into a plastic bag strapped to the leg.

Is there any treatment other than surgery for bladder tumors?

Yes. X-ray therapy can be used, although it is not very efficacious. Also, radium can be implanted into bladder tumors with occasionally successful results. More recently, radioactive materials, such as cobalt, have been used with encouraging results.

How long a hospital stay is necessary for operations upon the urinary bladder?

Operations for the removal of bladder stones, tumors, etc., usually require two weeks of hospitalization. Operations for removal of the entire bladder may require a much longer hospital stay.

Are blood transfusions necessary during operations upon the bladder?

Yes, if an extensive procedure is to be carried out.

Are special nurses needed for major bladder operations?

Yes, for several days.

What is the period of convalescence after a major bladder operation?

Approximately one month.

THE URETHRA

What is the urethra?

It is a tubular passageway leading from the bladder to the outside. Its sole function is to convey urine.

Is the female urethra very different in construction from the male urethra?

Yes. The female urethra is very short, leading from the bladder to its exit between the minor lips of the vulva. The male urethra extends the entire length of the penis.

What are the most common conditions affecting the urethra?

a. Strictures.

b. Caruncle.

c. Diverticulum.
d. Infections (gonorrhea).
e. Congenital deformities, such as hypospadias and epispadias.

Strictures

What is a stricture of the urethra?

An abnormal narrowing in the canal, usually caused by scar tissue formation.

What are the causes of strictures?

a. A birth deformity (congenital stricture).
b. Infection of the urethra, usually the end result of gonorrhea.

What are the symptoms of stricture of the urethra?

a. Reduction in the size and force of the urinary stream.
b. Retention of urine, if the stricture is extensive.
c. Recurrent attacks of cystitis.

How is the diagnosis of stricture made?

By noting the obstruction to the passage of an instrument through the urethral canal and by noting a narrowed urinary stream.

What is the treatment for urethral strictures?

a. Repeated dilatations by the passage of special instruments known as "sounds" or "bougies."
b. Cutting the stricture surgically.
c. In severe cases, plastic operations to reshape the urethra.

If a stricture cannot be cured by dilatation or operation, what procedure is recommended?

Since these cases are accompanied by obstruction to the outflow of urine, a cystotomy must be performed in order to drain the urine. In this event, the urine will drain abdominally through a rubber tube which is attached to a bottle. Fortunately, this situation does not often develop.

Caruncles of the Urethra

What is a caruncle of the urethra?

A small piece of overgrown tissue located at the opening of the urethra. It occurs exclusively in women and results from localized infection or chronic irritation.

What are the symptoms of a caruncle?

There may be no symptoms at all, or the patient may experience pain when the caruncle is touched or when urine passes over it. Frequency of urination with discomfort and bleeding occurs in some cases.

Is treatment always necessary for a caruncle?

No; only if it is large, painful, or causes symptoms.

What is the treatment for a caruncle?

It should be excised surgically or removed by means of an electrocautery. Very small caruncles may be cauterized with chemical agents such as silver nitrate.

Do caruncles have a tendency to recur?

Yes, but not after surgical removal.

Diverticulum of the Urethra

What is a diverticulum of the urethra?

It is a small outpouching of the urethral canal resulting from a birth deformity or secondary to infection in the wall of the urethra. It occurs almost exclusively in women.

What are the symptoms of an urethral diverticulum?

a. Recurrent attacks of bladder infection.
b. Obstruction to the passage of urine.
c. Painful intercourse.

d. After voiding, the patient finds that she can produce more urine by pressing on the region of the diverticulum.

What is the treatment for a diverticulum of the urethra?

Surgical removal, which will result in a cure.

Infections of the Urethra
(Gonorrhea, etc.)

Are infections of the urethra very common?

Yes.

What is the most common cause for an infection of the urethra?

Gonorrhea.

Can gonorrhea be contracted in any way other than by sexual contact?

This is an extremely rare occurrence, and when it does take place it occurs in the female, not in the male.

What are the symptoms of gonorrhea?

a. The appearance of a creamy urethral discharge about a week to ten days following unprotected sexual relations. This discharge appears from the orifice of the penis or from the vulva in the female.
b. Frequent, painful urination.
c. Pus and blood in the urine.
d. Pain and swelling in the region of the external genitals.

Does a discharge from the urethra always mean gonorrhea?

No. Other germs can also cause an infection in this area.

How is a positive diagnosis of gonorrhea made?

By actually visualizing the gonorrheal germ under the microscope. This is accomplished by taking some of the pus from the urethra.

Do gonorrhea and syphilis always occur together?

No, but when one of these conditions is present, a thorough search should be made for the other.

What is the treatment for gonorrhea?

The antibiotic drugs, if used promptly and properly, will bring about a cure within a few days.

How long does it take for the antibiotic drugs to work?

Their action is effective within twenty-four to forty-eight hours.

Is it safe for a patient with gonorrhea to administer treatment to himself?

Absolutely not. A chronic form of the disease may result if the patient attempts to treat himself by purchasing his own antibiotics. It is essential that these medications be given under the supervision of a physician.

Do all gonorrhea germs respond satisfactorily to all antibiotics?

No. The physician will frequently have to change the antibiotic in order to find the one which is most effective for the particular type of germ causing the infection.

What are the complications from the improper treatment of gonorrhea?

a. In men, a spread of the infection to the prostate gland, testicle, and/or epididymis.
b. A stricture of the urethra may result.
c. In women, a spread of the infection to the cervix, uterus, Fallopian tubes, and/or ovaries. Also, peritonitis may ensue from an extension of the infection to the abdominal cavity.

Can gonorrhea cause sterility?

Yes. In women, gonorrhea is the most frequent cause of sterility. In men, if the infection has involved the testicles or epididymis, sterility may sometimes take place.

How can one prevent sterility in cases of gonorrhea?

By prompt treatment by a competent physician.

Does gonorrhea often become chronic?

Yes. In inadequately treated cases, the germ may lie dormant within the genital tract for months or years, only to flare up from time to time.

Can chronic gonorrheal infection be cured?

Yes, by adequate treatment with antibiotics and, sometimes, by the performance of surgery to remove structures which have been destroyed by the gonorrheal infection, such as the Fallopian tubes, ovaries, etc.

Does gonorrhea cause impotence?

No.

Hypospadias and Epispadias

What are hypospadias and epispadias?

Birth deformities of the urethra, in which the urethra ends short of the tip of the penis. When the urethra ends on the under side of the penis, the condition is called hypospadias; when it opens on the top side, it is called epispadias.

Are there varying degrees of these deformities?

Yes. In certain cases the urethra ends right near the tip of the penis and no symptoms result. In the more severe types, the urethra may end near the very beginning of the penis; this will result in serious voiding difficulties.

What is the treatment for hypospadias or epispadias?

Minor deviations from normal require no treatment; others will require correction by plastic surgery. This is often carried out in several stages and constitutes complicated techniques necessitating the services of a competent urologist.

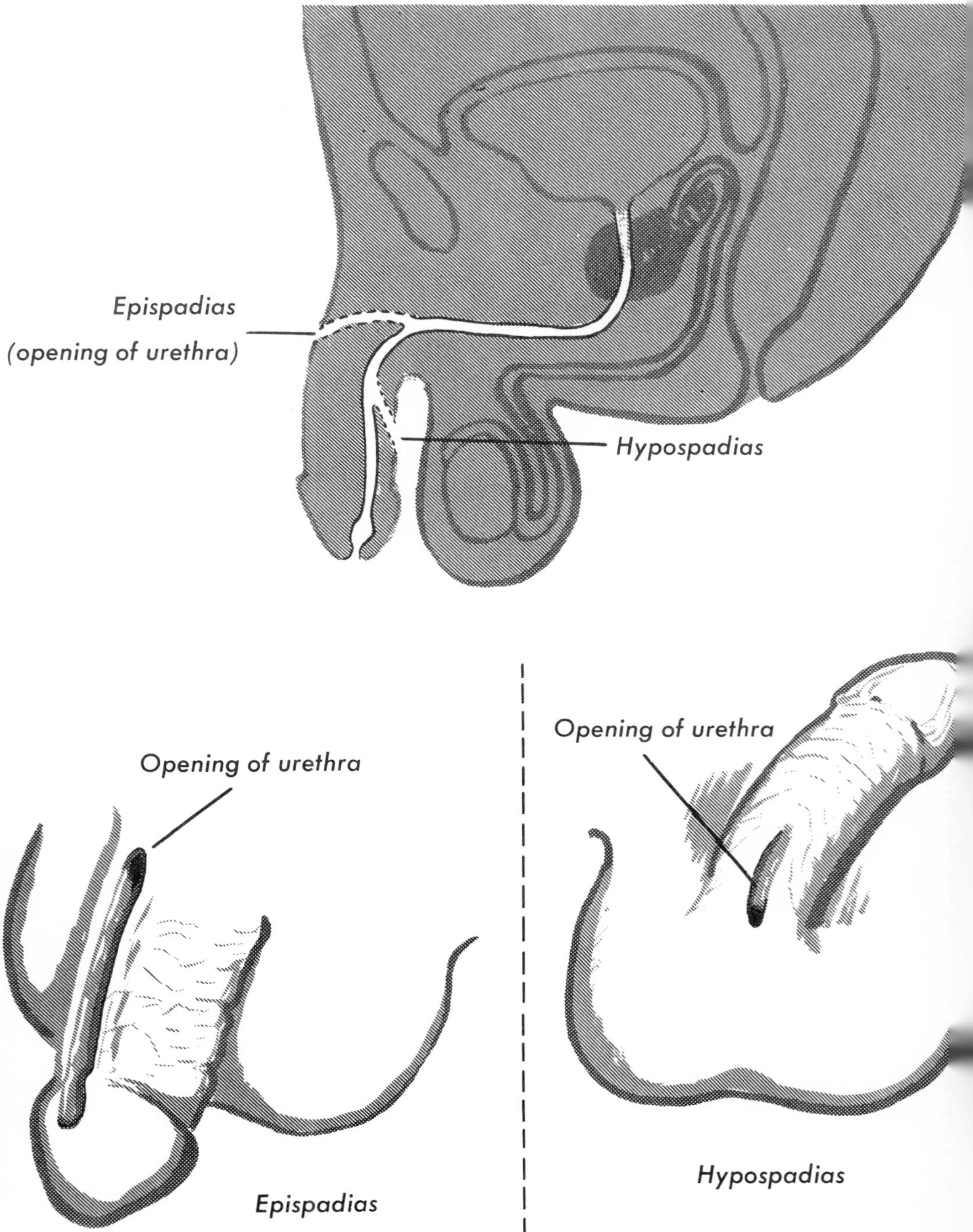

Epispadias and Hypospadias. These diagrams show birth deformities of the urethra. These abnormalities can be eliminated by plastic surgery upon the penis.

When is the best time to operate for hypospadias or epispadias?

During the first few years of life.

How successful are these operations?

In most cases good results are obtained. However, when the results are unsatisfactory, reoperation can effect a cure. Some of these reoperative procedures are carried out years later, when the tissues have grown considerably and are easier to handle surgically.

If the operations for hypospadias or epispadias are successful, will urinary and sexual function be normal?

Yes.

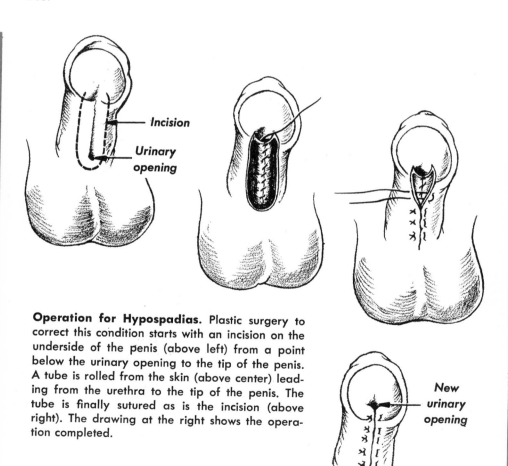

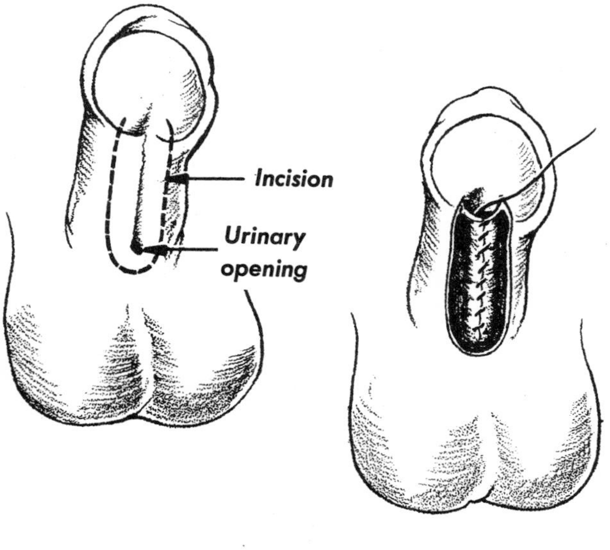

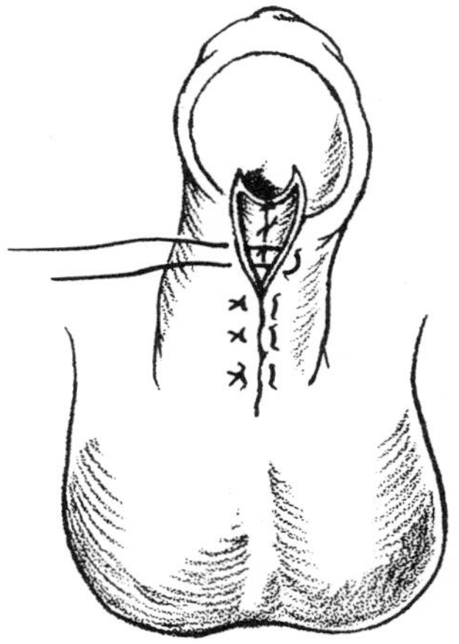

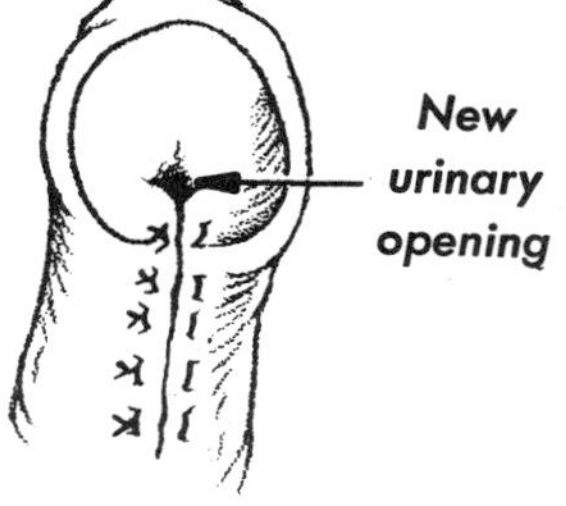

Operation for Hypospadias. Plastic surgery to correct this condition starts with an incision on the underside of the penis (above left) from a point below the urinary opening to the tip of the penis. A tube is rolled from the skin (above center) leading from the urethra to the tip of the penis. The tube is finally sutured as is the incision (above right). The drawing at the right shows the operation completed.

CHAPTER 73

Venereal Disease

(See also Chapter 24 on Female Organs; Chapter 39 on Male Organs; Chapter 64 on Sterility and Fertility; Chapter 72 on Urinary Bladder and Urethra)

What is a venereal disease?

A condition which is contracted as a result of sexual contact or exposure.

Is this the only way in which venereal disease can be contracted?

No. Kissing, nursing, or even the simple handling of infected materials may cause a venereal infection such as syphilis.

Can venereal diseases be contracted from unclean toilet seats?

This is theoretically possible, but with the exception of gonorrhea in the female, it is a very rare occurrence.

What venereal diseases are most prevalent?

a. Gonorrhea. (See Chapter 72, on the Urinary Bladder and Urethra.)
b. Syphilis.

What is the difference between gonorrhea and syphilis?

Although both are venereal diseases, there is very little similarity. Gonorrhea is caused by an organism which, in most instances, is localized to the genitals and is characterized by frequency of urination, painful swelling, and discharge from the region. Syphilis, on the other hand, is a disease which starts as a sore in the region of contact. It eventually spreads throughout the entire body and affects all the organs to a greater or lesser degree. In other words, gonorrhea is a localized disease; syphilis a generalized or systemic disease.

Which condition is more serious, gonorrhea or syphilis?

Syphilis is a much more serious condition, as it may ultimately produce grave damage to organs such as the brain, the heart, the liver, etc.

Does gonorrhea ever affect organs other than the genitals?

Yes. It may affect the eyes, and for this reason all newborns are given preventive eye drops at birth. Occasionally, if untreated, gonorrhea may affect the joints, causing a specific type of arthritis. Very rarely, it may involve the lining of the brain or spinal cord, thus causing a specific type of encephalitis or meningitis.

Will cleansing and taking a prophylactic treatment after exposure, prevent venereal disease in all instances?

No! The only sure way to avoid gonorrhea or syphilis is to avoid contact with infected individuals.

Are prophylactic treatments helpful at all in preventing venereal infection?

Yes, if taken properly, *immediately* after exposure. However, this procedure is never dependable.

SYPHILIS

What causes syphilis?

It is caused by a bacterial organism known as the treponema pallidum (a spirochete).

What is the incidence of syphilis in this country today?

Seventy-seven out of every hundred thousand people develop syphilis each year, according to the latest statistics.

Is syphilis on the decline?

It was until recently. Within the past year or two, however, there has been a marked increase in the incidence of syphilis due to carelessness and inadequate prophylactic precautions.

Does everyone who is exposed to syphilis develop it?

Not necessarily. There are factors, such as the state of activity of the disease, the type of exposure, contact, etc., which influence the likelihood of infection.

Is there any natural immunity to syphilis?

No.

Can syphilis be inherited?

Yes. Syphilis can be transmitted through the blood from parent to child.

How can one tell if he has syphilis?

A sore, called a chancre, will appear several weeks after the initial exposure. It may be located on the genitals or on any other region of the body where contact has taken place with an infected person.

Are there any other ways to tell whether one has syphilis?

Yes. There are several accurate blood tests which will indicate whether the patient is infected. (The most common test has always been the Wassermann test, but this has been replaced within recent years by other, more sensitive tests.)

What is a chancre?

It is the primary lesion of syphilis. It is a small painless sore, measuring no more than about one-half inch in diameter. The chancre will appear on the penis, the female genitals, or at any other point of contact, such as the lips, etc.

What happens to a chancre if it is permitted to go untreated?

It will persist for several weeks and then disappear spontaneously.

What happens after the chancre disappears?

A month or two later, a rash will appear on other parts of the body and a sore throat will develop. This is called the secondary eruption, or secondary stage of syphilis.

What happens to this rash and sore throat if permitted to go untreated?

This, too, will disappear spontaneously within a few weeks.

Does this mean that the patient is thereafter cured of his syphilis?

Emphatically not! The germs will live and travel throughout the entire body and may produce an active infection elsewhere at a later date, perhaps many years later.

Will the blood test be positive even when there is no obvious evidence of syphilis?

Yes.

Is there any way to prevent syphilis?

Yes, by avoiding exposure to a possible contact! Also, do not use personal utensils of unclean, potentially infected people.

Is there any entirely safe method of protection during sexual exposure?

No. If one has contact with a person suffering from active syphilis, the chances are great that one will acquire the disease.

Can a person have a positive blood test for syphilis without ever having had any signs whatsoever of the disease?

Yes. It is possible that a person might have inherited syphilis. This is one of the most potent arguments in favor of subjecting all people to a blood test for syphilis.

Is the blood test ever positive when the patient does not actually have syphilis?

Yes. This occurs only occasionally, in situations in which people have high fever, or in certain other diseases.

Is there any way of telling at birth whether a child has inherited syphilis?

Yes. A blood test can be taken from a sample of blood from the umbilical cord. More important, if neither parent has had the disease and their blood tests are negative, the child will not have the disease.

If one or both parents has had syphilis which has been treated successfully, what are the chances of their child having syphilis?

If the parents have been cured of the disease, their children will be free of the disease.

Are there any evidences during childhood that a child has inherited syphilis?

Yes. There are certain physical signs by which the physician will be able to make a diagnosis of inherited (congenital) syphilis.

Can syphilis in a newborn child be treated successfully?

Yes.

What are the dangers from untreated syphilis?

When untreated, syphilis will usually crop out years later with an active infection within a vital organ.

What organs are most frequently affected by late, or tertiary, syphilis?

a. The nervous system.
b. The heart.
c. The large blood vessels such as the aorta.
d. The liver.
e. The skin.

What diseases are caused by syphilitic infection of the nervous system?

a. A form of insanity known as paresis.
b. Tabes (locomotor ataxia), a condition in which there is loss of sense of position in the extremities, making it extremely difficult to walk.

What is the treatment for syphilis?

Syphilis can be treated very successfully today, if treatment is begun early in the course of the disease. Penicillin and other antibiotic drugs have been found to produce cures in the vast majority of cases.

Is it more difficult to cure syphilis in its secondary or tertiary stages?

Yes. Anyone with a primary lesion such as a chancre, should go for immediate treatment. Results are much better when treatment is started early.

Can the late complications of syphilis be treated effectively?

To a certain degree, but not nearly as effectively as in the early stages of the disease. Late complications can merely be arrested or prevented from getting worse.

How early in the development of syphilis will the blood tests register as positive?

By the time the chancre has appeared.

When is syphilis most contagious?

During its primary and secondary stages, when there is a chancre, rash, or sore throat.

Is syphilis contagious during the late stages (tertiary)?

Almost never, except that at any stage of the disease a syphilitic parent can transmit it to the unborn offspring.

Is hospitalization necessary in the treatment of syphilis?

Not during the initial stages of the disease, but it is sometimes advisable, for the purposes of isolation, to hospitalize those who are highly contagious and who will not use proper precautions to prevent its spread to others. Hospitalization is also necessary for the severe nervous system complications or the late heart complications.

By what method is penicillin given in the treatment of syphilis?

By injection into the muscles of the buttocks, by mouth, or by injections into the veins.

Should a patient who has had syphilis ever get married?

Yes, if the disease has been successfully treated and cured.

What are the chances of a syphilitic patient transmitting the disease to his or her mate?

If adequate treatment has been carried out, the chances are practically nil.

How long does it take for full recovery from syphilis when it has been thoroughly treated?

Before someone can be pronounced cured, he must be followed medically and found to be free of the disease for a period of at least two to three years.

How soon after treatment has begun does the contagious aspect of syphilis disappear?

Within a few days or, at the latest, weeks after penicillin injections have been started. Often, contagion disappears after the first few injections.

If a person eats in an ordinary restaurant, how can he be assured that the utensils are clean enough so that he will not contract syphilis?

The ordinary methods of cleansing plates and eating utensils are completely adequate to kill the germs of syphilis.

How long can the germs of syphilis live in the open air or on plates or eating utensils, etc.?

They die within a minute or two under such circumstances.

Can one contract syphilis a second time after having been "cured" of an initial infection?

Yes.

Are any medications other than the antibiotics effective in treating syphilis?

Yes. In the rare case, when an individual is sensitive to the antibiotics, treatment can be effectively carried out by the older methods of utilizing arsenic and bismuth injections.

Can arsenic and bismuth bring about cures in the average case of syphilis?

Yes, but the method of treatment with these medications takes much longer and is more painful than treatment with the use of the antibiotic drugs.

Can one return to a completely normal life after having been treated successfully for syphilis?

Yes.

Are there any permanent limitations on activity after an episode of syphilis?

No.

Does syphilis ever cause death?

Yes, particularly the late complications, such as syphilis of the brain or blood vessels.

Should a woman with syphilis permit herself to become pregnant?

Not until she has been fully treated and pronounced cured.

Is syphilis thought to be a cause for repeated miscarriage and for stillbirths?

Yes. Many physicians think that syphilis predisposes toward these conditions.

How often should one return to his physician for a checkup after having been discharged from treatment for syphilis?

At least once a year.

CHAPTER 74 *Vitamins*

(See also Chapter 5 on Aging; Chapter 20 on Diet; Chapter 31 on Infant Feeding; Chapter 54 on Pregnancy and Childbirth)

What are vitamins?

They are specific chemical compounds essential to normal body chemistry and health. They are not manufactured by the body itself but are obtained principally from foods.

Do vitamins add calories to food intake?

No.

Are vitamins essential to life?

Yes. However, people may live for long periods of time with insufficient vitamin intake before the deficiency diseases become apparent.

How can one tell if he needs vitamins?

The signs and symptoms of vitamin deficiency may be extremely difficult to diagnose. Certainly, the patient himself cannot make an accurate diagnosis of a vitamin deficiency and therefore should not undertake to medicate himself by taking vitamins indiscriminately.

Will the addition of vitamin pills to a normal diet increase the general resistance to disease?

No. If one's food vitamin intake is normal, and vitamin absorption by the body is normal, taking additional vitamins in the form of pills will not increase resistance to disease.

For how long a period of time must vitamins be taken in order to cure a deficiency?

If the deficiency has existed for a long time, it may take several weeks or longer for the body to attain a normal vitamin status. If the deficiency has been present for only a short time, adequate vitamin intake will probably start to have an effect immediately.

What are the causes of vitamin deficiency?

a. Inadequate food intake or unbalanced food intake.
b. Inadequate vitamin absorption due to intestinal dysfunction or disease.
c. Poor vitamin metabolism due to disease processes within various organs of the body.
d. Unusual vitamin demands, as would occur during sickness, during pregnancy, during periods of extraordinary growth, during periods of stress or special activity, and when the patient is undergoing surgery.

What diseases or conditions are caused by vitamin deficiency?

a. Vitamin A deficiency:
   1. Poor night vision.
   2. Dryness of the tissues of the eyes, skin, and respiratory tract.
   3. Poor formation of teeth and bones.
b. Vitamin B_1 or thiamin deficiency:
   1. Beriberi, a severe deficiency disease characterized by extreme degrees of weight loss, loss of muscle strength, neuritis, mental confusion, and impairment of heart function.
   2. Minor deficiencies in vitamin B_1 will lead to milder symptoms of weight loss, poor appetite, loss of strength, and damage to nerve tissues.
c. Vitamin B_2 or riboflavin deficiency:
   1. Cracking of the skin at the angles of the mouth, scaly lesions in the folds of the skin which extend from the angles of the nose to the lips. Also, irritation and redness of the lining of the mouth and tongue, with purplish discoloration.
d. Nicotinic acid deficiency:
   Pellagra, a severe deficiency disease characterized by sensitivity

of exposed skin surfaces to sunlight. This causes skin rashes. Pellagra is also accompanied by gastro-intestinal symptoms and mental instability and disorientation.

e. Folic acid deficiency:
This condition will cause severe anemia of varying types.

f. Vitamin B_6 or pyridoxine deficiency:
Gastro-intestinal symptoms, general weakness, nervousness, irritability, and nerve tissue damage can be caused by this vitamin deficiency.

g. Vitamin B_{12} deficiency:
This can create pernicious anemia and nerve tissue diseases such as neuritis.

h. Vitamin C or ascorbic acid deficiency:
Scurvy, a severe deficiency disease characterized by marked degrees of weakness, accompanied by bleeding tendencies. This is characterized by widespread bruising and bleeding from the gums or other organs.

i. Vitamin D deficiency:
Rickets, a severe deficiency disease in infants and children characterized by poor absorption of calcium from the diet with malformation of bone structures. This, in an advanced state, can lead to marked bowing of the legs or malformation of the pelvis or of the chest.

j. Vitamin E deficiency:
It is thought by some investigators that a Vitamin E deficiency tends to cause sterility, diseases of the heart and blood vessels, and diseases of muscles and nerves. The exact role of vitamin E has not yet been determined conclusively.

k. Vitamin K deficiency:
This vitamin is concerned with the manufacture of one of the important elements required in normal blood coagulation. Deficiency of vitamin K, as seen in cases of jaundice, may lead to severe hemorrhage from the various mucous membrane surfaces of the body.

l. Vitamin P deficiency:
There is insufficient data, at present, to classify this group of

compounds as to their exact function. Present evidence tends to indicate that they are concerned with capillary wall structure as well as the cement-like substance between tissue cells.

Do deficiencies of the above vitamins always produce the characteristic diseases?

No. The most common finding today is that one is only mildly deficient in these vitamins. Thus, the full-blown disease will not be evident but rather certain minimal symptoms of the disease may be present.

Is vitamin deficiency usually limited to one vitamin?

Generally speaking, isolated vitamin deficiency is the exception rather than the rule. When vitamin deficiency exists, multiple vitamin deficiency is usually the case.

Which foods are particularly rich in vitamin content?

a. Vitamin A:
Butter, eggs, milk, liver, fish, liver oils, green leafy vegetables, yellow vegetables.

b. Vitamin B_1 (thiamin):
Meat, whole grains, yeast, vegetables, liver, eggs.

c. Vitamin B_2 (riboflavin):
Dairy foods, meat, eggs.

d. Niacin:
Peanuts, liver yeast, organ meats, wheat germ.

e. Vitamin B_6 (pyridoxine):
Meat, fish, grains, vegetables, liver, yeast.

f. Vitamin B_{12}:
Meat, liver, eggs, dairy products.

g. Vitamin C:
Oranges, lemons, grapefruit and other citrus fruits, potato, cabbage, tomato, green pepper.

h. Vitamin D:
Fish liver oils, eggs, dairy products.

i. Folic Acid:
Green vegetables, yeast, liver, kidney.

j. Vitamin K:
A fat-soluble vitamin whose absorption depends greatly on normal fat absorption from the gastro-intestinal tract.

k. Vitamin E:
Wheat germ, whole grains.

What is meant by the minimum daily requirement of a vitamin?

The smallest amount which, when taken daily over a prolonged period of time, will prevent the development of a deficiency disease.

What is meant by "therapeutic formula" vitamins?

This term applies to a combination of all of the known vitamins in doses usually adequate to prevent and treat disease from most vitamin deficiencies. It usually contains many times the daily requirements of the body.

Should therapeutic formulas of vitamins be taken routinely wherever a deficiency seems to exist?

No. This practice is costly, wasteful, and without scientific logic.

Is it possible to take an overdose of vitamins?

Yes. Severe toxic effects and sometimes permanent damage can be caused by overdose of certain vitamins, particularly vitamins A and D.

Should all people routinely take vitamin pills to maintain good health?

No. They should be taken only when there is a known or strongly suspected vitamin deficiency or dietary deficiency.

Should people take vitamins on their own, or should they consult their physician before taking vitamins routinely?

Consult your physician. Most people, under the pressure of advertising, take an excess amount of vitamins. This is wasteful and, in some instances, may be harmful if an overdose is taken.

When is it necessary to give vitamins by injection?

a. When oral intake is not possible, such as after certain types of surgery or in severe cases of gastro-intestinal disorder.

b. When there is poor absorption of the vitamins from the intestinal tract.

c. When large initial doses are indicated in severe deficiencies and the physician wishes the patient to gain rapid absorption of large quantities of vitamins.

What vitamins are routinely given to newborns?

Newborns usually obtain a daily supplement of vitamins A, B, C, and D.

Do growing children normally require extra vitamin intake in the form of pills?

Not if they eat a well-balanced diet. Vitamins should be added to the diet only on the advice of one's physician.

Do aged people require extra vitamins?

Recent research would indicate that most aged people can well benefit from supplementary vitamins. This stems from the fact that their food intake of vitamin-rich substances is often reduced, their gastro-intestinal absorption is impaired, and their metabolic processes are inadequate.

What supplementary vitamins are usually given to pregnant women?

Because of increased needs for vitamins during pregnancy, it has become the practice to give expectant mothers vitamins A, C, D, and B complex. Sometimes, vitamins E, K, and P are added. Such vitamin intake should not be a substitute for a well-balanced diet.

Should people who are obese and who are undergoing strenuous dieting take vitamins?

Yes. It is wise for such people to take a multivitamin supplement containing most of the known vitamins.

Are vitamins of value in quieting nervous people?

Only if the nervousness is due to a vitamin deficiency. This is rarely the case.

Are vitamins valuable in treating anemia?

Very few types of anemia are caused by vitamin deficiency alone. However, where there is a vitamin deficiency along with anemia, vitamins may be given.

Will the taking of extra vitamins reduce the incidence of colds, grippe, or influenza?

There is insufficient scientific evidence to prove this. However, it is thought that people with vitamin deficiencies may be more susceptible to upper respiratory infection.

Does the regular taking of mineral oil interfere with the absorption of vitamins?

It is doubtful whether the taking of mineral oil results in serious interference with vitamin absorption. In order to insure that this does not take place, it is wisest to take the vitamins several hours before or after taking the oil.

Will taking vitamin A improve the eyesight?

No, unless the impaired eyesight is due to a proved vitamin A deficiency.

Does it make much difference which brand of vitamin one purchases?

All vitamin manufacture and distribution is regulated by the provisions of the Pure Food and Drug Act. It is safe to purchase any brand of vitamins as long as the quantities contained in the prescription are clearly marked on the label.

Are vitamins helpful in the so-called "general rundown condition"?

Only if there is an existing vitamin deficiency.

Will the taking of vitamins tend to make one gain weight?

Not unless the diet has been previously deficient in vitamins and such deficiency has in some way led to poor appetite and inadequate food intake.

CHAPTER 75 *X-ray*

(See also Chapter 14 on Bones, Muscles, Tendons, and Joints; Chapter 16 on Cancer; Chapter 26 on Gall Bladder and Bile Ducts; Chapter 34 on Kidneys and Ureters; Chapter 38 on Lungs; Chapter 43 on Neurosurgery; Chapter 62 on Small and Large Intestines; Chapter 65 on Stomach and Duodenum)

What are x-rays?

They are electromagnetic waves of very short length which are created by passing a high-voltage electric current through a vacuum tube equipped with a metallic target for the electrons to strike against. X-rays have a peculiar penetrative power through matter and living tissues. By passing these rays through the part of the body to be studied, shadows are created which can be recorded on photographic film. These shadows form certain patterns, varying according to the density of the particular tissue. The interpretation of these shadows is the task of the radiologist, who can, from his study, often make a specific diagnosis.

What is a radiologist?

A radiologist is a physician who has had special education and training and is qualified in the use of x-rays, radium, cobalt, and other radioactive substances, for the diagnosis and treatment of diseases and abnormalities of the human body.

What is an x-ray technician?

An x-ray technician is one who has had special training and experience in the use of x-ray apparatus for the purpose of taking x-ray films or giving x-ray therapy. He or she is also experienced in the technical processing of the exposed x-ray films.

Can all the tissues of the body be visualized by x-rays?

No. There are many soft tissues in the body which are not visualized by x-rays upon direct study. This is due to the fact that these tissues absorb the same amount of x-rays as the immediate surrounding tissues and therefore do not reveal contrast. However, with the aid of contrast media, such as opaque dye or air, almost all parts of the body can be visualized.

Is it safe for the x-rays to be taken by a technician?

Yes. The x-ray technician is a person who has been specially trained to do x-ray technical work, and he or she does this work under the supervision of the radiologist. Most states require certification, registry, or licensing of the x-ray technician.

Why do x-ray technicians stand behind screens or in another room when taking x-rays?

These screens, or room walls, have lead shielding to protect the technician from the effects of scattered radiation, which has a cumulative effect over a period of time, even though this radiation may be in small amounts at each exposure.

Is there any danger of getting a shock from an x-ray machine?

No. All present x-ray apparatus is fully shock-proof, as are the cables, etc.

Is an x-ray a true picture of the part of the body examined?

No. It is a projection of shadows as the x-ray beam goes through the various densities of the tissues. It is the interpretation of these shadows which makes the diagnosis.

Are x-rays that are recorded on paper as good as those made on film?

No. Better detail is obtained in x-ray studies upon film.

Are x-rays used only by the medical and dental professions?

No. They are also very valuable in research, industry, art-forgery detection, and law enforcement.

Can x-ray moving pictures be made?

Yes. These are known as cineradiograms or cinefluorograms.

Are x-ray films the property of the patient?

No. X-ray films are a part of the permanent record of a medical examination and, as such, are the property of the examining physician. State laws govern this factor. However, the patient is entitled to a report of the physician's findings or x-ray diagnosis.

Can x-ray films of different patients get mixed up?

This is almost impossible, as films are imprinted with the patient's name and a specific number.

What is a fluoroscope?

It is an x-ray apparatus which reveals the image of the parts of the body studied upon a fluorescent screen; it also shows the movements of these parts.

Why must the room be darkened during a fluoroscopic examination?

Because the images appearing upon the fluorescent screen will be much better visualized if the room is darkened to prevent light reflections upon the screen.

What is an image intensifier?

It is a unit which is attached to the fluoroscope and greatly increases the brightness and improves the visual acuity of the ordinary fluoroscopic image. It also permits fluoroscopy in room light.

Can photographs be taken from the fluoroscope?

Yes. Cinefilming and projection upon TV systems are also possible.

Why does the radiologist wear rubber gloves and a rubber apron when performing fluoroscopy?

Since he is constantly working in and around x-rays, the cumulative effect can be harmful unless he protects himself from overexposure. The apron and gloves protect him because they contain lead which is impervious to x-rays.

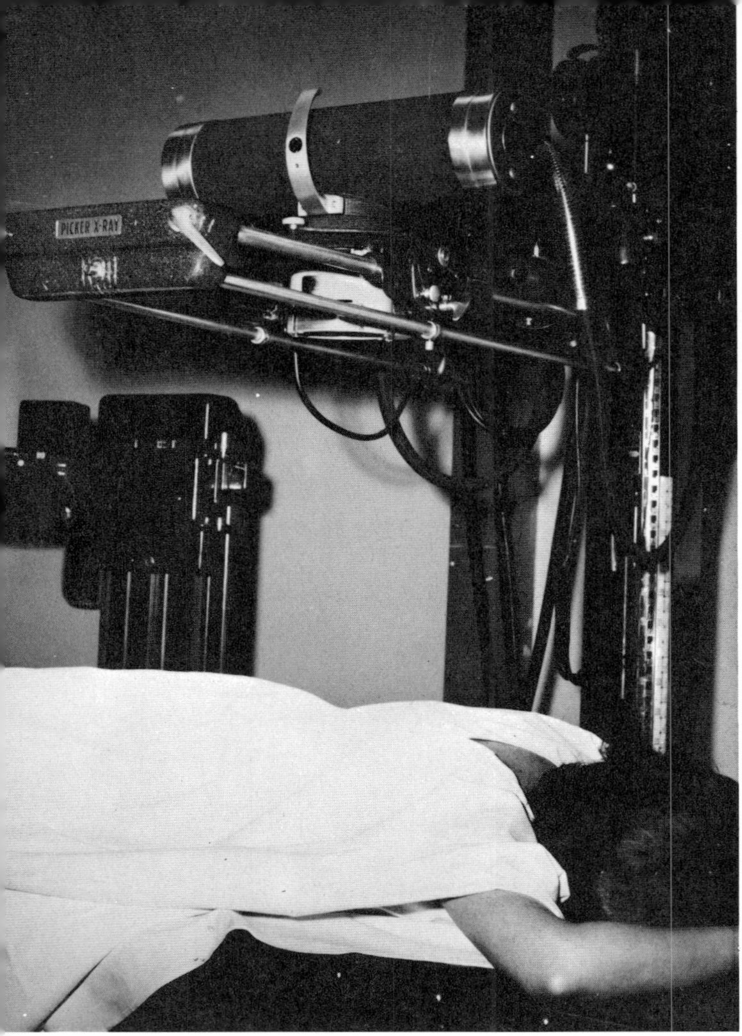

Diagnostic X-ray. This photograph shows an ordinary diagnostic x-ray being taken. There has been much agitation recently about people being subjected to too many x-rays. Patients should not worry about this, as their physician will safeguard them by ordering only those x-rays which are necessary.

Is it possible to undergo too many fluoroscopic examinations?

Yes. Overexposure is definitely bad for the patient. The amount of x-rays one can safely receive is determined by the radiologist. He will safeguard your welfare at all times.

Does one get an overdose of x-rays from the usual methods of examination?

No.

Is it safe for a child to be fitted for shoes by a fluoroscopic machine?

No. This is not advisable, as it may result in unnecessary exposure. Furthermore, there is no advantage to this method.

What are "contrast media"?

These are substances used to outline an organ or area in the body which has not sufficient density difference to be visualized by x-rays alone. One of the most frequently used contrast media is barium. This will demonstrate the outline of the entire gastro-intestinal tract.

Is it safe if repeated x-rays of the spine are taken?

No. When such x-rays are taken, there is a great deal of radiation directed toward the reproductive organs. The effect of this is cumulative and can be harmful if repeated too often.

What effect can an overdose of x-rays have upon the reproductive organs?

a. If given in very large doses directly over the female organs, radiation can cause a stoppage of menstruation. This effect may be temporary or permanent, and may cause sterility.
b. Small doses given repeatedly are thought to have an effect upon the eggs within the ovaries. Some investigators feel that this may lead to deformities in future offspring, even unto the second or third unborn generation.
c. An overdose in the region of the testicles may also cause sterility.

If a small metal pin has been swallowed, will it show up in the x-ray?

Yes. Any metallic foreign body will be visible by x-ray examination.

Can a piece of glass which has entered the body be seen on an x-ray film?

Yes, if the glass has sufficient opacity. A very tiny piece which has the same density as the surrounding tissues may not be visible.

Can wood which has entered the body be seen on an x-ray film?

Only if it has a greater density than the surrounding tissues. Small slivers and splinters usually cannot be seen.

Can air or other gases in various parts of the body be seen in the x-rays?

Yes, because they contrast with the denser surrounding tissues.

Can an entire section of the body be x-rayed at one time?

Yes. There is a special method of doing "body section" radiography with special x-ray equipment.

What special x-rays are employed to demonstrate the brain?

There is a special examination called pneumoencephalography. Fluid is removed from the spaces in and around the brain by performing a spinal tap. This fluid is replaced with air so that contrast will occur and thus demonstrate a tumor or other abnormality within the brain or the space around it. Angiography, injection of a contrast medium into the blood vessels, is also used.

Do x-rays often suggest the presence of a brain tumor?

Yes. Occasionally, direct studies will reveal evidence of a tumor. More often, the type of study mentioned above must be carried out.

Will a small foreign body in a bronchial tube show up on x-ray?

If the foreign body is opaque, it will be seen directly. If not, its presence may be suspected by changes in the normal x-ray appearance of the lungs.

What is a bronchogram?

It is a technique of visualizing the bronchial tubes by instilling an iodized oil into the trachea (windpipe). This oil is opaque to the x-rays and will therefore outline the tubes on film.

Are repeated routine chest x-rays safe to perform?

Yes. The amount of radiation received is very small and the amount of scattered radiation reaching the reproductive organs is negligible. However, the amount of radiation must be controlled by the radiologist.

Can an x-ray of the chest reveal tuberculosis even when there are no symptoms?

Yes. Therefore, it is advisable for everyone to have a periodic chest x-ray examination.

Can a chest x-ray show cancer of the lung?

It often will reveal the presence of a lung tumor long before there are any symptoms.

Can an x-ray determine the size of the heart?

Yes. It will show the size, contour, and position of the heart.

What is a kymogram?

It is an x-ray recording of the heart movements and is done with a special machine known as a kymograph.

Can the inside of the heart be seen by x-ray examination?

Yes, through angiocardiography. This is carried out by instilling an opaque substance into the chambers of the heart by injection. The injection is made not by putting a needle into the heart but by feeding a long tube from a vessel in the arm into the heart.

Can a deformity of the heart be seen on x-rays?

Some defects can be revealed by direct studies. Other defects can be demonstrated by angiocardiography, through the injection of an x-ray opaque contrast medium.

Can arteries be seen on x-ray films?

If they are hardened (sclerosed), they may be visible because of the accompanying calcium deposits. Most normal vessels are not opaque to the x-rays but can be visualized by arteriograms. These are special x-rays obtained by injecting an opaque substance directly into the arterial system.

Can veins be seen on x-rays?

No, but they can be visualized by injecting a substance which is opaque.

Can lymphatic vessels be seen merely by taking an ordinary x-ray?

No, but they *can* be visualized after injection of opaque contrast media directly into the lymph channel.

Why must a patient take a barium mixture when the gastro-intestinal tract is being x-rayed?

Barium is used to outline the mucous membrane lining of the tract. Disease or abnormality will show up as a deformity or variation from the normal pattern.

Why must the patient fast before stomach x-rays are taken?

If food is in the stomach, it will distort the pattern which will be seen on the films when the opaque barium mixes with it.

Why is it necessary to take so many views of the stomach?

The stomach and rest of the intestinal tract are in constant motion. It is therefore essential to take many films from many angles in order to gain full knowledge of the contour and action of the stomach.

Can a hernia of the diaphragm involving the upper end of the stomach be diagnosed by x-ray?

Yes.

Why is it sometimes necessary to take a laxative or an enema prior to x-ray examination?

This is done to eliminate gas or solid materials which might obscure the view of the organ to be studied.

Is the gall bladder seen on ordinary direct x-ray examination?

Usually not, unless it has calcium deposits in its wall.

Are gallstones usually visualized on direct x-ray examination?

The majority of them do not appear on the ordinary x-ray film. However, those that contain calcium are visualized.

How are the gall bladder and gallstones visualized by x-ray?

By a special test known as cholecystography. This consists of giving a special dye in the form of tablets the night before the x-rays are to be taken. The dye appears in the gall bladder the next day, unless disease is present. If the gall bladder fails to visualize on the x-ray film, it is diseased. Sometimes, when the gall bladder is visualized by the dye, it will demonstrate the presence of stones, which will appear as negative shadows.

If the gall bladder fails to visualize on x-ray film after the dye has been given, does this always indicate the presence of disease?

Yes. In more than 95 per cent of cases this indicates a diseased organ.

What is a cholangiogram?

It is the test used to visualize the bile ducts. It can be done by injecting certain dyes into the bloodstream; or, if the test is performed while the surgeon is operating upon the gall bladder, the dye is injected directly into the patient's ducts.

Why is it important to visualize the bile ducts?

To determine whether the bile ducts contain any gallstones that must be removed. Also, to learn whether any abnormalities of the ducts is present.

Can the kidneys be visualized on x-ray examination?

Yes, as they have sufficient density from the surrounding tissues to be revealed upon direct study.

What is an intravenous urography?

It is a study of the urinary tract after an opaque dye has been injected intravenously. This dye is excreted by the kidneys and therefore will cause the entire urinary tract to be visualized; by this method the diagnosis of malfunction, abnormality, or disease can be made.

Can kidney stones be seen in x-ray studies?

The stones which are opaque to the x-rays will be seen upon direct study. Those which are not opaque can be demonstrated in the urinary tract through intravenous urography, after which they may be seen as negative shadows.

What is a cystogram?

It is an x-ray study of the bladder after an opaque substance has been instilled into it.

Can a breast tumor be seen by x-rays?

Yes, in some instances. The process is known as mammography.

Can the uterus and Fallopian tubes be seen by x-ray examination?

Yes. This is done by instilling an opaque substance into these organs through the cervix.

What will an x-ray show during pregnancy?

The stage of development of the embryo, its position and size. If multiple pregnancy exists, this too will be demonstrated. Also, x-rays are quite accurate in showing the measurements of the maternal pelvis.

How early will x-rays show the presence of a pregnancy?

In about two and one-half to three months.

What is a pelvimetry x-ray?

This procedure is done to determine the measurements of the fetal head and maternal pelvis so as to ascertain whether a normal delivery will be possible. It may also demonstrate the need for a Cesarean section.

Will an x-ray show a fracture of any bone?

Yes, but it may require several different views or positions of the bone to reveal the fracture site. Such x-rays will also show the position of the fractured fragments of the bone.

Will an x-ray be able to demonstrate the presence of muscle sprains, ligament injuries, or torn cartilages?

Not muscle sprains. Ligament injuries and torn cartilages may be determined by x-ray with the aid of contrast media, such as air or opaque dye.

What is arthrography?

It is the visualization of a joint space by x-ray after the injection of a contrast medium into it.

Will a bone infection be seen on x-ray examination?

Not in the early stage of its development. However, it will be revealed when the bone cells show some destruction.

Will x-rays show a bone tumor?

Yes.

Why is it usually advisable to x-ray the opposite extremity after an injury?

To be certain that what appears to be an abnormality is not a normal deviation, such as an accessory bone.

What is myelography?

It is the x-ray examination of the spinal canal by means of introducing an opaque substance into the canal via spinal puncture. This will often demonstrate the presence or absence of a slipped disc or spinal cord tumor.

Can congenital heart defects be seen by x-ray examination?

Yes, after the injection of a contrast medium into the heart through the blood vessels. This is known as angiocardiography.

RADIATION THERAPY

(X-ray Therapy)

What is radiation therapy?

It is the treatment of diseases or tumors by the use of x-ray, radium, or radioactive substances.

What types of radiation therapy are used today?

X-rays, high energy electron beams, cobalt, radium, cesium, iridium, radioactive iodine, radioactive gold, radioactive phosphorus, etc.

Are newer types of radiation being discovered through development of atomic energy?

Yes. We can look forward to many new and beneficial types of radioactive substances and techniques of administration.

What are the most common forms of radiation therapy used?

X-rays of various voltages, radium and cobalt.

What is a kilovolt?

It is a thousand volts.

What does "Mev" mean?

It means a million electron volts, and usually is used to refer to multi-million volt x-ray apparatus.

What is an "r"?

It is a roentgen, which is a unit used in measuring ionizing radiation dosage.

What is a "rad"?

It is a unit of absorbed radiation dosage.

Why must so many treatments be taken in radiation therapy?

When a lesion is being treated, the amount of rays needed to affect the lesion must be divided into a number of smaller doses, so as not to damage the normal tissues surrounding the lesion.

Does radiation therapy cure?

Many conditions are completely cured by radiation therapy. In other cases, where the condition is beyond the stage of permanent cure, radiotherapy will often relieve the condition and extend life for many months or years. Pain and suffering are often relieved by the judicious use of radiation therapy.

Are there any hazards from exposure to the rays during radiation therapy?

There are some, but they are negligible when treatment is for conditions less serious than malignancies. In malignancies, the risk is minimized since the radiation is given under the care of a radiologist or radiation therapist.

Is radiation safe for the patient?

The radiologist or radiation therapist is an experienced and trained specialist, and under his care the patient is safe.

Is the effect of x-ray treatments in children the same as in adults?

No. The younger the child, the greater is the possible harmful effect from radiation. Such therapy should be used only when necessary and upon the explicit advice of the radiologist.

Is radiation therapy used for malignant conditions only?

No; it is of value and is used for many non-malignant diseases or lesions.

Does the patient feel any pain or discomfort while undergoing radiation therapy?

No. There is no sensation from the rays at the time of treatment.

Why does the skin get red after a period of radiation treatments?

Because the skin reacts to the rays in a manner similar to the way it reacts to the sun. The reaction in some people is greater than in others. The reaction will subside after the therapy is finished.

Does radiation therapy cause the hair in the area being treated to fall out?

If a large amount of therapy is given, the hair will fall out. In many cases, the hair will grow back.

What is radiation sickness?

Some patients develop nausea, weakness, loss of appetite, and possibly vomiting after a series of treatments. This is called radiation sickness. It is controlled readily by appropriate medication and, if necessary, by adjusting therapy radiation dosages and frequency.

How long does radiation sickness usually last after therapy has been discontinued?

Usually not longer than several days.

Does radiation therapy destroy the normal cells around the diseased cells?

The diseased cells are more sensitive to the rays than the normal cells and the therapy is so given as to destroy only the diseased cells. Normal cells recover from the temporary damaging effect of radiation.

Can radiation therapy shrink a large thyroid gland which causes pressure in the neck?

It may diminish the size of the gland to some degree, but treatment by other medical or by surgical means is preferable.

Is x-ray therapy helpful for an enlarged thymus gland in an infant?

Yes. However, it should be used only when other methods, medical or surgical, fail.

Can x-ray therapy help inflammation of the breasts which sometimes follows childbirth?

Yes.

Can fibroids of the uterus be treated successfully by radiation therapy?

Surgery is the best method of treatment in such cases.

Can a cyst within the abdomen be treated effectively with x-ray therapy?

No. The cyst should be removed surgically.

Can x-ray therapy remove warts?

Some can be treated adequately by means of x-ray; others will require surgical removal. Nonirradiation methods are preferable.

Can x-ray therapy reduce the size of a keloid (an overgrown scar)?

Yes, in many instances. However, if treatment is to be effective, it must begin soon after the appearance of the keloid.

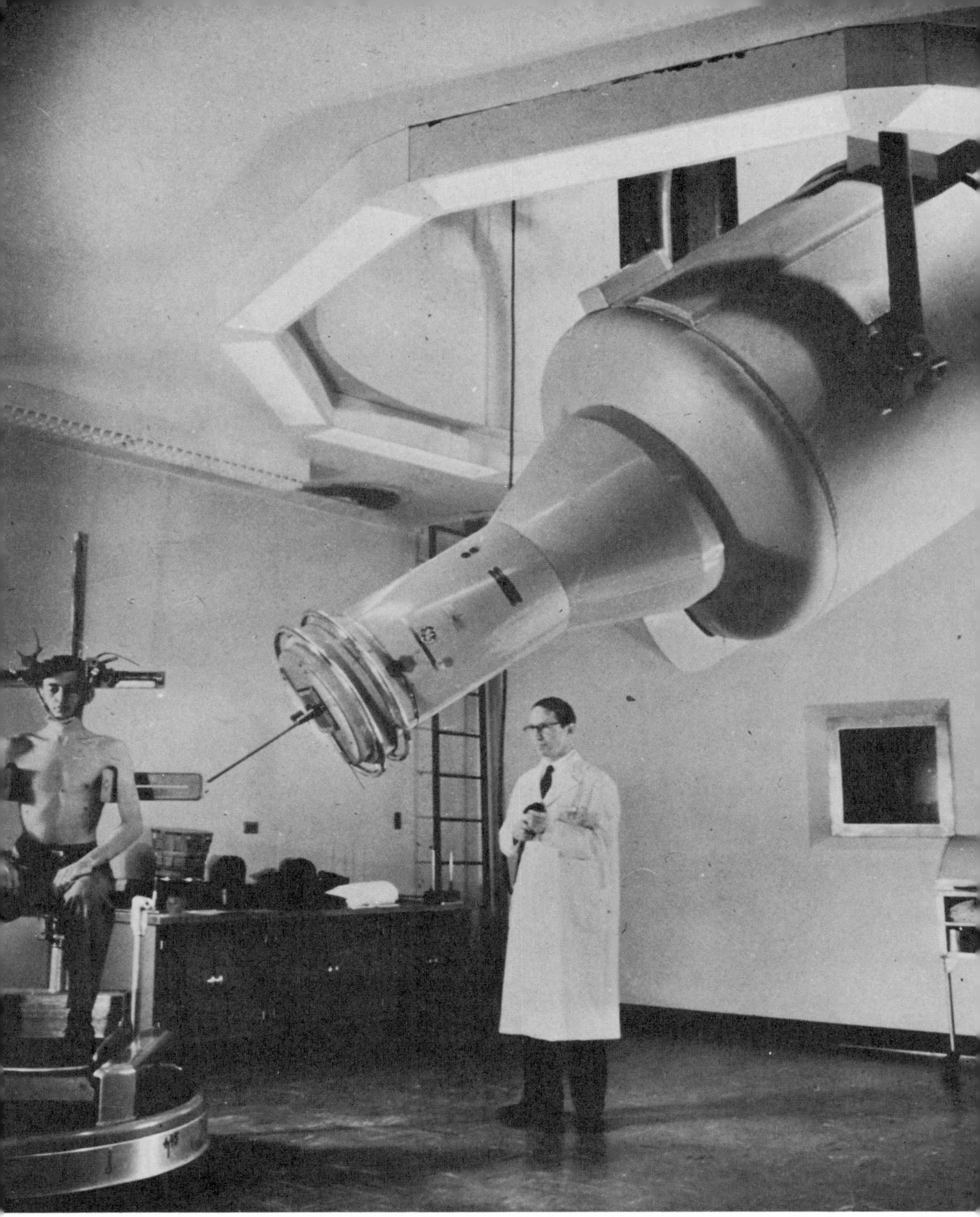

Rotation Radiation. This method of treating deep-seated cancer combines the application of multi-million-volt x-rays with a rotational system of therapy. As the chair rotates, the cancer gets the maximum x-ray dosage while the surrounding tissues receive a fraction of the radiation.

Will radiation therapy remove a "strawberry" birthmark?

Radium is the form of radiation therapy used. However, other non-radiation methods are effective and should be used.

Is there danger in the use of radium to remove a birthmark?

There is no danger when a competent specialist is in attendance. However, if the birthmark is near a gland, as for instance on the neck, irradiation is not advisable.

Can x-ray therapy aid the patient with acne?

In certain carefully selected cases, it is beneficial.

Will x-ray therapy clear the pockmarks in acne?

No. These marks are scars resulting from the acne and are best treated by other methods.

Can x-ray therapy relieve obstruction of the Eustachian tubes which extend from the inside of the throat to the ears?

If such obstruction is caused by enlarged lymphoid tissue, x-ray or radium therapy often shrinks such tissue and relieves the obstruction of the ears. However, surgery would be more advisable than irradiation for children.

Is x-ray therapy used to treat arthritis?

Radiation therapy has proved valuable for some types of arthritis by reducing inflammation and relieving pain.

Is x-ray therapy of value for the treatment of bursitis?

Yes, in certain cases. It will reduce the inflammation and relieve the pain.

Can x-rays affect the reproductive system so that birth deformities may be more likely to occur in one's children or grandchildren?

Yes. This is a distinct possibility in a small number of cases when excessive doses of x-ray are given. The chances of such an eventuality are minimal when x-rays are controlled by competent radiologists.

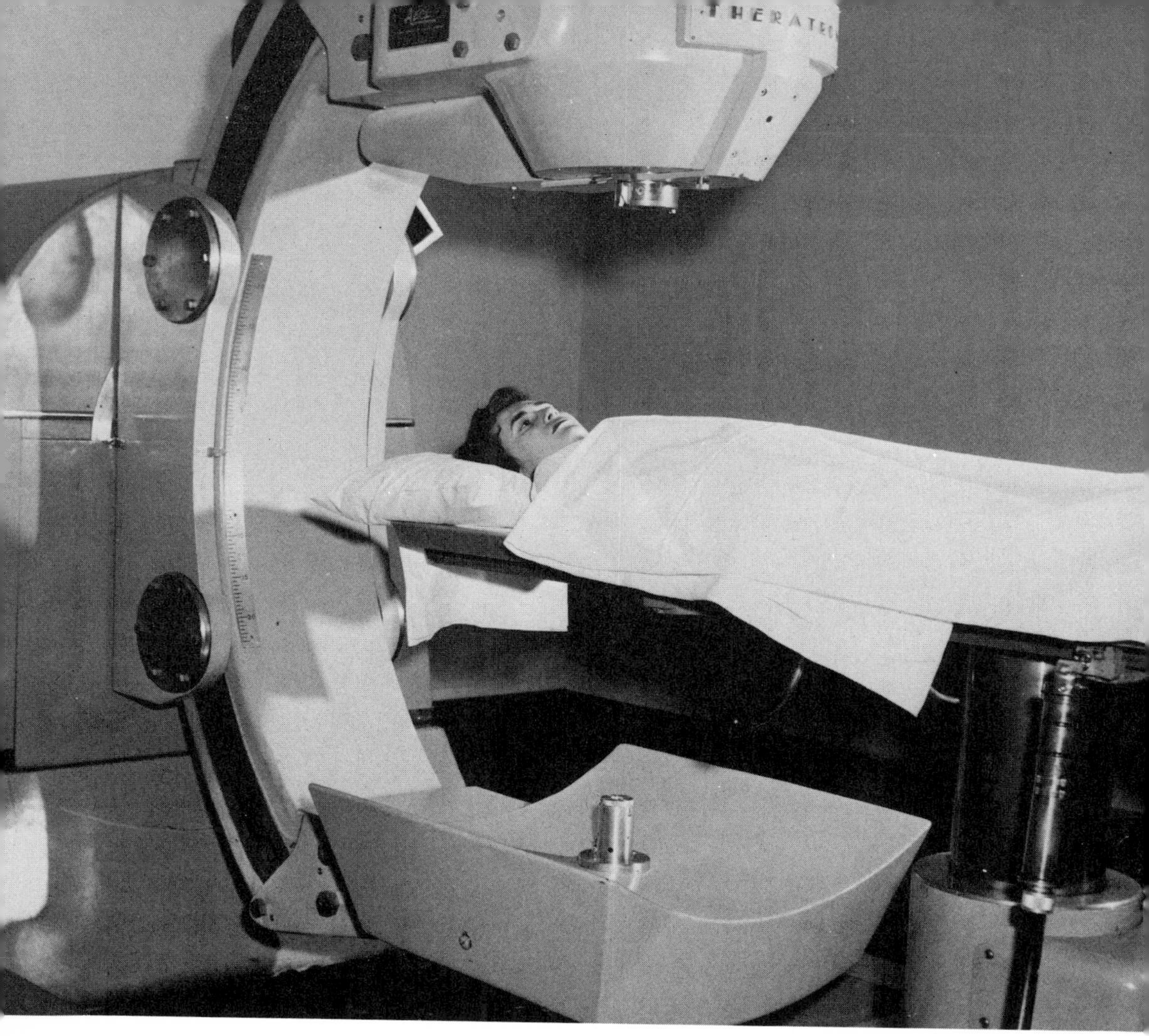

Cobalt Irradiator. This C-shaped machine rotates completely around the patient as it emits pinpoint radiation equivalent to that of a three-million-volt x-ray machine.

How is radium applied?

It is placed in tubes, needles, flat applicators (plaques), and is used as a gas which is sealed in hollow gold containers ("seeds").

What is radon?

It is a gas given off by radium when it breaks down. This gas is usually encapsuled in small gold "seeds," which are then implanted in tumors so as to produce maximal radiation effect locally.

Is the effect of atomic fallout upon the human body similar to that of x-rays or radium?

Yes.

What are isotopes?

These are substances which had been made radioactive in atomic piles and are used as tracer chemicals or for radiation therapy.

How many radioactive isotopes are in existence today?

There are more than nine hundred known isotopes.

Are radioactive isotopes dangerous to handle?

Yes, very much so, and many precautions are taken to safeguard all personnel involved in the production, transportation, and use of all radioactive materials.

What is meant by "tagging" with an isotope?

Combining a substance such as a food or drug with a radioactive product so that the isotope can then be traced in the body with a radiation-detection apparatus.

Do isotopes lose their power in time?

Yes. Some are radioactive for a period of hours and others for days, months, or years. The half-life period for some of the radioactive isotopes used in radiation therapy is as follows: gold, 64.6 hours; iodine, 8.1 days; iridium, 2.48 months; cobalt, 5.3 years.

Are radioactive isotopes used in industry?

Yes. They are used for purposes of tracing and testing. They are used in agriculture to produce better plant types.

Which are the more commonly used isotopes?

Iodine 131, cobalt 60, gold 198, iron 59, phosphorus 32, cesium 137, and strontium 90.

What is Cobalt 60?

It is chemical cobalt which has been made radioactive in an atomic pile; it gives off gamma rays similar to those from radium.

What are the uses of the iodine isotope?

Iodine 131 has an affinity for the thyroid gland and is used as a tracer. In cases of overactivity of the thyroid, it will sometimes suppress its secretion and return the gland to a less active state. It is also used in certain cases of thyroid cancer, and has been known to effect an occasional cure.

What are the uses of phosphorous isotopes?

Phosphorus 32 is used as a tracer in much the same manner as other radioactive drugs. It has also proven effective in the treatment of certain blood diseases, such as leukemia and polycythemia.

What is photoscanning?

It is the radiation scanning from the isotope tracer used for the particular gland or organ in which this isotope will settle. It will reveal either a normal outline or an abnormality.

How is this done?

By means of a scintillation counter apparatus which is affected by the local radiation coming from the isotope contained in the gland or organ.

Definitions of Medical Terms

A

abdominal cavity That portion of the body extending from beneath the diaphragm down to the pelvis. It contains all of the abdominal organs.

abducens The sixth cranial nerve, which controls outward rotation of the eyeball.

aberration Any deviation from normal.

abnormal Not conforming to standard.

ABO incompatibility A rare type of blood incompatibility.

abortion A miscarriage. The spontaneous or induced passage of a non-living embryo during the early stages of development.

abrasion A scratch or scrape.

abruptio placenta Premature separation of the placenta from the wall of the uterus, occurring during the latter part of pregnancy.

abscess A localized collection of pus in the skin or in any organ.

a.c. On a prescription, means "before meals."

accommodation Adjustment of the eye, as to dark or light.

acetabulum The hip socket.

acetone A chemical found in patients with diabetic acidosis.

achalasia Constriction of the lower end of the esophagus due to inability of the muscles to relax.

Achilles tendon The heel tendon.

achlorhydria Absence of hydrochloric acid in the stomach.

Achromycin An antibiotic drug.

acidosis Intoxication caused by faulty metabolism and inability to eliminate excess acids from the body.

acne A pustular skin condition seen on the face, chest, and back in adolescence.

acoustic nerve The eighth cranial nerve, which supplies the ear.

acquired characteristic A trait developed rather than inherited.

acromegaly A bone-distortion disease resulting from overactivity of the pituitary gland.

acromion The bone at the tip of the shoulder.

ACTH A hormone (adrenocorticotropic) produced by the pituitary gland.

acute Rapid; sudden; severe. The opposite of chronic.

adaptation disease Any disease associated with stress.

addict One who is dependent on a drug.

Addison's disease A serious disease associated with malfunction of the adrenal glands.

adenitis Inflammation of a lymph gland or node.

adenocarcinoma Cancer originating in a gland.

adenoid Lymph tissue located in the throat behind the nose.

adenoidectomy Removal of the adenoids.

adenoma A tumor in which the cell arrangement appears glandlike.

adenopathy Swelling or disease in a lymph gland.

adhesion A fiber or band, often seen following inflammation in the abdominal cavity.

adipose tissue Fat tissue.

adolescence The period between puberty and maturity.

adrenal glands Two hormone-producing glands in the upper part of the abdomen above the kidneys.

adrenalin (epinephrine) One of the hormones secreted by the adrenal glands.

Aëdes aegypti The mosquito that transmits dengue fever and yellow fever.

afebrile Without elevation of temperature above normal.

afferent Going toward the center, as an afferent nerve.

afterbirth The placenta and membranes that connect a newborn child to the mother's womb.

agammaglobulinemia A condition in which less than a normal amount of antibodies circulate in the blood.
agent A substance causing a reaction.
agglutination The joining together of separate particles; often refers to the clotting of blood.
aggression A hostile attitude or hostile action.
agranulocytosis An acute dangerous condition in which there are too few white blood cells in the blood.
ague Malaria.
air embolus Air getting into the bloodstream and interfering with the flow of blood.
albinism Lack of pigment in the skin, as occurs in albinos. An inherited condition.
albumin One of the main protein components of all living animal tissue.
albuminuria Albumin in the urine.
alcoholism Poisoning by alcohol. The results of the excessive and prolonged drinking of alcohol or alcoholic beverages.
alimentary tract The food track, beginning with the esophagus (food pipe) and extending for 20 to 25 feet to the rectum and anus.
alkaline The opposite of acid.
alkalosis Too much bicarbonate in the blood; the opposite of acidosis.
alkaptonuria An inherited and metabolic disturbance seen in children.
allergen Any substance that causes an allergic condition.
allergic rhinitis Inflammation of the nasal passages due to an allergy.
allergist A physician who treats allergies.
allergy An altered response to an allergen; also, hypersensitivity to irritating substances.
alopecia A skin condition characterized by patchy or total loss of hair.
Alternaria A mold that causes a form of hay fever.
altitude sickness Dizziness and shortness of breath, or fatigability caused either by a flight to a high altitude or by travel in high altitudes.
alveolus The bony socket of a tooth; also, an air cell in the lungs.
amaurosis Blindness.
amaurotic familial idiocy An inherited disease characterized by mental deterioration, blindness, and death by the age of two years.
ambidextrous Able to use both hands equally well.
ambisexual Feelings and reactions which are neither typically male nor female, but which have traits of both sexes.
ambivalent Feeling both love and hate for the same person or thing.
amblyopia Diminished sight.
ambulation, early Getting out of bed soon after a surgical operation or illness.
ambulatory Not bedridden.
ameba A one-celled organism, some species of which cause dysentery.
amebiasis Infection with the *Endamoeba histolytica.*
amebic dysentery A diarrheal disease caused by a specific ameba germ (*Endamoeba histolytica*).
amelioration Improvement in the course of a disease.
amenorrhea Failure of menstruation.
amino acids A large group of organic compounds, many of which are essential to life. They represent the end product of protein metabolism.
aminuria Ammonialike chemicals in the urine.
amnesia Loss of memory.
amnion The membranous sac surrounding the embryo in the womb.
amniotic fluid The fluid surrounding the embryo in the womb.
amorphous Without shape or structure.
amputation The surgical removal of a part of the body.
amylase An enzyme that acts in the digestion of sugar.
amyloid degeneration The deposit of amyloid in tissues and organs that are degenerating.
amyotonia Absence of muscle tone.
anacidity Total lack of hydrochloric acid in the stomach.
anaerobe A germ which can grow and multiply in absence of air or oxygen.
anal Pertaining to the anus.
analgesic drugs Pain-relieving medications such as aspirin.
anaphylaxis A state of shock caused by an extreme allergy or sensitivity.
anastomosis The joining together of two or more hollow organs.
androgen The male sex hormone.
anemia Insufficiency of red blood cells, either in quality or in quantity.
anesthesia Loss of sensation, usually produced in order to permit surgery without pain.
anesthesiologist A physician who specializes in the administration of anesthesia.
aneurysm An abnormal dilatation of a portion of the wall of an artery.
angina pectoris Pain in the chest, sometimes radiating to the left arm, caused by a spasm of the coronary artery of the heart.
angiocardiography X-ray visualization of the chambers of the heart and the large blood vessels that enter or leave the heart.
angioma A benign tumor composed of lymph and blood vessels.
angioneurotic edema Localized swellings, commonly about the face, caused by emotional factors or allergy.
ankle The joint connecting the leg and the foot.
ankylosis Fusion of a joint so that it cannot move.
anomaly A deviation from the normal, such as a birth defect.
Anopheles The mosquito that transmits malaria and sometimes other diseases.
anorectal Pertaining to the anus and rectum.
anorexia Lack of appetite.
anoscope An instrument used

for the internal examination of the anus and rectum.
anoxemia Lack of sufficient oxygen in the blood.
anoxia Inadequate oxygen supply.
antacid A medication used to relieve excess acidity.
antepartum Before childbirth.
anterior Located in the front; the opposite of posterior.
anterior pituitary gland The portion of the pituitary that produces ACTH and the growth hormones.
anthrax A serious infection in sheep or cattle which is sometimes transmitted to humans.
anthropology The science of man.
antiallergics The antihistaminic drugs.
antibacterial Preventing the growth and multiplication of bacteria.
antibiotic drugs Those drugs composed of extracts of living organisms, such as molds, that have the ability to destroy or stop the growth of bacteria.
antibody A substance produced in the blood that is capable of producing a specific immunity to a specific bacteria or virus.
anticoagulant A substance that prevents blood clotting.
antidote A substance given to counteract a poison.
antigen Any substance that stimulates the formation of an antibody.
antihistamine A medication that tends to counteract an allergic condition.
antipruritic A medication given to relieve itching.
antipyretic A drug that tends to lower body temperature.
antiseptic An agent that inhibits or destroys bacteria.
antispasmodic A medication used to relieve or prevent spasm.
antitoxin A substance that neutralizes the effects of a poison released by bacteria.
antivenin An antidote to snake poison.
antrum A bony cavity that forms the sinus in the cheek.
anuria Lack of urination due to kidney failure.
anus The outlet of the gastrointestinal tract.
aorta The large artery that originates from the left ventricle of the heart.
aortography A technique that outlines the aorta on x-ray films.
aperture An opening.
Apgar test A test performed on newborns to give some indication of the state of the child immediately at birth.
aphthous stomatitis Sore throat and mouth associated with many small white blisters and ulcerations.
aplasia Failure of an organ or part to develop.
apnea Temporary stoppage of breathing.
apoplexy Hemorrhage into the brain. A stroke.
appendectomy Surgical removal of the appendix.
appendix The small outpouching of the cecum (the first portion of the large bowel).
applicator A wooden stick with a cotton tip.
apposition A fitting together; the act of placing one thing next to another.
aqueous humor The fluid in the anterior chamber of the eye.
arrest The halting or checking of a disease process.
arrhythmia Lack of rhythm, applied mainly to irregularities of heartbeat.
arterial system The network of arteries which supplies blood to the various parts of the body.
arteriography X-ray visualization of arteries.
arteriosclerosis Hardening of the arteries.
artery A blood vessel that carries blood from the heart to the tissues.
arthritis Inflammation of a joint.
arthrography X-ray of a joint.
arthrotomy A surgical incision into a joint.
artificial insemination A procedure whereby a physician takes the live sperm of a husband, or donor, and places them, by syringe injection, at the entrance to the cervix of the uterus.
artificial respiration The process of restoring breathing in one who has ceased breathing.
Ascaris A worm that sometimes infests the intestinal tract.
Aschoff's bodies Cells seen in a child afflicted with heart disease caused by rheumatic fever.
ascites An accumulation of fluid in the abdominal cavity, seen in cirrhosis of the liver.
ascorbic acid Vitamin C.
asepsis A sterile state in which no bacteria are present.
Asiatic influenza Infection of the respiratory tract caused by a specific influenza virus.
asphyxia Suffocation.
aspiration Sucking up a fluid or solid into the respiratory tract (wind pipe or lungs).
aspirin Acetylsalicylic acid, an effective pain-relieving medication.
asthenia Weakness.
asthma An allergic condition of the respiratory tract accompanied by wheezing, coughing, and the collection of mucus sputum in the bronchial tubes.
astigmatism Irregularity in the curvature of the front portion of the eye.
astragulus The anklebone.
astringent A medication that contracts or constricts tissues.
astrocytoma A malignant brain tumor.
asylum An obsolete term for an institution caring for those unable to care for themselves.
asymmetry Lacking equal proportions in corresponding parts.
asymptomatic Without symptoms.
ataxia Lack of muscle coordination.
atelectasis A partially or fully collapsed condition of a lung or part of a lung.
atherosclerosis Hardening of the arteries; (the same as arteriosclerosis).
athetosis Purposeless motion of the limbs.

athlete's foot A fungus infection.
athlete's heart An out-of-date expression referring to a strained or overworked heart.
atom The smallest amount of an element that can exist alone.
atony Lack of tone, as in a muscle.
atopy Allergy.
atresia A failure of development of an opening in an organ.
atrial fibrillation Irregularity of the heartbeat, originating in an auricle of the heart.
atrium The upper chamber of the heart; the auricle.
atrophy The withering of an organ that has previously been normal.
atropine A medication that tends to dry up secretions, dilates the pupil of the eye, and relaxes spasms, especially in the intestinal tract.
atypical Not typical.
audiogram An instrument to test hearing.
aura A premonition, such as a warning that an epileptic seizure is about to take place.
auricle The external portion of the ear; also, an upper chamber of the heart.
auricular fibrillation Atrial fibrillation.
auscultation The detection of sounds by use of a stethoscope.
auto- Pertaining to oneself.
autoeroticism Self-stimulation or masturbation.
autogenous vaccine A vaccine manufactured from bacteria taken from the body of the patient.
autograft The graft of tissue from one part of a patient's body to another.
autoimmunization Immunity resulting from a substance developed within the patient's own body.
autointoxication A poisoning brought about by an upset in metabolism or by a substance produced within the patient's body. (An outmoded term.)
automatism An act not under voluntary control, such as sleepwalking.
autonomic imbalance Lack of normal function of the involuntary nervous system.
autonomic nervous system The portion of the nervous system over which there is no voluntary control.
autopsy Examination of the body after death.
avascular Bloodless.
avitaminosis A disease brought on by lack of vitamins.
avulsion Tearing away of a piece of tissue.
axilla The armpit.
axon The extension of a nerve cell.
A-Z test Pregnancy test, utilizing the urine of the pregnant woman.

B

bacillary dysentery A diarrheal disease caused by a specific bacillus.
bacilli Bacteria shaped in the form of rods.
bacteremia Bacteria circulating in the bloodstream.
bacteria Germs.
bacterial endocarditis An infection of the valves of the heart.
bactericide A substance that kills bacteria.
bacteriology The study of bacteria and germs in general.
Baker's cyst A cyst formation in the back of the knee.
balance A state of equilibrium, such as fluid balance.
balanitis An inflammation of the tip of the penis.
band An adhesion composed of fibrous tissue.
Banti's disease A disease characterized by enlargement of the liver and spleen, anemia, and a tendency to hemorrhage.
barbiturates A group of drugs that calm nerves and induce sleep.
barium An opaque substance that will show up on x-ray films. It is used to demonstrate the intestinal tract.
barium enema The giving of a fluid mixture containing barium through the rectum in order to outline the large bowel for x-ray.
barium meal The swallowing of a mixture of barium to outline the stomach and small intestines for x-ray.
Bartholin glands Two small glands located near the entrance to the vagina. They often become infected, especially in a patient with gonorrhea.
basal metabolic rate (BMR) The amount of energy expended when a person is at rest, measured by a special breathing test.
BCG A vaccine given to immunize against tuberculosis.
b.d. On a prescription, means "to be taken twice daily."
beading of the ribs A beadlike feel to the ribs encountered in rickets.
bedwetting Enuresis; involuntary urination during sleep.
Bell's palsy Paralysis of one side of the face due to inflammation of the facial nerve.
benign Not malignant.
benzoin A substance often used as an inhalant with steam in cases of croup or bronchitis.
beriberi A vitamin-deficiency disease caused by lack of thiamine (vitamin B_1).
bezoar A ball of hair, sometimes found in the stomach as a result of pulling out and eating one's own hair.
bicarbonate The alkali reserve in the blood.
biceps The strong muscle in the front of the upper arm that flexes the forearm.
bicuspid Teeth containing two cusps (points).
b.i.d. On a prescription, means "take twice daily."
bilateral Pertaining to both sides.
bile The yellow liquid secreted by the liver into the intestinal tract. It aids in the digestion of fats.
bile acid An acid formed from bile in the liver.
bilirubin A bile pigment.
biliuria Bile in the urine, seen in patients with jaundice.
bimanual An examination carried out with two hands.

biochemistry The chemistry of living tissue.
biopsy The surgical removal of tissue in order to determine the exact diagnosis.
biparous Giving birth to twins.
bisexual Having male and female sex organs.
bismuth A chemical often used in stomach and intestinal upsets.
blackhead A plugged oil gland in the skin.
blackout Loss of consciousness.
blackwater fever Malaria.
black widow spider A female black spider that has an hourglass-shaped red area on its abdomen and is poisonous.
bladder An organ that acts as a container of fluid, such as the gall bladder or urinary bladder.
blastomycosis A disease caused by a yeast-like organism.
bleb A blister.
bleeder One who bleeds excessively even after a trivial injury, as a hemophiliac.
blepharitis An inflammation of the eyelids.
blepharospasm Uncontrollable winking of the eyelids.
blister A collection of blood or serum beneath the superficial layers of the skin.
blood The liquid that travels throughout the body in the veins, arteries, and capillaries, bringing nutrients and oxygen to all cells and removing carbon dioxide and waste products from them.
blood bank A laboratory which collects donor blood and holds it available for immediate transfusion.
blood coagulation Blood clotting.
blood compatibility The ability of a donor's blood to mix with a recipient's blood without clotting.
blood count A microscopic test to determine the number of red and white blood cells in the circulation.
blood culture The placing of a sample of blood in a culture medium in order to permit the growth of bacteria that might be circulating in the bloodstream.
blood group Blood falls into four distinct groups: A, B, AB, and O. If some of these groups are mixed, clotting and destruction of red cells will ensue.
blood pressure The force exerted by the heart in pumping blood from its chambers.
blood type A microscopic test to determine a subject's blood group.
blood vessels The channels through which blood flows; arteries, capillaries, and veins.
blood volume The quantity of blood circulating through the blood vessels.
blue baby Baby born with defects of the heart or major blood vessels.
BMR *See* basal metabolic rate.
Boeck's sarcoid *See* sarcoidosis.
boil An abscess of the skin and subcutaneous tissue.
bolus A lump of food.
bone Skeletal tissue; the framework of the body.
bone marrow The soft tissue inside the long bones that forms blood cells.
booster shot An additional vaccination or inoculation given after the original injection.
boric acid A mildly antiseptic acid used in compresses or ointments.
botulism An often fatal form of food poisoning caused by a specific bacterium.
bowel The intestine.
bowlegs Outward curving of the legs, usually caused by rickets.
BP Blood pressure.
brachial plexus The group of nerves in the base of the neck and armpit that supply the arm and shoulder region.
brain The origin of the central nervous system; the part that occupies the inside of the skull.
branchial Referring to the gills that are present during early embryonic development.
branchial cyst A deformity in which the gill slits fail to close off completely.
breast The mammary gland.
breastbone The bone in front of the chest to which the ribs are attached; the sternum.
breech delivery The birth of a child feet first.
bregma The spot on the skull where the two frontal bones fuse with the parietal bones.
Bright's disease Chronic nephritis; kidney inflammation.
Brill's disease Typhus fever.
bromhidrosis Body odor.
bromides Drugs used to calm excess emotional disturbance.
bronchial Relating to the bronchial tubes.
bronchiectasis Dilation of the small bronchial tubes associated with chronic inflammation and infection within the lungs.
bronchioles The small bronchial tubes in the lungs.
bronchitis Inflammation of the bronchial tubes.
bronchogram X-ray of the bronchial tubes.
bronchopneumonia Inflammation of the bronchial tubes and the lungs. A common form of pneumonia.
bronchoscopy The passage of a bronchoscope into the bronchial tubes.
bronchospasm Spasm and constriction of the bronchial tubes.
bronchus A bronchial tube.
brucellosis Malta fever, a disease caused by a germ transmitted by goats, cattle, and hogs.
bruit A murmur or sound heard when a stethoscope is placed over the heart or over an artery.
buccal Referring to the mucous membrane lining the inside of the cheek.
Buerger's disease A chronic inflammatory disease of the arteries and veins of the lower extremities. (Thromboangiitis obliterans.)
buffer A substance that preserves the balance of acidity and alkalinity in a solution.
bulbar poliomyelitis That type of infantile paralysis affecting the base of the brain and

usually associated with paralysis of the breathing muscles.

bulla A large blister.

BUN Blood urea nitrogen, a test of the adequacy of kidney function.

burn First-degree involves only the superficial layers of the skin, as in sunburn. Second-degree involves all but the deepest layer of the skin. Third-degree involves all layers of the skin and possibly tissues beneath the skin.

bursa A small soft-tissue sac located between parts that move against each other.

bursitis Inflammation of a bursa.

buttock That portion of the body behind the hips upon which one sits.

C

cachexia An emaciated state.

cadaver A dead body.

caked breasts Breasts hardened and swollen with milk.

calamine lotion A medication used locally to treat some skin conditions.

calcaneus The heelbone.

calcemia Excessive calcium in the blood.

calcification The deposit of calcium in tissues of the body.

calcium A chemical normally found in the body's tissues, especially in bones, teeth, and in blood plasma.

calculus A stone, such as a kidney or gall-bladder stone.

callus New bone that develops at the site of a fracture; also, markedly thickened skin.

calorie A unit of heat.

cancer A malignant tumor of any type.

cancer smears Cells obtained by swabbing tissues which might contain extruded cancer cells. Such cells are smeared on a glass slide and examined under a microscope.

canine teeth The sharp teeth located just in front of the premolars.

canker sore An ulceration of the tongue or gums.

canthus The angles formed by the eyelids.

capillaries Very small blood vessels from which oxygenated blood and nourishment go directly to the tissues of the body.

capsule A sheath or covering.

carbohydrate Sugar or starch.

carbuncle A large abscess that discharges pus from several openings.

carcinogen A substance that stimulates the formation of cancer.

carcinoma Cancer.

cardia The upper end of the stomach where it joins the esophagus.

cardiac Relating to the heart.

cardiac arrest Stoppage of the heart during an operation.

cardiac failure A condition caused by inadequate heart function.

cardiac massage An emergency measure to start a heart that has stopped.

cardiogram A recording of the heart's pulsations.

cardiologist A physician who specializes in diseases of the heart.

cardiopulmonary Referring to the heart and lungs.

cardiovascular Referring to the heart and blood vessels.

carditis Inflammation of the heart.

caries Cavities in the teeth.

carotid arteries The large arteries on either side of the neck that supply blood to the head.

carpal Referring to the wrist or one of its bones.

carrier A healthy person who harbors or carries germs that can infect and cause disease in others.

cartilage The elastic semihard tissue covering the surfaces of some bones and joints.

cascara A laxative.

casein The protein found in large quantities in milk.

cast 1. A term used for crossed eyes (strabismus). 2. A plaster cast; a mixture of gypsum and water used to immobilize fractures. 3. Renal casts; abnormal forms in the urine that denote kidney disease.

castor oil A powerful laxative.

castration Removal of the testicles.

catalepsy A mentally disturbed state characterized by trance-like immobility.

catalyst An agent that hastens and stimulates a chemical reaction.

cataract An opacity of the lens of the eye.

catarrh Irritation of a membrane, especially of the respiratory tract, associated with the production of large quantities of mucus.

catgut A suture material used in surgery. Actually made from sheep intestines.

cathartic A laxative.

catheter A rubber, glass, or plastic tube inserted into the bladder in order to withdraw urine; also, a plastic tube passed into any structure for the purpose of injecting or withdrawing a fluid.

catheterization Withdrawal of fluid through a catheter.

caudal Toward the tail; downward.

cauterization Burning by application of a caustic, heat, or electric current.

cavity A hollow in an organ.

cc. Cubic centimeter (equals approximately 15 drops of a fluid from an eyedropper).

cecum The beginning of the large bowel.

celiac Referring to the abdomen.

celiac disease A disease of early infancy associated with intestinal difficulties, anemia, malfunction of the pancreas, and retarded growth.

celiotomy Any operation in which the abdominal cavity is opened.

cell The unit of protoplasm containing a nucleus and cytoplasm.

cellulitis Inflammation of connective tissues, usually tissues just beneath the skin.

centigrade scale A temperature scale. Water boils at 100°C. and freezes at 0°C.;

normal body temperature is 37°C.

centimeter Approximately two-fifths of an inch.

central nervous system The brain and spinal cord and the nerves originating from them.

cephalic Relating to the head.

cerebellum The lower part of the brain, located beneath the cerebrum.

cerebral Referring to the cerebrum.

cerebral palsy *See* palsy.

cerebrospinal fluid The fluid surrounding the brain and spinal cord.

cerebrovascular accident Apoplexy; a stroke.

cerebrum The higher brain cells; the chief portion of the brain controlling conscious thought and action.

certifiable disease A contagious disease that must be reported to the local board of health.

cerumen Wax in the ear canal.

cervical region The neck.

cervix The entrance and lower portion of the uterus (womb).

Cesarean section Delivery of a child surgically through an abdominal incision.

chafing Irritation.

Chagas' disease A parasitic disease found in South America.

chalazion An inflamed cyst of an eyelid.

chancre The primary sore of syphilis.

change of life Menopause. The time of life when a woman's menstrual periods cease.

chapped Roughened, cracked.

charley horse A muscle strain associated with hemorrhage and tearing of muscle fibers.

cheilosis Splitting of the skin at the corners of the mouth, usually due to vitamin-B_2 deficiency.

chemotherapy Treatment of an infection with the use of chemicals.

chicken-breasted Having a pointed breastbone.

chickenpox A highly contagious virus disease characterized by pocklike eruptions on the body.

chigger A mite that bites and burrows beneath the skin and causes severe itching.

chilblain Swelling and congestion of the skin caused by exposure to cold.

chloral hydrate A medication often used to combat convulsions in children.

chlorination Disinfecting by the addition of chlorine.

Chloromycetin A powerful and effective antibiotic drug.

chlorosis A type of anemia seen most frequently in young girls.

Chlortrimeton A patented antihistaminic drug used against allergies.

cholangiogram An x-ray taken following the administration of a dye to visualize the bile ducts.

cholangitis Inflammation of the bile ducts.

cholecystitis Inflammation of the gall bladder.

cholecystography X-raying the gall bladder after the administration of a dye.

cholecystostomy A surgical operation that makes an opening into the gall bladder in order to drain its contents.

choledochitis Inflammation of the common bile duct.

choledochotomy An operation that makes an opening into the common bile duct, usually performed to remove stones.

cholelithiasis Stones in the gall bladder.

cholemia Bile in the blood, usually secondary to failure of the liver to get rid of its bile and bile products.

cholera A serious infectious disease associated with vomiting, diarrhea, and dehydration.

cholesterol A normal chemical component of animal oils and fats.

chologogue A drug that stimulates increased bile flow.

choluria Bile in the urine.

chondral Relating to cartilage.

chondritis Inflammation of cartilage.

chondrocostal Referring to the junction of the ribs and the cartilage.

chondroma A benign tumor of cartilage.

chordae tendinae Strands of tissue attached to the muscles of the ventricles in the heart and extending to the valves between the atria and ventricles.

chordee Curvature of the penis.

chorditis Inflammation of the spermatic cord.

chordoma A very rare tumor located at the base of the spine.

chorea St. Vitus' dance. A nervous disease characterized by purposeless, involuntary movements of the muscles of the limbs and face.

chorion A membrane surrounding the embryo within the womb.

choroid A membrane of the eyeball containing blood vessels.

choroid plexus A group of small blood vessels and covering membranes that project into the fluid-filled spaces within the brain.

choroiditis Inflammation of the membrane within the eyeball.

Christian-Schüller disease A rare disease of infants in which there are abnormal deposits of fatty substances and eventually softening of the skull and other bones.

Christmas disease A hereditary disease having many of the characteristics of hemophilia.

chromaffin Cells of the adrenal and other glands that stain deeply with a chromium dye.

chromatin The dark-staining substance within the nucleus of a cell.

chromosomes The bodies within a cell that contain the genes.

chronic Of long duration; the opposite of acute.

chyle Partially digested fat that is being transported from the intestine through lymph channels.

chyme Food that has been acted on by stomach juices but has not yet passed into the intestines.

chymotrypsin An enzyme in the small intestine that aids in the digestion of proteins.

cicatrix Scar tissue.

cilia Eyelashes or other hair-like structures.
ciliary body The muscles that dilate and contract the pupil of the eye.
circulation The passage of blood from the heart to all parts of the body and its return from the tissues to the heart.
circulation time The rate at which the blood flows.
circumcision The removal of the foreskin of the penis.
circumoral Surrounding the mouth.
cirrhosis An inflammatory disease of the liver associated with the replacement of liver cells by inert fibrous tissue.
cirsoid aneurysm A group of dilated capillaries, arteries, and veins beneath the skin of the scalp that forms a large mass and may require surgery.
claudication Cramplike pains in the legs due to insufficient arterial blood supply to the muscles. Seen in association with hardening of the arteries of the legs.
claustrophobia A morbid fear of confined spaces.
clavicle The collarbone.
clawfoot A foot with an exceptionally high arch (pes cavus).
clawhand A deformity of the hand produced by paralysis of the nerves to the middle, ring, and little fingers.
clearance test A kidney-function test that analyzes the rate at which a substance passes through the kidneys.
cleft palate A birth deformity in which the palate in the roof of the mouth fails to fuse along the midline.
climacteric The menopause. Change of life.
clinical Relating to the course of a disease.
clitoris Part of the external female genitals. It contains erectile tissue and is the female counterpart of the penis.
clonic Referring to jerky muscle contractions or spasms.
closed reduction Setting a fracture by manipulating the bones.
clostridium A group of spore-bearing bacteria that live without oxygen. Members of the group cause tetanus, lockjaw, gas gangrene, and other infections.
closure The suturing of a wound.
clot Solidification of blood or lymph.
clotting time The length of time it takes blood to coagulate.
clubbed fingers A rounding out of the tips of the fingers, seen in chronic lung conditions or chronic heart disease.
clubfoot A congenital deformity in which the front portion of the foot is turned inward.
clumping Agglutination; the grouping together and adhesion of cells.
cm. Centimeter. Approximately two-fifths of an inch.
coagulation The formation of a clot, as in blood coagulation.
coarctation of the aorta A birth deformity in which there is a narrowing of the passageway through the artery.
cobalt A mineral element that when radioactive can be used in the same manner as x-rays in the treatment of disease.
coccidioidosis A lung disease caused by the repeated inhalation of spores of a certain fungus. Also called desert fever or San Joaquin Valley fever.
coccus A bacterium with a round shape, such as a staphylococcus or streptococcus.
coccyx The last bone in the spinal column, sometimes referred to as the vestigial tail.
cochlea The internal ear, which harbors the main organ of hearing. It is also concerned with the sense of balance.
codeine A derivative of opium, effective in relieving pain.
cod-liver oil An oil obtained from the livers of certain fish; extremely rich in vitamin D.
coitus Sexual intercourse.
cold The common cold; an inflammation of the mucous membranes of the nose caused by a virus; coryza.
cold sore A crusted sore of the lip seen in people who have recovered from a cold or high fever.
colectomy Removal of a portion of the large bowel.
colic Severe abdominal pain thought to be caused by excessively strong contractions of the intestines.
colitis Inflammation of the large bowel (colon).
collarbone The clavicle.
collateral Secondary; often used to refer to collateral circulation, blood vessels that carry the blood when the main vessel is blocked.
Colle's fracture A fracture of the wrist involving a break in the radius and ulna bones.
coloboma A birth deformity of the iris (colored portion) of the eye.
colon The large bowel.
colony A growth of bacteria.
color blindness The inability to distinguish colors. It is an inherited characteristic seen only in males.
colostomy An operation in which the large bowel is brought to the abdominal wall and opened.
colostrum The first substance that comes from the mother's breast following childbirth.
colpitis Inflammation of the vagina.
colposcopy Examination of the vagina with an instrument (speculum).
columella The tissue between the nostrils.
coma Unconsciousness.
comedo A blackhead.
comminuted fracture Fracture in which the bone is broken in several places.
commissurotomy An operation upon the heart in which a deformed heart valve is cut so as to permit a more normal flow of blood.
compatibility In blood grouping, the ability of blood from two different people to mix without clotting.
compensate To make up for or counterbalance a defect.
complication An unforeseen situation occurring during the course of a disease.
compound fracture Fracture

in which the skin overlying the bone is cut or punctured.

compress A poultice.

compression Strong pressure, often applied to control superficial bleeding.

compulsion An uncontrollable impulse to do something.

compulsive neurosis State in which the person is compelled to follow a certain pattern of behavior.

concave Hollowed out.

conceive To become pregnant.

concentration The degree of dilution of a solution.

conception Pregnancy.

concha The hollow portion of the outer ear.

concretion A stone, such as a kidney stone or a gallstone.

concussion A blow; a sudden head injury associated with momentary unconsciousness.

condensation The transformation of a gas into a liquid.

conditioning Obtaining a new reaction to a familiar stimulus, or an old response to a new stimulus.

conduction The passage of electrical, heat, or sound waves along nerves.

conduction system of the heart The mechanism by which impulses to contract are transmitted to the muscles of the heart.

condyles The rounded portions of bones at the joints.

condyloma A warty growth around the anus.

confinement Giving birth, or the lying-in period.

conflict In psychology, the coexistence of two or more opposed wishes or desires.

congenital defects Birth deformities; anomalies.

congestion An excessive amount of blood in an area, such as in the mucous membrane of the nose when a cold exists.

conjunctivitis Inflammation of the covering membrane of the eye.

connective tissue Tissue that connects and holds together the cells of an organ; also, tissues that lie between various structures.

consanguinity Blood relationship.

conscious Mentally aware.

consolidation The appearance of a lung involved in pneumonia.

constipation Difficult bowel evacuation.

constitutional disease One that originates because of the particular makeup of the individual.

constriction Narrowing.

contact lenses Lenses to aid vision which fit directly on the anterior surface of the eyeball.

contagion The spreading of disease from one individual to another.

contamination Soiling; permitting infected material to touch clean surfaces.

contiguous Bordering on; adjacent.

contraceptive An agent used to prevent conception (pregnancy).

contractility The ability of tissue to shorten or contract.

contraction The temporary shortening of a muscle fiber or muscle.

contracture The permanent shortening of a muscle, tendon, or other structure so that it cannot relax or be straightened out.

contraindicated Not advisable.

contralateral Opposite, referring to the opposite side of the body.

contrast medium An opaque substance, such as barium, given to visualize a part of the body on x-ray examination.

contusion A bruise.

convalescence The recovery period after an illness.

conversion hysteria An unconscious mental maneuver in which an emotional problem is turned into a physical disability, such as is seen in hysterical paralysis.

convex Protruding outward.

convolution One of the folds of the brain tissue in the cerebrum.

convulsion A violent, uncontrolled muscle spasm, sometimes accompanied by unconsciousness.

convulsive disorder Any disease associated with recurring convulsions, such as epilepsy.

Cooley's anemia An anemia seen among people who dwell in the Mediterranean areas or who come from that area.

coordination The ability of structures or organs to function properly in relation to one another.

coprophagy The eating of feces, encountered occasionally in infants.

coprophobia Morbid repugnance to defecation and to feces.

copulation Sexual intercourse.

coracoclavicular Referring to the point where the scapula meets the clavicle.

cord presentation The appearance of the umbilical cord at the outlet of the vagina during labor. Unless delivery is rapid, the child may suffocate.

corium The deepest layer of the skin.

corn A thickening of the skin on the toes.

cornea The transparent membrane on the surface of the eyeball.

coronary arteries Arteries supplying the heart muscle.

coronary occlusion Closure (thrombosis) of a coronary artery.

coronary thrombosis Clotting of a coronary artery in the heart.

corpuscle A cell with a rounded shape, as a red blood cell.

corpus luteum The yellow area in an ovary found at the site where an egg has formed and burst from the gland preparatory to menstruation.

cortex The surface layer of an organ.

corticosteroid A chemical having the properties of hormones secreted by the cortex of the adrenal gland.

cortisone A hormone secreted by the cortex of the adrenal gland.

coryza A common cold.

cosmetic surgery Surgery performed to beautify or improve the looks of a patient.

costal arch The arch formed by the ribs in the front of the body.
costal cartilage The cartilage that connects the long ribs to the breastbone.
counterirritant A substance applied to the skin to produce an irritation, such as a mustard plaster.
cowpox The reaction caused by vaccination against smallpox.
coxa valga A deformity of the thighbone in the hip region in which the angle between the neck and the shaft is increased.
coxa vara A deformity of the thighbone in the hip region in which the angle between the neck and the shaft is decreased.
Coxsackie disease An infectious disease with symptoms resembling meningitis or poliomyelitis, but which clears up without aftereffects within a few days.
cramps Painful muscle contractions.
cranial nerves The 12 paired nerves originating from the brain and exiting through openings in the skull.
craniotabes Thinning of various spots in the bones of the skull, found in infants with rickets or syphilis.
craniotomy A surgical opening made in the skull in order to expose the brain.
cranium The skull.
cretinism Severe thyroid deficiency present from birth.
cricoid cartilage The cartilage of the larynx in front of the neck.
crisis The turning point in a severe illness such as pneumonia.
cross-matching The process of mixing a sample of a donor's blood with that of the recipient's blood in order to be certain that they are compatible and will not clot.
cross section A slice of tissue to be examined microscopically.
croup An inflammation of the larynx associated with coughing, fever, and difficulty in breathing.
crypt A small cavity or sac, as in a mucous membrane.
cryptorchidism Undescended testicle.
cryptozygous Having a narrow face and a wide skull formation.
cubital Referring to the elbow or forearm.
culture Usually, a colony of bacteria that are artificially grown in a laboratory.
curettage Scraping the interior surface of an organ with an instrument. Usually in reference to the scraping of the cavity of the uterus.
curvature of the spine Scoliosis or kyphosis; improper alignment of the spinal column.
Cushing's disease Overactivity or overgrowth of the cortex of the adrenal gland, characterized by obesity, high blood pressure, and streaks on the abdominal wall.
cuspid A tooth with a single cusp (point); canine tooth.
cutaneous Referring to the skin.
cutis The skin.
cyanosis Bluish discoloration of the skin and mucous membranes.
cyclic therapy Hormone treatment carried out intermittently, according to the phases of the menstrual cycle.
cyclopropane A nontoxic anesthetic agent given by inhalation.
cyst A sac containing fluid, blood, sweat-gland secretions, or other material.
cystadenoma A nonmalignant tumor composed of glandular tissue and cysts.
cystic duct The tube connecting the gall bladder to the common bile duct.
cystitis Inflammation of the urinary bladder.
cystocele A hernia of the bladder resulting in its protrusion into the vagina.
cystogram An x-ray of the urinary bladder.
cystolithiasis Stones in the urinary bladder.
cystoscope An instrument used to examine the interior of the urinary bladder.
cystotomy An operative incision into the urinary bladder, usually performed when there is obstruction to the outflow of urine from the bladder.
cytology The science dealing with the nature of cells.
cytopathology A branch of pathology in which diagnoses are made by the microscopic examination of cells.
cytoplasm The portion of a cell that does not contain the nucleus.

D

"D and C" operation Dilatation and Curettage; scraping of the interior of the uterus.
dacryocystitis Inflammation of the tear sac of the eye.
dacryostenosis Obstruction of the tear duct leading from the eye to the nose.
dactyl A finger or toe.
dactylomegaly Overgrown toes or fingers; a birth deformity.
Darwin's tubercle A small projection of cartilage in the upper portion of the external ear; a not unusual birth deformity.
daymare A nightmare occurring during the day.
deaf-mute One who is unable to talk because he was born deaf.
deafness Inability to hear.
debility Weakness.
débridement Surgical removal of devitalized tissue in a wound.
decalcification Loss of calcium from bone.
decibel A unit of measurement of sound or hearing.
deciduous teeth First teeth; baby teeth.
decompensation Failure of circulation due to poor heart function.
decompression The removal of excess pressure.
decubitus ulcer Bedsore.
dedentition Loss of teeth.
deerfly fever Tularemia.
defecation Bowel evacuation.
defense mechanism A reaction by which one protects himself

from blame, sense of guilt, shame, or anxiety.

deficiency disease Disease associated with a lack of vitamins or minerals, such as scurvy or rickets.

deformity A deviation from normal.

degeneration Deterioration of tissue with loss of function.

deglutition Swallowing.

dehydration Loss of water from the body.

delayed union Failure of the ends of fractured bones to knit.

delinquency Antisocial, unacceptable behavior.

delirium Mental confusion or excitement, as in a disease with high fever.

delivery The act of giving birth.

delusion A false belief.

demi- Half.

demineralization Loss of mineral salts from the body, such as salt loss from excessive perspiration.

demulcent A medicated ointment.

dendrite The part of a nerve cell that receives impulses and transmits them to the center of the nerve cell.

dengue fever A virus disease transmitted by the bite of a mosquito and characterized by high fever and severe pain in muscles, bones, and joints.

dentition The breaking through the gums of teeth.

denude To strip bare.

depressant drugs Ones that lower the functional activity of an organ or organs.

depression Dejection; a melancholy state.

derma Skin.

dermabrasion Scraping off the surface layers of the skin with a specially constructed instrument; performed by skin specialists to remove skin scars due to acne.

dermatitis Inflammation of the skin.

dermatologist A physician who specializes in diseases of the skin.

dermatophytosis Athlete's foot; ringworm.

dermographia An allergic condition of the skin wherein the skin becomes raised and red wherever it is irritated or lightly scratched.

dermoid cyst A hollow sac (cyst) whose structure resembles that of skin.

desensitization A process in which an individual loses sensitivity to an irritant.

desert fever Valley fever; San Joaquin Valley fever; a chronic lung infection.

desquamation The shedding of the superficial layers of the skin.

detoxication The process of purification or rending a poisonous substance harmless.

devascularize To cut off blood supply.

deviated septum A crooked or deflected wall separating the two nostrils.

dextrocardia A birth deformity in which the heart is located on the right instead of the left side of the chest.

dextrose A form of sugar.

diabetes insipidus A metabolic disease in which there is marked thirst and the passage of huge quantities of urine; not related to diabetes mellitus.

diabetes mellitus A chronic disease characterized by inability to utilize sugars that are ingested. It is caused by insufficient production of insulin by the pancreas.

diagnosis The determining of the nature of an illness or disease.

diaper rash A rash caused by irritation from the diaper or by soap used in cleaning the diaper.

diaphoresis Perspiration; sweating.

diaphragm The thick muscular partition separating the chest and abdominal cavities.

diaphysis The shaft of a long bone.

diarrhea Increased frequency and liquid consistency of stool.

diastasis Separation of parts that are normally in contact.

diastole The relaxed phase of heart action.

diastolic pressure The blood-pressure level during the time the heart muscle is relaxed.

diathermy The application of heat to body tissues through the use of a machine which generates an electric current of high frequency.

diathesis A tendency toward or susceptibility to the development of disease.

Dick test An obsolete skin test to discover an individual's susceptibility to scarlet fever.

differential diagnosis The distinguishing of one disease from another.

digestion The process of breaking down food so that it can be absorbed through the lining of the intestines.

digit A toe or finger.

digitalis A drug used in the treatment of heart disease.

Dilantin A drug used in the treatment and prevention of epileptic seizures.

dilatation Distention, or the process of stretching.

dilution Weakening the strength of a solution.

diopter A unit of measurement for the power of the lens of the eye.

diphtheria A contagious disease characterized by sore throat and the formation of a membrane on the larynx that interferes with breathing.

diplomate A physician who has received his diploma; more specifically, a diploma from the American Specialty Boards; a qualified specialist.

diplopia Double vision.

dipsomania A compulsion to drink excess quantities of alcoholic beverages.

discharge A secretion or emission, as of pus or blood.

discrete Separate; not joined together.

disease A disturbance in the structure or function of an organ or organs.

disgerminoma A tumor of the ovary composed of primitive cells.

disoriented Mentally confused.

dissect To cut tissues.

disseminated sclerosis Multiple sclerosis, a chronic disease of the nervous system.

dissemination The spreading or scattering of a disease process throughout the body.
dissolve To break down when put into a solution.
distal Away from the center; out toward the end.
distention The condition of being inflated or dilated.
distortion A deformed state.
diuresis Increased flow of urine.
diuretic A medication that causes increased flow of urine.
diverge To go in opposite directions, as in divergence of the eyes.
diverticulitis An inflammation of a diverticulum of the bowel.
diverticulosis The presence of many diverticula in the large bowel.
diverticulum An outpouching from the wall of an organ, such as the esophagus, bowel, or urinary bladder.
DNA Deoxyribonucleic acid, a primary constituent of chromosomes.
dolichocephalic Having a long narrow head.
dominant characteristic Trait that tends to be inherited; the opposite of a recessive characteristic.
donee One who receives transfused blood or a graft.
donor One who gives blood, an organ, or a graft.
dorsal Referring to the back or back part of an organ.
dorsiflexion Bending the foot toward the upper surface.
dorsum The back of an organ or part.
dosage The amount of a medication or drug to be administered.
douche Cleansing of the vaginal canal by use of a syringe and stream of water.
drainage A method of evoking a discharge, as in the drainage of pus from an abscess.
dram One-eighth of an ounce.
dream Mental activity during sleep.
dressing Bandages, gauze, or other material applied to protect a wound.
dropsy Swelling of the ankles secondary to heart disorders.
duct A channel or tube.
ductless glands The endocrine glands, such as the pituitary, adrenal, thyroid, parathyroid, testicles, or ovaries. They secrete hormones directly into the bloodstream.
ductus arteriosus A blood vessel present in the embryo connecting the pulmonary (lung) artery and the aorta. Normally, this duct closes off by the time the child is born.
duodenal ulcer Ulcer of the duodenum.
duodenojejunostomy An operation to construct an artificial opening between the duodenum and jejunum.
duodenum The first portion of the small intestine, commencing immediately after the stomach.
dura The thick outer covering of the brain and spinal cord.
dwarfism A condition in which an individual is of smaller than normal size. Often caused by inadequate function of the pituitary gland in the base of the skull.
dyscrasia An abnormal condition.
dysembryoplasia A deformity that develops within an embryo.
dysentery An inflammation of the large bowel associated with diarrhea and abdominal cramps.
dysfunction Malfunction.
dysmenorrhea Painful menstruation.
dysostosis Impaired bone formation.
dyspareunia Difficult or painful sexual intercourse.
dyspepsia Indigestion.
dysphagia Impaired swallowing.
dysphemia Stuttering.
dyspituitarism Abnormal function of the pituitary gland.
dysplasia Impaired growth processes.
dyspnea Shortness of breath.
dystocia Impaired labor, often due to disproportion between the size of the child and the diameter of the birth canal.
dystrophy Abnormal development.
dysuria Impaired ability to urinate; also, painful urination.

E

eardrum The membrane located at the end of the ear canal. Sound waves vibrate against the eardrum.
ear, external The outer ear, or the part that protrudes from the side of the head, and the canal to the eardrum.
ear, inner The part containing the organ of hearing, including the nerve of hearing and the organ controlling the sense of equilibrium.
ear, middle The earbones (incus, stapes, and malleus), the ear cavity, the eustachian tubes leading to the throat, and the mastoid bone cells.
early ambulation Getting a patient out of bed soon after surgery or some confining illness.
Ebstein's disease A birth deformity of the heart associated with displaced heart valves and abnormal connections between the two sides of the heart.
ecchymosis Purple discoloration of the skin because of hemorrhage beneath it; a bruise.
ECG Electrocardiogram.
echinococcus cyst A cyst caused by infestation with a worm carried by dogs.
ECHO virus A virus often causing an upper-respiratory infection associated with severe headache, stiffness of the neck, and other symptoms suggestive of poliomyelitis or meningitis.
eclampsia A convulsive disorder that may occur during the last three months of pregnancy.
ECS Electroshock therapy.
ectoderm The tissue in the embryo that goes to form the skin, the nervous system, and the intestinal tract.
-ectomy A suffix meaning surgical removal.

ectopic pregnancy One taking place in the Fallopian tube.

ectropion The turning out of an eyelid so that it does not lie close to the surface of the eyeball.

eczema An inflammatory condition of the skin.

edema A swelling caused by excessive accumulation of fluids in the tissues.

edentulous Without teeth.

EEG Electroencephalogram.

efferent Leading away from, as an efferent nerve.

effluent An outflow.

effluvium Body odor.

effusion The flowing out of liquid from a part of the body.

egg Ovum; the female germ cell.

ego The conscious realization of oneself; the self.

ejaculation An emission, such as takes place during orgasm.

EKG Electrocardiogram.

electrocardiography The recording of the electrical impulses of the heart.

electrocautery The burning of tissue with an electric current.

electrocoagulation The coagulation and destruction of tissue by use of an electric current.

electroencephalography The recording of brain waves.

electrolysis A procedure for removing hair.

electrolyte A substance that can, when in solution, convey an electrical impulse.

electron microscope An electrical apparatus that makes it possible to see very small objects, such as chromosomes, that cannot be seen through an ordinary microscope.

electroshock therapy The causing of convulsions by use of an electric shock. Helpful in the treatment of some psychiatric states.

elephantiasis Huge enlargement of the legs due to obstruction of the lymph channels.

emasculation Removal of the testicles; castration.

embolism The obstruction of an artery by an embolus, usually a piece of clotted blood.

embolus Something that breaks off in one part of the body and travels through the bloodstream to another part.

embryo The developing child during the first few months of pregnancy. During its later development it is called a fetus.

embryology The study of the embryo and its growth.

emesis Vomiting.

emetic A medication given to stimulate vomiting.

emollient A soothing skin ointment.

emotion An intense feeling.

emphysema A condition in which air spaces in the lungs are enlarged and dilated.

Empirin A patented medicine similar to aspirin and other pain-relieving drugs.

empyema Pus in the cavity surrounding the lungs.

emulsion Particles of one fluid suspended in another fluid, as oil in water.

encanthis A tumor involving the inner corner of the eye.

encapsulated Having a capsule.

encephalitis Inflammation of the brain.

encephalogram A special x-ray technique for seeing the various parts of the brain.

encephalomeningitis An infection of the brain and its coverings.

encephalomyelitis Inflammation or infection of the brain and spinal cord.

encephalon The brain.

encephalopathy Disease of the brain.

encysted Covered by a capsule or sheath.

Endamoeba A type of ameba that causes dysentery.

endarteritis Inflammation of the inner layer of an artery.

endemic A disease, usually contagious, occurring in one locality such as a town or city.

endocarditis Inflammation of the valves or the lining membrane of the heart.

endocardium The membrane lining the chambers of the heart.

endocrine glands Glands that secrete their hormones directly into the bloodstream; ductless glands, such as the pituitary, thyroid, parathyroid, and adrenal.

endocrinology The study of the endocrine glands.

endogenous Originating within the body; opposite of exogenous.

endometriosis The presence of cells which ordinarily line the uterus in unusual places, such as in the bladder or intestinal wall.

endometritis Inflammation of the lining of the uterine cavity.

endometrium The mucous membrane lining the uterus.

endomorph An individual whose bodily constitution is round, soft, and fat.

end organ The end of a nerve fiber and the point where it enters the skin, muscle, or other structure.

endothelium Cells that form the inner lining of blood vessels, lymph channels, and other body cavities.

endotoxin A poison formed within bacteria that is not released until the bacterial cells die.

end product The final product following the breakdown of a complex chemical into its most basic components.

enema An injection of fluid into the rectal canal.

enervation Weakness; loss of energy.

engorged Filled with blood.

ensiform cartilage The lowest tip of the breastbone.

enteritis Inflammation of the intestinal tract.

enterococcus A type of streptococcus found in the intestinal tract.

enterocolitis Inflammation of the small and large intestines.

entoderm Primitive tissue found in the embryo that goes to form the inner lining of the intestinal tract.

entropion A turning in of the eyelid, causing eyelashes to rub against and scratch the eyeball.

enuresis Bedwetting; involuntary urination during sleep.

enzyme A substance produced

by living tissue that stimulates specific chemical actions.
eosinophil A type of white blood cell that has a reddish color when stained and examined under the microscope.
eosinophilia An abnormally large number of eosinophils in the circulating blood, sometimes seen in allergies and in parasitic infestations.
eosinophilic granuloma of bone A rare disease of bone.
eosinophilic tumor A tumor of the pituitary gland in the base of the skull.
ephedrine A chemical with many of the same actions as adrenalin.
ephemeral Fleeting; lasting but a short time.
epicanthus An extra fold of skin covering the inner portion of the eyes, seen in Orientals.
epicondyle A protrusion of bone in the region of the joint.
epicranium The coverings of the skull.
epicrisis The period of an illness after the crisis has passed.
epidemic A disease that simultaneously affects large numbers of people in one or more communities.
epidemiology The study of the occurrence and prevalence of disease, often applied to the study of the manner of spread of contagious diseases.
epidermis The outer layer of the skin.
epidermoid tumor A tumor containing elements of skin.
epidermomycosis A fungus infection of the skin.
epididymis The portion of the seminal tube located immediately above the testicle. It collects sperm from the testicle.
epidural The space just beyond and around the dura covering the brain.
epigastric Referring to the space in the abdomen just below the ribs in the midline; the pit of the stomach.
epiglottis The cartilage in the throat that guards the entrance to the windpipe (trachea).
epilepsy A brain disorder accompanied by periodic convulsions and loss of consciousness.
epinephrine The hormone secreted by the inner portion of the adrenal gland; also called adrenalin.
epiphora An excessive flow of tears.
epiphysis The portion of a bone between the main shaft and the cartilage. It is the main point of bone growth.
epiphysitis Inflammation of the epiphysis.
epiploon The great omentum, a large pad of fat that covers the intestines like an apron.
episiotomy An incision made between the vaginal outlet and the anus during childbirth to avoid excess tearing of tissue as the baby's head is delivered.
episode An attack of an illness.
epispadias A birth deformity in which the urethra ends short of the tip of the penis and opens along the shaft.
epistaxis Nosebleed.
epithelium The tissue cells composing the skin; also, the cells lining the passages of the hollow organs, such as the respiratory, digestive, and urinary tracts.
eponychium The cuticle of the nails.
Epsom salts Magnesium sulfate; used as a laxative or as a poultice for wounds.
epulis A tumor of the jawbone.
equilibrium Balance.
equinocavus A foot deformity in which there is an abnormally high arch.
equinovarus A foot deformity in which there is a turning in of the front of the foot.
Erb's palsy Paralysis of nerves (brachial plexus) supplying the arm, resulting from injury during childbirth.
erection The hardening of the male organ due to engorgement with blood.
erosion The eating away of the surface of a structure, as an erosion of the lining of the stomach that will cause an ulceration.
erupt To break out, as in a rash.
erythema Redness of the skin.
erythroblast A primitive red blood cell.
erythroblastosis Anemia of the newborn, occurring when the mother is Rh-negative and develops antibodies against the unborn child, who is Rh-positive. Also called Rh-factor disease.
erythrocyte A red blood cell.
esophagogram An x-ray of the esophagus.
esophagoscopy Examination of the esophagus by passing a specially designed instrument through the mouth.
esophagus Foodpipe. It goes from the back of the throat to the stomach.
estrogen The female sex hormone produced by the ovaries.
ether A volatile vapor used as an anesthetic agent.
ethmoidectomy Surgical removal of the ethmoid cells because of infection. The ethmoid cells are sinus cells back of the nose.
ethnic Relating to races and peoples.
ethyl chloride A very volatile chemical used as a local anesthetic. It freezes the surface of the skin when it comes into contact with it.
etiology The study of the cause of disease.
eugenics The science of improving the species or race.
euphoria An exaggerated state of well-being.
eustachian tube The tube leading from the back of the throat to the ear.
euthyroid Denoting a state of normal thyroid function.
evacuate To empty.
eversion Turning outward of a part or structure.
evisceration The accidental opening of an abdominal surgical wound with spillage of intestines onto the abdominal wall.
evolution The process by which complex animal life has developed from primitive forms.
Ewing's tumor A cancerlike malignant growth of the long bones.

exacerbation Flare-up of a disease; relapse.

exanthem subitum A childhood disease characterized by a light reddish rash and fever. It lasts only a few days and disappears spontaneously.

exchange transfusion A method used to save the lives of newborns with erythroblastosis (Rh-factor disease). Most of the infant's blood is removed and donor blood is substituted.

excise To cut out surgically.

excrement Feces; stool.

excrete To expel.

exenteration operations Operations performed upon far advanced cancer patients in an attempt to prolong life. It often involves removal of many organs, including the bladder and rectum.

exhale To breathe out.

exhaustion Extreme fatigue.

exocrine glands Glands that secrete through ducts (tubes) rather than directly into the bloodstream. The salivary glands are exocrine glands.

exogenous Originating outside the body; opposite of endogenous.

exophthalmos Bulging of the eyeballs seen in some cases of overactivity of the thyroid gland.

exostosis A nonmalignant tumor of bone characterized by a bulging at one or more sites.

exotoxin Poison secreted by living germs.

expectorant Any medication given to promote the secretion of mucus from the lungs or bronchial tubes.

expiration Breathing out; exhalation.

exstrophy of the bladder A birth deformity of the urinary bladder in which the anterior wall of the bladder is missing and the urine empties onto the abdominal wall.

extradural Located outside the dural covering of the brain.

extrasystole A heartbeat occurring before its normal time. Commonly referred to as a skipped beat.

extremity A limb, such as an arm or leg.

exudate Inflammatory fluid, such as serum or pus.

eye The organ of sight.

eye ground The retina, or back of the inside of the eyeball.

eyeteeth The sharp canine teeth in the upper jaw.

eyewash A solution used to bathe inflamed eyes.

F

face presentation A position of the unborn child during labor in which the face appears at the outlet of the vagina.

facial artery The main artery to the face.

facial nerve The seventh cranial nerve, supplying the muscles and surfaces of the tongue, ear, and face.

Fahrenheit scale A temperature scale commonly used in the United States. Water freezes at 32°F. and boils at 212°F.; normal body temperature is 98.6°F.

fainting A momentary loss of consciousness.

Fallopian tube The uterine tube on either side of the uterus. The egg (ovum) moves from the ovary to the uterus through this tube.

Fallot's tetralogy A birth deformity of the heart involving defects in the blood vessels and walls of the heart chambers.

familial disease A disease occurring in several members of the same family.

familial tendency A tendency for a condition to occur in several members of the same family.

fantasy Imagination.

farsightedness An eye condition in which the eyeball is abnormally short, thus causing light rays to focus behind the retina. Distant objects are seen more clearly than near objects.

fascia Connective tissue.

fatigue Weariness; exhaustion.

fatty degeneration Degeneration of an organ with the replacement of its normal structure by fat.

febrile Feverish; having an elevated temperature.

fecalith A hard ball of feces (stool) within the bowel or appendix.

feces Stool.

fecundation Fertilization.

feeblemindedness A mental state below normal but above that of an imbecile or idiot.

felon An abscess of the fingertip.

feminism The appearance of female traits in a male.

feminizing tumor A tumor of the ovary that results in the exaggeration of female sex characteristics. If this occurs in a female child, it may lead to breast development and the onset of menstruation at a very early age.

femur The thighbone between the hip and knee.

fenestration operation An operation performed to relieve deafness.

fertility The ability to bear children.

fertilization The entrance of the male sperm cell into the female ovum (egg).

fester To form an abscess; to discharge pus.

fetal Referring to the unborn child.

fetal rickets Rickets having its onset before birth.

fetology The study of the child while still within the mother's uterus.

fetus The unborn child during the later part of pregnancy. (Before the third month, it is called an embryo.)

fever Elevation of body temperature above 98.6°F.

fiber A threadlike tissue or structure.

fibrillation An irregular heart action due to abnormal spread of impulses from one portion of the heart to another.

fibrocystic disease of bone Cyst formation in bone due to overactivity of the parathyroid glands in the neck.

fibroid A nonmalignant, benign tumor of the uterus composed largely of fibrous tissue.

fibroma A noncancerous tumor composed of fibrous tissues.

fibrosis Replacement of the normal components of a structure by fibrous tissue.

fibrous Containing fibers.

fibula The smaller of the two legbones, extending from the knee to the outer side of the ankle.

filariasis A parasitic infestation associated with great swelling of the legs.

finger cot A rubber sheath for a finger, used by physicians in performing examinations of different body openings.

first aid Emergency medical care given before professional help arrives.

fissure A cleft or crack, such as a fissure of the anus (fissure in ano).

fistula An abnormal canal or connection, often occurring in or about the anus (fistula in ano).

fit A convulsion or seizure.

flank The loin; the area on the side of the body extending from the lowermost rib down to the hipbone.

flatfoot Flattening of the normal arch of the foot; pes planus.

flatus Gas in the lower intestinal tract.

flexion A bending motion, such as when one bends the arm at the elbow.

flu Grippe. A respiratory infection caused by a virus and accompanied by inflammation of the respiratory passages.

fluke A worm that causes disease in organs such as the intestines, liver, and lungs, and in the bloodstream.

fluoridation of water The adding of a fluoride compound to drinking water at its source. This is advocated as a means of cutting down tooth decay among children.

fluoroscopy X-raying a part of the body and recording the rays on a special (fluorescent) screen. This is done in order to view the motion of organs.

focus The main site of a disease process.

folic acid A normal chemical constituent of the body necessary for growth and maintenance of health.

fontanel The soft space in between the bones of the skull, found in newborns and children under a year or two of age. These areas fill in with bone during the first two years of a child's life.

food allergy Sensitivity to a food. Food allergy may evidence itself by nausea, vomiting, diarrhea, or by a skin rash with hives.

food poisoning An intestinal upset caused by toxins or bacteria in ingested foods.

foramen An opening, such as in the bones of the skull.

forceps . delivery Childbirth aided by the application of an instrument known as a forceps to the sides of a child's head.

forearm The arm below the elbow.

forefinger The index finger.

forefoot The front portion of the foot.

foreskin The skin over the head of the penis; the prepuce.

formative The early stages of development.

formula A prescription; also, the ingredients of a child's diet during the first few months or year of his life.

fracture Any break in a bone.

freckle A circumscribed, flat, pigmented area on the skin, often brought on by exposure to sunlight.

frenum A fold of skin or mucous membrane that limits the motion of a structure, such as the frenum beneath the tongue with which some children are born.

Friderichsen-Waterhouse syndrome Blood poisoning associated with a meningitis infection. It leads to hemorrhage within the adrenal glands, collapse, and death.

Friedreich's ataxia A hereditary disease in which there is paralysis of the lower limbs and marked curvature of the spine.

frigidity Absence of sexual desire in women.

Froehlich's syndrome Inactivity of the pituitary gland in children, resulting in marked obesity and underdevelopment of the genital organs.

frontal sinuses The air spaces (sinuses) in the skull located directly above the eyes.

frostbite A burn resulting from extreme cold.

frozen section A technique whereby tissue removed in surgery is submitted to microscopic examination within a few minutes after its removal.

frustration The blockage of a strong desire accompanied by a sense of lack of completion.

full-thickness graft A skin graft made up of all the layers of the skin.

fulminating The rapid progression of disease.

functional disease A disease with an upset in function rather than a change in structure; the opposite of an organic disease.

functional disorder An upset in function rather than a disease process.

fungus A form of plant life sometimes causing infection in humans, such as athlete's foot.

funnel chest A deformity of the breastbone due to rickets. There is a depression of the sternum.

furuncle A boil or abscess.

fusion Union.

G

gait The way one walks.

galactocele A milk cyst in a breast.

galactose The sugar in breast milk.

gall Bile; the material secreted by the liver.

gall bladder A hollow, pear-shaped organ that stores and concentrates bile and is located beneath the liver.

gallstones Stones within the gall bladder.

gamete A sperm or an egg; the sex cells that unite to form an embryo.

gamma globulin A substance containing antibodies. It is often injected after exposure to certain infections in order to make the disease milder.

ganglion A group of nerves alongside the spinal cord; also, a cyst of the sheath of a tendon, frequently appearing on the upper surface of the wrist in children.

gangrene Death of tissue.

gargle To rinse the mouth.

gas gangrene A serious form of gangrene caused by a specific gas-forming germ.

gastrectomy Surgical removal of part or all of the stomach.

gastric Referring to the stomach.

gastric analysis Examination of the secretions of the stomach, performed by the passage of a tube from the mouth or nose into the stomach.

gastric lavage Washing out the stomach.

gastritis Inflammation of the lining of the stomach.

gastrocnemius The large calf muscle in the back of the leg.

gastroenteritis Inflammation of the stomach and intestines associated with abdominal cramps and diarrhea.

gastrointestinal Relating to the stomach and the intestines.

gastroscope An instrument that is passed through the mouth and esophagus down into the stomach.

gastrostomy An operation to establish an artificial opening of the stomach on the abdominal wall.

Gaucher's disease A chronic disease in which there is anemia and enlargement of the liver and spleen.

gauze Wound coverings made of cheesecloth.

generation The interval between the birth of a child and the birth of the child's child.

genes The units responsible for inheritance.

genetics The science dealing with heredity.

genitals The organs of reproduction. In the female: the vulva, vagina, uterus, Fallopian tubes, and ovaries. In the male: the penis, testicles, and prostate gland.

genitourinary Referring to the urinary system and the sex organs.

geriatrics The study of conditions affecting old people.

germ Any bacteria or microorganisms that cause disease.

germ cell A gamete; an ovum or sperm.

germinate To grow from a cell or seed into a mature form.

gestation Pregnancy.

Ghon tubercle The primary tuberculosis infection in the lungs of children, visible as a shadow on x-rays. It is not usually associated with an acute infection.

giantism Abnormally large size.

gigantism Same as giantism.

gingiva The gums; the tissue surrounding the teeth.

gingivitis Inflammation of the gums.

glabella The portion of the skull located just above the bridge of the nose.

gland An organ that manufactures a chemical that will be utilized elsewhere in the body.

glandular fever Infectious mononucleosis; a subacute infectious disease characterized by sore throat, weakness, swollen glands, and atypical blood count.

glans The head of the penis.

glaucoma An eye disease associated with increased pressure within the eyeball.

glioma A tumor originating from the tissue that surrounds the brain and spinal cord.

globulin A protein found throughout the body's tissues in various forms, such as gamma globulin, serum globulin, etc.

glomerulonephritis An inflammation of the kidneys.

glossa The tongue.

glossitis Inflammation of the tongue.

glossopharyngeal nerve The ninth cranial nerve, which supplies the tongue and throat.

glottis The vocal cords and the opening between them.

glucose A form of sugar.

glucose-tolerance test A blood test performed to determine the ability of the body to utilize and store sugar. A specific test for diabetes mellitus.

glycogen Sugar as it is stored in the liver and held ready for release to other parts of the body.

glycosuria Sugar in the urine. This is frequently evidence of diabetes.

gm. Gram.

goiter An enlargement of the thyroid gland.

gonad A sex gland; testicle or ovary.

gonococcus The germ causing gonorrhea.

gonorrhea A venereal infection of the lining of the vagina or penis.

gout A type of arthritis or inflammation about a joint caused by excess uric acid in the blood. It occurs in sudden attacks and brings on great pain. The big toe is a favorite site.

graft Tissue to replace a defect that is taken from another part of the same body or from another body.

grain A unit of weight. (480 grains equal 1 ounce.)

gram The equivalent of 1 cc. or 15 drops.

grand mal A major epileptic seizure.

granulation tissue Freshly formed tissue composed of capillaries and connective tissue, seen very often during the process of healing.

gravid Pregnant.

gray matter A common term referring to the higher brain cells; the cerebrum.

greenstick fracture A break in an oblique direction that does not go all the way through the bone.

grippe Mild influenza.

groin The line of division between the thigh and the abdomen; often referred to as the inguinal region.

growth hormone The hormone secreted by the anterior part of the pituitary gland.

guinea-pig inoculation An injection of a specimen taken from a patient's sputum or urine into a guinea pig in order to determine whether the patient has tuberculosis.

gums Gingiva; the mucous membrane around the teeth.

gynecologist A physician who specializes in diseases of the female organs.

gynecomastia Enlargement of the male breast, usually due to overgrowth of breast tissue.

gyrus A portion of the cerebrum.

H

habit Fixed behavior produced by repetition.

habituation Addiction, as to a narcotic drug.

hacking cough A dry cough.

Hadfield-Clarke syndrome A condition present from birth in which the pancreas fails to develop fully or to function normally.

hair follicle The tiny sac out of which a hair grows.

halitosis Bad breath.

Haliver oil Oil from the liver of a halibut, which is rich in vitamin D.

hallucination A false sense perception.

hallux The big toe.

harmartoma A growth made up of excessive amounts of normal tissue cells.

hammer toe A toe that is bent and cannot be extended or straightened.

hamstring muscles The muscles in the back of the thigh.

Hand-Schüller-Christian syndrome A congenital disease in which there is a deposit of yellow xanthoma cells throughout the organs and tissues.

hangnail A piece of loose skin near the base of the fingernail.

Hansen's disease Leprosy.

harelip A birth deformity in which there is a cleft in the upper lip.

haustra The normal pouchlike bulges in the wall of the large intestine.

hay fever An allergic condition of the nasal passages caused by sensitivity to ragweed pollen.

Hb Hemoglobin.

HCl Hydrochloric acid.

heart The hollow muscular organ in the chest that pumps blood throughout the body.

heartbeat The rhythmic contraction and relaxation of the heart as it pumps blood.

heart block A disorder in the transmission of the heartbeat from the atrium to the ventricle.

heartburn Indigestion associated with a burning pain in the lower chest or upper abdomen.

heart failure A general term used to define inadequate function of the heart.

heart rate The number of heartbeats per minute.

heart sounds The sounds heard through a stethoscope and the impulses felt when the heart muscles contract and relax.

heat cramps Muscle cramps following marked perspiration with loss of salt from the body.

heat prostration A condition characterized by elevated temperature, poor heart action, and a shocklike state; heat exhaustion.

heat rash Prickly heat; small pink and red spots on the skin associated with perspiration in intensely hot weather.

heat stroke Sunstroke.

helix The rounded portion of the external ear.

helminthiasis Any disease caused by infestation with worms.

hemagglutination The clumping together of red blood cells.

hemangiectasia Dilatation of blood vessels, usually small capillaries, in the skin or in the lining of the intestinal tract.

hemangioma A nonmalignant tumor of blood vessels.

hemangiosarcoma A malignant tumor originating from blood vessels.

hemapoiesis The production of red blood cells, such as the process that takes place in the bone marrow.

hemarthrosis Blood in a joint secondary to hemorrhage.

hematemesis The vomiting of blood.

hematin The iron constituent of hemoglobin.

hematinic A medication given to increase the amount of hemoglobin in the blood.

hematocolpos A collection of blood within the vagina, particularly in females whose vaginal outlet is blocked by an intact maidenhead (hymen).

hematocrit test A test on blood to determine the relative proportion of red blood cells to plasma.

hematologist A physician who specializes in diseases of the blood and blood-forming organs.

hematolysis The destruction of red blood cells and the release of hemoglobin from the cells.

hematoma Hemorrhage under the skin or in deeper tissues with the formation of a blood clot.

hematopoiesis The formation of blood.

hematoporphyrinuria Blackish urine due to the presence of porphyrin. It is caused by the breakdown of red blood cells and the release and decomposition of hemoglobin.

hematuria Blood in the urine.

hemi- Half.

hemiatrophy Degeneration limited to one side of the body.

hemic Pertaining to blood.

hemicolectomy Removal of part of the large bowel.

hemicrania Headache on one side of the head only, as in migraine.

hemihypertrophy Overgrowth of one side of the body or one organ on one side of the body.

hemiplegia Paralysis of one side of the body.

hemisphere One half of the brain.

hemo- Referring to blood.

hemochromatosis A disease in which there is cirrhosis of the liver, diabetes, and deposition of iron pigments in the skin and various other tissues throughout the body.

hemoconcentration Concentration of the blood as a result of loss of body fluid or plasma.

hemodialysis The separation, as in use of the artificial-kidney machine, of poisons and wastes from the circulating blood.

hemodilution The opposite of hemoconcentration.

hemodynamics The study of blood flow, blood pressure, and blood volume.

hemoglobin The pigment in the red blood cells. It carries oxygen to the tissues.

hemoglobinemia A type of anemia in which, although there are a sufficient number of red blood cells, the cells are deficient in hemoglobin.

hemoglobinuria Hemoglobin in the urine.

hemolysis Destruction of red blood cells and the escape of hemoglobin in the bloodstream.

hemolytic anemia An anemia caused by the destruction of red blood cells.

hemopericardium A collection of blood in the pericardial sac surrounding the heart.

hemoperitoneum Blood in the abdominal cavity.

hemophilia An inherited disease in which the blood clots improperly. Hemophiliacs are almost invariably males; they are called bleeders.

hemopneumothorax A collection of blood and air in the pleural cavity surrounding the lungs.

hemoptysis The coughing up of blood.

hemorrhage Escape of blood from the blood vessels. It may be either external or internal.

hemorrhoids Varicose veins of the rectum and anus; piles.

hemostasis A surgical term denoting the fact that bleeding has been stopped.

hemostatic An agent that stops hemorrhage.

hemothorax A collection of blood in the chest cavity.

Henoch's purpura A children's disease characterized by bleeding into the tissues of the body, particularly beneath the skin.

hepar The liver.

heparin An anticoagulant given to prolong blood-clotting time.

hepatectomy Removal of part of the liver.

hepatic Referring to the liver.

hepatitis Inflammation of the liver.

hepatoma A malignant tumor of the liver seen in children.

hepatomegaly Enlargement of the liver.

hepatosplenomegaly Enlargement of both the liver and the spleen, as in Gaucher's disease.

heredity The passage of bodily characteristics or disease from parent to offspring.

hermaphrodite An individual born with structures of both sexes. Usually underdeveloped.

hernia A rupture; a weakness in the musculature allowing the protrusion of tissues normally contained within the abdominal cavity.

herniate To rupture.

hernioplasty An operation to repair a hernia.

herniorrhaphy An operation to repair a hernia.

herniotomy Opening the sac of a hernia before its surgical repair.

herpes Acute inflammation of the skin, caused by a virus. It is characterized by the formation of small pustular areas.

heterogenous Dissimilar; different.

heterophil A white blood cell.

heterophil test A blood test that, when positive, indicates the presence of infectious mononucleosis (glandular fever).

heterosexuality Sexual feelings for one of the opposite sex.

heterotoxin A poison or toxin originating outside the body.

heterotropia Cross-eye; squint.

hexachlorophene A powerful germicide.

hexadactylism Six fingers or toes on an extremity.

hiatus An opening.

hiatus hernia A hernia of the diaphragm taking place through the opening where the esophagus passes.

hiccough A sudden spasm of the diaphragm.

hidrosis Excessive perspiration.

hilar lymph nodes The lymph nodes at the base of the lung.

hip The joint where the upper end of the thighbone and the pelvic bones meet.

hippus A jerky movement of the pupil of the eye.

Hirschsprung's disease Megacolon; dilatation of the large bowel, present at birth, caused by constriction of the large bowel in the region of the rectum.

hirsutism Excessive growth of hair.

histamine A breakdown product of protein metabolism. It stimulates the secretion of gastric juice and the secretions from other glands. It also causes dilatation of small blood vessels.

histology The study of cells and organs by microscopic examination.

histoplasmosis A serious fungus disease that results in anemia, emaciation, and high fever.

history The record of symptoms and the sequence of events in an illness.

hives Urticaria; an allergic reaction of the skin secondary to a sensitivity characterized by itchy red blotches or welts.

H_2O Water.

H_2O_2 Hydrogen peroxide.

Hodgkin's disease A malignant disease of the lymph nodes, usually ending fatally.

homeostasis Stability of all body functions at normal levels.

homo- The same.

homogenous Similar in structure.

homograft A graft of tissue taken from the body of another being of the same species.

homolateral On the same side of the body.

homologous Corresponding to the same type.

homologous serum jaundice Inflammation of the liver (hepatitis) following the receipt of a blood transfusion, a plasma injection, or certain serum injections.

homosexuality Sexual feelings for one of the same sex.

homunculus A dwarf.

hookworm disease A parasitic

disease caused by the hookworm.

hordeolum Sty; an abscess or boil on the eyelid.

hormone A chemical produced by a gland and secreted into the blood. Hormones affect the function of distant organs or cells.

hornification Callus formation of the skin.

horseshoe kidney A birth deformity in which the two kidneys are fused, usually at their lower poles, thus assuming the shape of a horseshoe.

host One who harbors a germ, a parasite, or a growth.

Huhner test A test for sterility, whereby sperm are examined from the vagina one hour after intercourse.

humerus The bone of the upper arm.

Huntington's chorea An inherited disease in which there are purposeless muscle movements of the face, arms, and legs, along with speech defects and progressive degeneration of brain tissue.

hyaline-membrane disease A disease of premature babies in which there is respiratory failure due to a membrane covering the air cells.

hyalinization The replacement of a functioning tissue by an amorphous, inert material known as hyaline.

hybrid A mixed type.

hydatid of Morgagni A cyst occurring just above the testicle.

hydramnios A condition in which excess fluid surrounds the unborn child in the womb.

hydrarthrosis Fluid in a joint; "water on the knee."

hydrate To add water.

hydremia Excessive fluid content of the blood.

hydro- Referring to water.

hydrocele A collection of fluid in a sac surrounding the testicle.

hydrocelectomy Surgical removal of a hydrocele.

hydrocephalus A condition coming on shortly after birth in which the child's head enlarges as a result of the accumulation of fluid around the brain. Also known as giant head.

hydrochloric acid An acid secreted by the cells lining the stomach. This acid aids in digesting foods.

hydrocortisone A cortisone medication.

hydronephrosis A condition in which there is obstruction of the outflow of urine from a kidney.

hydrophobia Rabies; a disease fatal to humans and animals, caused by the bite of an infected animal.

hydropneumothorax A condition in which fluid and air occupy the chest cavity surrounding the lungs.

hydrotherapy Treatment of muscles, bones, or tendons by the application of water, as in whirlpool baths.

hygiene Observation and practice of health and sanitation standards.

hygroma A cyst formed out of lymph channels. It is sometimes seen in the neck region in children.

hymen The maidenhead; the membrane covering the entrance to the vagina.

hymenotomy The surgical cutting of the maidenhead.

hyoid bone The bone located beneath the chin in the upper part of the neck. The tongue muscles are attached to it.

hyoscine Scopolamine.

hyper- Excessive.

hyperacidity Excessive acidity.

hyperalgesia Extreme sensitivity to pain.

hypercalcemia Excessive calcium in the blood.

hyperchlorhydria Excessive hydrochloric acid in the gastric juice.

hyperemia An increased amount of blood in an area, as seen where inflammation exists.

hyperesthesia Excessive sensitivity.

hyperextension Overstraightening.

hyperflexion Overbending.

hyperglycemia Excessive sugar in the blood, a frequent finding in diabetes.

hypergonadism Excessive secretion of hormones by the testicles or ovaries.

hyperhidrosis Excessive perspiration.

hyperinsulinism Too much insulin, often resulting in too little sugar in the blood.

hyperkalemia Excessive amounts of potassium in the blood.

hyperkeratosis Overgrowth of the corneal tissue covering the pupil of the eye.

hyperkinetic Relating to excessive movements of muscles.

hypermetropia Farsightedness.

hypermotility Overactivity.

hypernatremia Excessive amounts of sodium in the blood.

hypernephroma A tumor of the kidney.

hyperopia Farsightedness.

hyperparathyroidism Excessive secretion by the parathyroid glands, characterized by loss of calcium from the bones, cyst formation within the bones, bone deformities, and kidney stones.

hyperperistalsis Overactive contractions of the intestines.

hyperpituitarism Overactivity of the pituitary gland, leading to gigantism or acromegaly.

hyperplasia Overgrowth of tissue.

hyperpnea Exceptionally deep and rapid breathing.

hyperpotassemia Excessive potassium in the blood.

hyperpyrexia High fever.

hypersalivation Drooling; the excessive secretion of saliva.

hypersensitivity Excessive sensitivity, as in an allergic condition.

hypersplenism A set of diseases associated with excessive activity of the spleen.

hypertension High blood pressure.

hyperthyroidism Overactivity of the thyroid gland.

hypertonic Excessively tense; overactive.

hypertrophy Increase in the size of an organ.

hyperventilation Excessively deep breathing.

hypervitaminosis A condition

caused by the excessive intake of vitamins.

hypesthesia Decreased sensitivity.

hyphemia Hemorrhage in the eyeball.

hypnosis A trance induced by the repeated suggestions of a hypnotist.

hypnotic A medication that produces sleep.

hypo- Too little.

hypoacidity Too little acid.

hypoadrenalism An exhausted, depressed state characterized by low blood pressure, low metabolism, and inadequate function of the adrenal glands.

hypocalcemia Too little calcium in the blood.

hypochlorhydria Too little acid in the stomach.

hypochondriac One who thinks he is afflicted with diseases that are not present.

hypodermic Beneath the skin.

hypofunction Lessened function.

hypogastrium The region of the abdomen extending down from the navel to the pubic bone.

hypogenitalism Underdevelopment of the sex organs.

hypoglossal Under the tongue.

hypoglossal nerve The 12th cranial nerve, which supplies the muscles of the tongue.

hypoglycemia Too little sugar in the blood.

hypogonadism Diminished function of the sex glands.

hypokalemia Too little potassium in the blood.

hyponatremia A diminished amount of sodium in the blood.

hypoparathyroidism Inadequate function of the parathyroid glands.

hypopharynx The area between the back of the throat and the larynx.

hypophysis Scientific name for the pituitary gland.

hypopituitarism Insufficient secretion of the pituitary hormones.

hypoplasia Underdevelopment of an organ or tissue.

hypopotassemia Too little potassium in the blood.

hypoproteinemia Insufficient protein in the blood.

hyposensitivity Diminished reaction to stimulation.

hypospadias A birth deformity in which the urethra ends before it reaches the tip of the penis.

hypotension Low blood pressure.

hypothalamus A part of the brain below the higher brain centers.

hypothenar The fleshy part of the hand in the region of the ring and little fingers.

hypothermia A lower than normal body temperature, sometimes produced artificially to slow bodily processes during operations on the heart.

hypothyroidism Underactivity of the thyroid gland.

hypotonia Lessened muscle tone.

hypoventilation Less air and oxygen in the lungs than normal.

hypovitaminosis A deficiency of vitamins.

hypoxia Inadequate oxygen in the lungs and in the blood.

hysterectomy Surgical removal of the uterus.

hysteria An extremely emotional state.

hysterotomy Surgical incision into the uterus.

I

iatrogenic Caused by a physician.

icteric Referring to jaundice (yellow discoloration of the skin).

icterus *See* jaundice.

ichthyoid Fishlike.

ichthyosis Scaly skin giving the appearance of fish scales. In some instances this condition is inherited.

id The unconscious force responsible for instinctive impulses.

idea A thought or belief.

idealization The process by which one gives excessive values to a loved object.

identification The process of recognizing a person or thing by its characteristics.

idiocy A condition in which mental development is restricted to less than that of a three-year-old child. Idiots have an I.Q. of less than 25.

idioglossia The jabbering of an infant before he is old enough to talk.

idiopathic Of unknown origin or cause.

ileitis Inflammation of the lower portion of the small intestine.

ileocecal valve The muscular mechanism at the junction of the small and large intestines in the lower-right portion of the abdomen.

ileocolic Referring to the ileum and the colon.

ileocolitis An inflammation of both small and large intestines.

ileostomy A surgical procedure in which the ileum is brought out onto the abdominal wall and opened.

ileum The lower portion of the small intestine, terminating in the cecum (large intestine).

ileus Obstruction of the small intestine because of paralysis or mechanical obstruction.

ileus, meconium A disease of the newborn in which the fecal contents of the small intestine cause obstruction.

iliac Referring to the ilium, the winglike portion of the hipbone.

ilium The flank; the upper portion of the hipbone.

illegitimate Born out of wedlock.

illusion A false impression.

I.M. Infectious mononucleosis (glandular fever); also, intramuscular.

image The picture that is recorded by the retina in the back of the eye.

imbalance Lack of balance; upset.

imbecility A state of mental development in which the I.Q. is between 25 and 50; one grade above idiocy.

immobilize To render a part immovable, as by applying a plaster cast or a splint.

immune Protected against a disease.
immunization The process of making one immune to a disease.
immunohematology A branch of medicine that deals with both the blood cells and the antibodies and antigens in the blood.
immunotransfusion A blood transfusion from a donor who is immune to the disease from which the recipient is suffering.
impacted Firmly wedged in.
impacted cerumen Wax hardened in the ear canal.
impacted feces Stool hardened in the rectum.
impalpable Not able to be felt with the hands.
imperforate Not perforated; lacking a normal opening.
impetigo A highly contagious, pustular inflammation of the skin, seen in infants and young children.
implant A fragment of tissue that grows in an area other than its usual one.
impotence Inability to have sexual intercourse.
impregnate To make pregnant.
inanition The condition resulting from starvation.
inarticulate Unable to express oneself.
inborn Congenital; inherited.
incarcerated Hemmed in; stuck. An incarcerated hernia is one in which the herniated parts are firmly lodged in the hernial sac.
incest Intercourse between two members of the same immediate family.
incidence A term denoting the frequency with which a condition occurs.
incipient Early; beginning.
incise To cut surgically.
incision A surgical cut.
incisional hernia A hernia occurring through the site of a previous operative wound.
incisor teeth The front cutting teeth.
inclusion cyst A cyst composed of skin and lying beneath the normal surface of the skin.
incompatible Not capable of existing together.
incompetent Not functioning adequately.
incontinence Involuntary passage of urine or stool.
incoordination Lack of coordination.
incrustation Scab formation.
incubation period The interval between exposure to a disease and its appearance.
incubator A heated and humidified container for a newborn child.
incubus A nightmare.
incus One of the small bones of hearing in the middle ear.
indication Something pertaining to a disease that points the way toward treating it. (Pus may be an indication for surgical incision and drainage.)
indigestion Dyspepsia. Disturbed digestion.
indolent Inactive; not progressing.
induction The beginning stages of anesthesia.
induration Thickening.
inertia Failure to move or contract; lack of activity.
infant A child below the age of two years.
infantile paralysis Poliomyelitis.
infantilism Childish characteristics in an adult.
infarct An area of tissue deprived of its blood supply because of a clot within its artery.
infection The presence and growth of bacteria, viruses, or parasites within the body.
infection, airborne The spread of infection by coughing or sneezing (droplet infection).
infection, concurrent Two distinct infections occurring at the same time in one person.
infection, cross Infection in a hospital as a result of transmission from one patient to another.
infection, focal An infection localized to a specific tissue from which bacteria may spread throughout the body.
infection, mixed One in which two or more bacteria are present.
infection, secondary An infection superimposed upon another infection.
infectious disease A disease caused by bacteria, funguses, or parasites.
infectious hepatitis An inflammation of the liver caused by a virus.
infectious mononucleosis Glandular fever, characterized by sore throat, swollen glands, weakness, and an abnormal blood count.
inferiority complex An outmoded term applied to a state of mind in which one feels inadequate.
infertility Sterility.
infestation Invasion of the body by mites, insects, worms, or ticks.
infiltration The passage of cells or fluid into tissue spaces usually free of such elements.
infirmity A weakness.
inflammation The reaction of tissues to injury or invasion by bacteria or viruses, manifested by heat, pain, redness, and swelling.
influenza A virus infection of the upper respiratory tract; grippe; flu.
infradiaphragmatic Pertaining to the area beneath the diaphragm.
infraorbital Pertaining to the area below the floor of the eye.
infrapatellar Pertaining to the region beneath the kneecap.
infrared rays Invisible rays of an exceptionally long wavelength. They are used to supply deep heat to an injured part of the body.
infusion The injection of a solution into a vein or beneath the skin.
infusion reaction Fever and chills following the administration of fluids into a vein.
ingest To eat.
inguinal region The groin.
inhalant A medication administered by inhalation.
inhalation The act of breathing in.
inhalation burn A burn of the respiratory passage and lungs

caused by inhaling steam or an irritating gas or vapor.

inherent Inborn.

inherited Handed down from the parents by genetic transmission.

inhibition Restraint of a process or action.

inhibitor A substance that offsets or stops the effect of another substance.

injection The act of forcing a substance into a part of a body through a needle and syringe.

innervation The nerve supply to an organ or part.

innocuous Harmless.

inoculation The act of injecting a vaccine or other substance for the purpose of inducing immunity.

inoperable Unable to be corrected or improved by surgery.

inorganic Not organic.

insanity A legal term referring to an individual who is unable to control his life, unable to maintain socially accepted conduct, and unable to distinguish right from wrong.

inseminate To ejaculate sperm into the vagina.

insensible Lacking in sensation.

insight The ability to understand.

in situ In place.

insoluble Not capable of being put into solution.

insomnia Sleeplessness.

inspiration The breathing in of air into the lungs.

inspissated Thickened; hardened.

instability Emotional imbalance.

instep The arch of the foot.

instill To introduce a liquid.

instinct The primitive unconscious driving forces that motivate certain reactions.

insufficiency The condition of being inadequate for a given function.

insufflate To blow a powder or vapor into a part of the body.

insulin A hormone produced in the cells of the pancreas. When secreted into the bloodstream, it permits the metabolism and utilization of sugar. Inadequate insulin leads to diabetes. Too much insulin leads to a condition known as hypoglycemia.

insulinoma A tumor of the insulin-producing cells of the pancreas.

insult Damage to an organ or part.

integration The process by which various functions are coordinated.

integument The skin.

intellect The reasoning faculty.

intelligence quotient (I.Q.) The ratio of an individual's mental age to his chronological age, determined by giving certain psychological tests.

intensity The degree of strength of a process.

inter- Between.

intercellular tissue The area between the cells.

intercostal The area between the ribs.

intercurrent disease A disease occurring during the existence of another disease.

interdiction Prohibiting a patient from doing something.

interdigitate To dovetail.

interlabial Between the lips.

intermenstrual Between menstrual periods.

intermittent Starting and stopping.

intermural Between the walls of a structure.

intermuscular Located between muscles.

internal Within the deep structures of the body.

intern(e) A medical graduate serving in a hospital in order to train and to treat patients under the supervision of the medical staff.

internists Physicians who specialize in internal medicine and in the diagnosis of medical diseases.

interosseous muscles Small muscles located between the bones of the hand.

intersex Someone with a developmental defect of sex differentiation, such as a hermaphrodite.

interspace The space between two similar organs or structures.

interstitial Relating to small gaps or intervals between tissues or structures.

intertrigo An inflammation in the folds of the skin.

intervertebral Between the vertebrae.

intestine The part of the digestive tract that extends from the exit of the stomach to the termination of the rectum.

intima The inner lining of a blood vessel.

in-toeing Pigeon-toed.

intolerance Inability to take a medicine because of sensitivity.

intoxication A poisoned state.

intra- Inside.

intra-abdominal Within the abdominal cavity.

intra-atrial Within an atrium of the heart.

intracapsular Within the capsule surrounding a joint.

intracellular Located within the cells.

intracranial Within the skull.

intracutaneous Within the skin.

intradermal Within the dermal layer of the skin.

intraluminar Within a hollow structure.

intramural Within the wall of an organ.

intramuscular Within a muscle.

intranasal Within the nose.

intraocular pressure The pressure within the eyeball.

intraoral Within the mouth.

intrapleural Within the chest cavity.

intraspinal Within the spinal canal.

intrauterine Within the cavity of the uterus.

intravenous Within a vein.

intrinsic Inherent.

introitus The entrance to the vagina.

introspection The examination of one's own thoughts.

introvert An individual whose thoughts dwell on himself and his problems.

intubation The passage of a tube.

intussusception The telescoping of one loop of intestine into another.

inunction An ointment that is rubbed into the skin.

in utero Unborn; within the uterus.

invagination The process of folding in tissue to form a hollow space.
invalid One whose illness interferes with his ability to care for himself.
invasive Referring to a tumor or infection that grows and invades other parts of the body.
inversion State of being upside down.
in vitro Within a test tube.
in vivo Within a living organism.
involuntary Not under the control of the conscious mind.
involution The process of deterioration.
iontophoresis A technique whereby electrically charged ions are passed into mucous membranes or skin in an attempt to treat a local condition.
ipecac A medication that increases secretions and thus promotes the production of phlegm. Also used to stimulate vomiting.
ipsilateral On the same side of the body.
I.Q. Intelligence quotient.
iridectomy The surgical removal of part of the iris of the eye.
iridocyclitis Inflammation of the iris and ciliary body of the eye.
iris The colored portion of the eye.
iritis Inflammation of the iris.
iron An element normally found in the blood. It is present in large quantities in the oxygen-carrying hemoglobin of the red blood cells.
iron lung A respirator used for patients who have paralysis of the muscles of breathing.
irradiation Treatment of a disease with radiation.
irreducible hernia Hernia in which the contents of the hernial sac cannot be replaced in their normal position.
irreversible Unable to be remedied, as irreversible shock.
irrigate To flush or wash out.
irritant A substance administered to produce an irritation, such as a mustard plaster.
ischemia Lack of blood supply to an organ or part caused by obstruction or spasm in the artery supplying it.
ischiopubic bones The bones in which the pubic bones and ischial bones are joined.
ischium The bone on which one places one's weight when sitting.
island A group of cells.
islet-cell tumor A tumor within the cells of the pancreas that secrete insulin.
islets of Langerhans The cells in the pancreas that secrete insulin.
isoimmunization Immunizing a member of a species with antigens derived from the same species.
isolation The confinement and separation of a patient from others.
isolette A heated incubator in which a premature newborn is placed.
isoniazid An antituberculosis drug.
isotonic solution A solution that is compatible with body tissues.
isotope A substance having the same atomic number as another substance but a different atomic weight.
isthmus A narrow portion of an organ or structure.
-itis A suffix meaning "inflammation."
i.v. Intravenous.

J

Jacksonian seizure A convulsive attack in which the convulsion is limited to one side of the body.
Jackson's membrane A film of tissue, present in some people, that binds the appendix and first portion of the large intestine to the side wall of the abdomen.
jaundice Yellow discoloration of the skin and eyes, caused by the presence of bile pigments in the blood.
jaundice, obstructive Jaundice caused by blockage of the flow of bile into the intestines.
jaws The bones that form the mouth. The upper jaw is the maxilla; the lower jaw is the mandible.
jejunum The upper portion of the small intestine, about eight feet in length, extending from the duodenum to the ileum.
jerk A muscular reflex, such as the knee jerk.
joint The place at which two or more connecting bones are joined.
joint fusion A surgical procedure performed for the purpose of joining bones that make up a joint.
joint mouse A loose calcified body found floating in a joint.
jugular vein The large vein on either side of the neck that drains blood from the head to the heart.
juice The secretions of the stomach, intestines, or one of the glands, such as the pancreas.
junction The point where two or more structures come together.

K

Kahn test A blood test for syphilis.
kalemia The presence of potassium in the blood.
Kaopectate A patented medication given in some cases of diarrhea to solidify the feces.
karyokinesis Mitosis, or cell division.
keloid An overgrowth of scar tissue.
keratin The main component of tissues such as the nails and hair.
keratitis Inflammation of the cornea of the eye.
keratoiritis Inflammation of the cornea and the iris.
keratoplasty An operation for transplantation of the cornea.
kernicterus The discoloration and degeneration of the brain and other nerve structures, seen in newborns suffering from a certain type of jaundice.
ketogenesis The process of forming acetone (ketone)

bodies. This leads to acidosis and is seen often in diabetes.

ketonuria The presence of ketone bodies in the urine.

ketosis Acidosis.

kidneys Organs lying in the upper posterior portion of the abdomen. They remove waste products and water from the bloodstream.

kilogram 1,000 grams, about 2⅕ pounds.

kinesthesia The sensation of muscle movements.

kinetics The science of motion.

kleptomania An uncontrollable desire to steal.

Kline test A test for syphilis.

knee The joint between the thigh and the calf.

kneecap The patella; the bone overlying the knee joint.

knee jerk The muscle movement normally found when the tendon below the knee is struck sharply.

knit To heal.

knock-knee A condition in which the knees are together while the ankles are not.

knuckles The joints of the hands.

Koplick spots Whitish spots on the mucous membrane of the mouth that herald the onset of measles.

kyphosis Curvature of the spine in an anterior-posterior direction.

L

labia majora The major lips (folds of skin) of the external female genitals.

labor Childbirth.

labor, false The onset of contractions of the uterus several days before real labor.

labor, induced Labor brought on by the physician.

labor, instrumental Delivery of a child with forceps.

labor, missed A situation in which a dead embryo is retained within the uterus and labor does not begin normally.

labor pains The periodic abdominal pains caused by the contractions of the uterus.

labor, precipitate A childbirth that comes on suddenly, usually before the mother can receive medical assistance.

labor, premature A childbirth taking place before the usual length of pregnancy.

labor, spontaneous A normal childbirth without the use of instruments.

laboratory The site where clinical tests are performed.

labyrinthitis Inflammation of the inner ear, often associated with dizziness and an upset in the sense of balance.

laceration A cut or wound.

lachrymal glands The tear sacs.

lachrymation Crying.

lactalbumin Proteins contained in milk.

lactase A chemical that digests the sugar found in milk.

lactation The secretion of milk from the breast.

lacteals The lymph channels originating in the intestines that carry chyle (fat absorbed from partially digested food).

lactic acid A chemical that helps in the digestion of milk and is therefore occasionally added to formulas.

lactobacillus A species of helpful bacteria found in the intestinal tract. They produce lactic acid.

lactose Milk sugar.

la grippe Influenza.

laity All people outside a profession.

lallation Gibberish; sounds made by infants.

lambda The L-shaped area in the back of the skull where the bones come together.

laminectomy An operation for the removal of the vertebral arch. Usually done in order to approach the spinal cord and for removal of a tumor.

lance To incise.

lanugo The fine hair found on newborn children. It is replaced as the child grows older.

laparotomy An incision through the abdominal wall into the abdominal cavity.

laryngitis Inflammation of the vocal cords and voice box (larynx).

laryngoscope An instrument used for examining the larynx.

laryngospasm Severe spasm and occlusion of the larynx.

larynx The voice box, situated between the base of the tongue and the windpipe (trachea).

Lassar's paste An ointment used in the treatment of eczema and other skin conditions.

lassitude Tiredness; weakness.

latent Not obvious.

lateral Out to the side.

laudanum A tincture of opium, sometimes given to relieve colic.

lavage Washing out the stomach.

laxative A purge.

L.E. Lupus erythematosus.

lead poisoning A disease caused by the ingestion of substances containing lead. It is characterized by severe abdominal cramps, weakness, anemia, black stippling dots in the red blood cells, and discoloration of the gums.

leiomyoma Fibroids of the uterus.

leishmaniasis A disease caused by a parasite and transmitted by the bite of certain flies.

lens The portion of the eye lying behind the pupil that focuses light rays on the retina.

leprosy A chronic infection occurring in tropical countries and associated with loss of sensation in certain parts of the body.

lesion A change in tissue structure due to injury or disease.

lethal Deadly.

lethargic encephalitis Sleeping sickness secondary to an infection of the brain.

lethargy Inactivity; drowsiness.

leukemia A group of malignant, fatal diseases of the white blood cells and blood-forming organs.

leukemoid reaction The presence of blood cells usually seen in the blood in leukemia but actually caused by other factors.

leukocytes White blood cells.

leukocytosis An increase in the number of circulating white blood cells. This occurs during infections and toxic conditions.

leukopenia A lower than normal number of white blood cells in the circulating blood.

leukoplakia A disease with thickening and overgrowth of mucous membrane, sometimes leading to cancer. Seen frequently in the mouth, tongue, or vagina.

leukorrhea A whitish discharge from the vagina.

levulose Fruit sugar.

libido Sexual desire and sex drive.

lichen planus A common skin condition associated with reddish-purple spots on the skin.

lien The spleen.

lienitis Inflammation of the spleen.

ligament The tough connective tissue that holds bones together.

ligation Tying off.

ligature Thread for tying off a blood vessel or other structure.

lightening The change in sensation accompanying the descent of the unborn child into the lower part of the pelvis during the last weeks of pregnancy.

ligneous Hard or woody.

limb An arm or leg.

limbus of the eye The circular area where the colored portion of the eye meets the white of the eye.

linear In a straight line.

lingual Referring to the tongue.

lipase An enzyme produced in the pancreas that aids in the digestion of fats.

lipectomy The surgical removal of excess fat.

lipid Referring to fats and fatlike substances.

lipodystrophy A metabolic disorder in which fat disappears from beneath the skin.

lipoid diseases A group of diseases in which fatlike deposits occur in the spleen, liver, and other organs. Niemann-Pick disease and Gaucher's disease are lipoid diseases.

lipoma A benign fatty tumor.

liposarcoma A malignant tumor originating from fat tissue.

liquefaction Degeneration of a solid into a fluid or semifluid mass.

liter A liquid measure representing 1,000 cc., or 1.056 quarts.

lithiasis The formation of stones within the body.

lithopaxy A procedure whereby a stone in the urinary bladder is crushed and washed out of the bladder. This is performed through a cystoscope.

Little's disease Cerebral palsy in infants.

liver The largest gland in the body, occupying the upper-right and part of the upper-left portions of the abdominal cavity.

lobe A rounded segment or portion of an organ.

lobectomy An operation for the removal of a diseased lobe (one portion) of a lung.

lobotomy An operation performed upon the front portion of the brain in an attempt to relieve certain forms of insanity.

lobule A small portion or small lobe.

local Confined; not widespread.

localized Limited; not generalized.

lockjaw Tetanus.

locomotion The ability to move.

locus A spot; a localized area.

loin The flank; the area just below the ribs in the back of the body.

longitudinal Along the long axis of the body; lengthwise.

lop ears Ears bent over on themselves.

lordosis Excessive arching of the back.

lotion A medicated solution applied to the skin.

Ludwig's angina An infection of the floor of the mouth extending down along the neck toward the larynx.

lues Syphilis.

lumbar puncture The insertion of a needle through the back and into the spinal canal to permit withdrawal of spinal fluid.

lumbar region The lower back.

lumbodorsal Referring to the lower back and part of the chest.

lumbrical muscles Small muscles in the hands and feet.

lumen The passageway inside a hollow organ.

lump A mass or swelling.

lungs The organs of breathing.

lupus erythematosus An acute or chronic disease of the skin and other organs, accompanied by a characteristic butterfly-shaped rash on the skin of the face.

lupus vulgaris Tuberculosis of the skin.

lycine An essential amino acid.

lymph The fluid that is derived from connective tissue and tissues between organs. Lymph travels through lymph channels.

lymphadenitis Inflammation of a lymph node (gland).

lymphadenopathy Any disease of lymph glands.

lymphangioma A benign tumor of lymph tissue.

lymphangitis Inflammation of a lymph channel.

lymphatics The vessels or channels that carry lymph.

lymphoblastoma A malignant tumor of a lymph gland.

lymphocyte A type of white blood cell.

lymphocytosis Increase in the number of lymphocytes in the circulating blood.

lymphoma A tumor composed of lymph-node tissue.

lymphomatosis *See* Hodgkin's disease.

lymphosarcoma A malignant tumor of the lymph nodes.

lysis The receding and decline of symptoms and fever; also, the cutting of adhesions during an operation.

lyssa Rabies.

M

McBurney's incision An oblique incision in the lower-right part of the abdomen, used most commonly when removing the appendix.

macerated Softened as a result of being soaked.

macrocyte An exceptionally large red blood cell.
macrodactyly Marked enlargement of one or more fingers or toes.
macrodontia Overenlargement of the teeth.
macroglossia Enlargement of the tongue.
macromastia Enlarged breasts.
macroscopic Of sufficient size to be seen by the naked eye.
macrostoma A birth deformity in which there is an abnormally large mouth.
magnesium In certain compounds, this element acts as a mild laxative and as an antacid.
magnification Enlargement.
maidenhead The covering tissue of the entrance to the vagina; the hymen.
maimed Crippled.
malacia Softening of an organ or part of an organ as a result of degeneration.
maladjusted Unable to fit into the environment in which one lives.
malady An illness.
malaise A feeling of being ill.
malar bone The cheekbone.
malaria A chronic parasitic disease transmitted by the bite of infected mosquitoes.
malformation A birth deformity.
malignancy Cancer; deadliness.
malignant Dangerous to life; cancerous.
malleable Easily molded.
malleolus Rounded projection of the ankle.
malleolus, lateral The lower end of the fibula on the outer side of the ankle.
malleolus, medial The lower end of the tibia on the inner side of the ankle.
malleus One of the three small bones of the middle ear that transmit sound waves.
malnutrition Undernourished state.
malocclusion Improper meeting of the upper and lower teeth.
malposition Abnormal position.
malpractice Improper or negligent treatment.
Malta fever A chronic infection caused by a germ found in goat's milk; brucellosis; Mediterranean fever.
maltose An intermediate product in the breakdown of starches into simpler sugars.
malunion Poor healing or uniting of the fragments of broken bones.
mammary glands The breasts.
mammilla Nipple of the breast.
mandible The lower jawbone.
maneuver A manual procedure or manipulation.
mania A form of insanity in which there is wild behavior.
manic-depressive A form of psychosis (insanity) associated with periods of great elation and great depression.
manipulation Curing or improving a condition by use of one's hands.
manometer An instrument used to measure the pressure of liquids, such as is used to measure the pressure of spinal fluid.
Mantoux test A skin test for sensitivity to tuberculosis.
manubrium The upper part of the breastbone.
manus The hand.
marasmus Extreme undernourishment.
marble bones A condition in which the bones become much harder than normal.
marrow The soft tissue inside long bones that forms blood cells.
marsupialization An operation in which the walls of a hollow cyst are stitched to the skin.
masculinization The development of male characteristics in a female.
masculinizing tumor of the ovary A tumor that produces male characteristics in a female.
masking of symptoms Concealment of a condition.
masochism An abnormal mental state in which one derives pleasure from being treated cruelly.
mass A lump or tumor.
massage, cardiac An emergency measure carried out when the heart stops beating during an operation.
masseter muscle The main muscle of chewing.
mastectomy An operation for removal of a breast.
masticate To chew.
mastitis Inflammation of the breast.
mastodynia Pain in the breasts.
mastoid bone The bone in back of the ear. It is filled with air cells, which are sometimes infected following a severe infection of the middle ear.
mastoidectomy An operation for the removal of infected mastoid–bone cells.
mastoiditis Inflammation of the mastoid-bone cells behind the ear.
masturbation Obtaining a sexual climax by self-stimulation.
maternal Referring to the mother.
maternity Motherhood.
matrix The basic tissue of an organ.
maturate To ripen or mature.
maturation The process of developing fully.
maturity Full development.
maxillary bone The upper jawbone.
maxillary sinus The antrum; the sinus located in the cheekbone.
maximum The greatest possible quantity.
Mazzini test A reliable test for syphilis.
M.D. Doctor of medicine.
measles A highly contagious virus disease characterized by inflammation of the mucous membranes of the respiratory passages along with high fever and a typical rash.
meatitis Inflammation of the opening of the urethra.
meatotomy Cutting and enlarging an opening, usually having reference to incising the opening in the tip of the penis in a newborn.
meatus An opening.
Meckel's diverticulum An outpouching of part of the wall of the small intestine.
meconium The contents of the intestinal tract of unborn and newborn infants.

media The middle layer of the wall of an artery or vein.
medial Toward the midline of the body; the opposite of lateral.
mediastinitis Inflammation of the tissues in the mediastinum.
mediastinum The space beneath the breastbone containing the heart, aorta, vena cava, trachea, and thymus gland.
medicated Containing a medicine.
medication The giving of a drug or medicine in the treatment of a disease.
medicine The art or science of healing.
medicine, physical The application of physical means to rehabilitate and restore sick or injured people.
medicine, preventive The branch that concentrates on preventing disease.
medicine, psychosomatic The branch dealing with conditions of emotional origin.
medicine, social The branch that concentrates on the social implications of illness.
medicine, tropical The branch dealing with diseases found in tropical countries.
Mediterranean fever *See* Malta fever.
medium The substance in which bacteria are grown in a laboratory.
medulla oblongata The lowermost portion of the brain, just above the beginning of the spinal cord.
medulloblastoma A cancer of the brain.
megacardia Enlargement of the heart.
megacolon Hirschsprung's disease; huge dilatation of the large bowel.
megakaryocyte A very large primitive cell found in bone marrow that eventually forms blood platelets.
megalo- Denotes excessive enlargement of an organ or part.
megaloblast A large primitive cell.
megalocyte A very large primitive red blood cell.
megalomania A mental illness in which the patient has delusions of grandeur.
Meibomian glands Small glands in the eyelids.
melancholia A mental depression.
melanin Dark-brown pigment in the skin, hair, eyes, and other tissues.
melanoblastoma A malignant tumor of the skin originating from primitive pigment cells.
melanocyte A pigment cell containing melanin.
melanoma A cancer derived from cells containing pigments, usually a mole.
melena Black, tarry stools caused by the presence of altered blood following bleeding higher up in the intestinal tract.
melotia A birth deformity in which the ear is displaced onto the cheek.
membrana tympani The eardrum.
membrane A thin layer of tissue.
membrane, fetal Tissue surrounding the embryo within the uterus; the chorion, amnion, and allantois.
membrane, mucous Tissue that secretes mucus. It lines the nose, throat, and lungs, and intestinal, urinary, and genital tracts.
membrane, placental Tissue that separates the blood circulation of the mother and that of the unborn child.
membrane, serous A thin layer of cells lining body cavities.
membrane, synovial A thin layer of tissue lining joints.
membrane, tympanic The eardrum.
menarche The beginning of menstruation.
Mendelian law The law of heredity that certain characteristics are distributed in offspring on the basis of their dominance or recessiveness.
Ménière's disease A disease caused by upset in sodium metabolism, characterized by intense dizziness and vertigo.
meningeal Referring to the membranes covering the brain and spinal cord.
meninges The three membranes (pia, arachnoid, and dura mater) covering the brain and spinal cord.
meningioma A tumor composed of the tissues that cover the brain or spinal cord.
meningismus Inflammation of the coverings of the brain and spinal cord secondary to some disease such as measles, whooping cough, or pneumonia.
meningitis Inflammation and infection of the membranes covering the brain and spinal cord. This serious disease may be caused by any number of different germs, such as the meningococcus, pneumococcus, or streptococcus.
meningocele A birth deformity in which there is a hernia around the covering of the brain or spinal cord through a defect in the bones of the skull or vertebral column.
meningococcus A germ that causes inflammation of the coverings of the brain and spinal cord.
meningoencephalitis Inflammation or infection of the brain, the spinal cord, and their covering membranes.
meniscus The crescent-shaped cartilage lying on the tibia within the knee joint. It is frequently injured during athletic activities.
menopause Change of life. The climacteric. That time of life when a woman's menstrual periods cease.
menorrhagia Excessive bleeding during menstruation.
menorrhea Excessive menstruation.
menses Menstruation.
menstrual cycle The rhythmic preparation of the uterus to receive a fertilized egg and the discharge of the uterine lining, usually at monthly intervals, when no fertilized egg enters the uterus.
menstruation The discharge, at regular intervals, of blood and fluid from the vagina.
menstruation, anovular Periodic vaginal bleeding without the passage of an egg from the ovary.

mental retardation Arrested mental development; feeble-mindedness.
mercury A chemical element useful as a medication when combined with other substances.
mercury, ammoniated An ointment used to treat various skin conditions.
mercury, bichloride of A solution used to kill germs.
mesenchyme Embryonic tissue that eventually forms connective tissue, blood, blood vessels, and the heart.
mesenteric arteries Two large blood vessels, the superior and inferior, that originate from the abdominal aorta and supply blood to the intestines.
mesentery The tissues that connect the intestine with the posterior wall of the abdominal cavity.
mesial Toward the midline of the body; medial.
mesoderm The primitive tissue of the embryo that goes to form connective tissue, muscles, kidneys, and other organs.
mesomorph A body type characterized by great strength and large muscles.
metabolism The process by which foods are transformed into basic elements that can be used by the body.
metacarpal bones The bones of the hand to which the bones of the fingers are attached.
metaplasia A change in the structure of a tissue into that of another tissue.
metastasis The traveling of a disease process from one part of the body to another.
metatarsal bones The long bones of the foot to which the bones of the toes are attached.
meter A unit of measure, approximately 39⅓ inches.
methemoglobin A form of hemoglobin that is incapable of combining with oxygen and is therefore useless.
methionine An amino acid essential for normal growth.
metrorrhagia Uterine bleeding between menstrual periods.
micrencephalon An abnormally small brain.
micro- Abnormally small.
microbes Bacteria; germs.
microbiology The study of bacteria, viruses, etc.
microcephaly An abnormally small head resulting from premature hardening of the skull and closure of the fontanels.
microcyte An exceptionally small red blood cell.
microdactylia A birth deformity in which the fingers or toes are abnormally small.
micromastia Abnormally small breasts.
micrometer One-millionth of a meter.
microorganisms Bacteria and viruses.
microphotograph A photograph of cells or tissues seen through a microscope.
microscopic So small that it can only be seen under the magnification of a microscope.
microsurgery Surgery performed with special instruments through a microscope on minute structures.
microtome A cutting apparatus that slices extremely thin pieces of tissue so that they can be prepared for microscopic examination.
micturition Urination.
mid In the middle.
midget A dwarf whose bodily parts are in normal proportion to each other.
migraine Severe headache, often associated with spots before the eyes, nausea, and vomiting.
migration The traveling of an egg that has burst forth from the ovary. It migrates to the Fallopian tube and down through the tube to the uterus.
milaria Prickly heat.
miliary The size of a millet seed; less than one millimeter in size.
miliary tuberculosis Tuberculosis that has spread throughout the lungs and is characterized by innumerable small lesions.
milk, acidophilus Milk containing special cultures of a beneficial bacterium known as the *Lactobacillus acidophilus.*
milk, albumin Milk containing large amounts of protein and fat but small quantities of sugar and salt.
milk, casein Same as albumin milk.
milk, certified Extra-pure, rich milk, certified by authorities as meeting high standards.
milk, condensed Milk from which a certain proportion of water has been evaporated and sugar has been added.
milk crusts Scabs on the scalp of a baby with eczema.
milk, dialyzed Milk with the sugar removed.
milk, evaporated Canned milk with approximately half its water removed.
milk fever An old term for fever occurring following childbirth.
milk, fortified Milk to which vitamins, cream, albumin, or other substances have been added.
milk, homogenized Milk treated so that the cream is broken down into tiny particles and therefore does not separate.
milk, modified Milk altered so that its ingredients are in similar proportion to those in mother's milk.
milk, mother's Breast milk.
milk, pasteurized Milk that has been heated for 40 minutes at 60° to 70°C.
milk, protein Milk high in protein and low in sugar and fat content.
milk, skim Milk from which the cream has been taken.
milk, sour Milk that has been acted on by bacteria normally present within the milk itself.
milk, witch's Milk from the breast of a newborn child.
milli- One thousand or one-thousandth.
milliequivalent (**mEq**) The weight of a substance contained in one cubic centimeter of a normal solution.
milligram One-thousandth of a gram.
milliliter One cubic centimeter; about 15 drops.
millimeter One-thousandth of a meter.
min A drop of water.
minim One drop of water.

miosis Contraction of the pupil of the eye.
miscarriage The expulsion of a dead embryo or child.
miscegenation Sexual intercourse between persons of different races.
miscible Able to go into solution.
mites Ticks.
mitosis The division of a living cell.
mitral commissurotomy An operation in which the constricted mitral valve is cut or stretched. Performed to relieve mitral stenosis.
mitral stenosis Deformity of the mitral valve of the heart, usually secondary to rheumatic fever.
mitral valve The valve on the left side of the heart between the upper atrium and lower ventricle.
mittelschmerz Pain in the lower abdomen occurring between menstrual periods.
mixed tumor of the salivary gland A most frequently encountered growth within a salivary gland.
ml. Milliliter; one-thousandth of a liter; 1 cubic centimeter.
mm. Millimeter.
mobilization Freeing an organ from its attachments; also, loosening a stiff joint.
molar One of the large back teeth used for chewing.
molding The overlapping of the bones of the unborn child's skull as it passes through the pelvic outlet in childbirth.
mole A tumor of the skin, often pigmented brown or bluish-black.
molecule The smallest particle of a substance that exhibits all its properties.
molluscum contagiosum A chronic skin condition in which there are isolated, raised, rounded, pea-sized lumps of yellowish-pink hue.
mongolian spot A bluish discoloration of the skin found in the lower back at birth. It usually decreases in size or disappears entirely early in life.
mongolism A form of idiocy, caused by a chromosomal abnormality, in which the facial features resemble those of an Oriental.
moniliasis A fungus infection often seen in the vagina.
mono- One; single.
monocyte A type of white blood cell.
mononucleosis *See* infectious mononucleosis.
monozygotic Developed from one egg.
monster A markedly deformed newborn incapable of sustaining life.
morbid Unhealthy.
morbidity rate The ratio of the number of sick people to the number in the total population.
morbilli Measles.
morcellate To break into fragments.
moribund Dying; unconscious or semiconscious.
moron A mentally deficient person with an I.Q. between 50 and 75.
morphine A chemical compound derived from opium.
morphology The science of anatomy.
mortality The death rate.
motility The ability to move.
mouth-to-mouth breathing Artificial respiration carried out by placing the mouth against the mouth of the patient and forcefully blowing air into it. This is done rhythmically about 20 times per minute until the patient resumes breathing on his own.
movement, bowel Evacuation of stool.
mucocele A cavity filled with mucous secretions.
mucocutaneous junction The areas where skin meets mucous membrane, as at the lips of the mouth or at the margin of the anus and the skin of the buttocks.
mucous Relating to mucus.
mucous membrane A surface membrane composed of cells that secrete various forms of mucus, as the lining of the respiratory and gastrointestinal tracts.
mucous patches The eruptions seen within the mouth and about the lips during the second stage of syphilis.
mucus A thick liquid secreted by mucous glands.
multi- Many.
multipara A woman who has given birth to one or more children.
multiple sclerosis Disseminated sclerosis; a chronic disease of the nervous system leading to partial paralysis.
mumps Epidemic parotitis; a highly contagious virus disease causing swelling of the parotid glands at the angles of the jaw.
murmur An abnormal heart sound heard when listening to the chest with a stethoscope.
muscle Tissue composed of fibers that have the ability to elongate and shorten, thus causing bones and joints to move.
musculoskeletal system The bones, muscles, ligaments, tendons, and joints of the body.
mutation A change in the characteristics of an organism as a result of changes in genes or other hereditary factors.
mutilate To maim.
mutism Dumbness; absence of speech.
myalgia Pain in muscles.
myasthenia gravis A serious chronic debilitating disease associated with wasting of muscles, especially those muscles which enable a patient to swallow.
myatonia Lack of muscle tone.
mycoid Resembling a fungus.
mycology The study of funguses.
mycosis An infection caused by a fungus.
mydriasis Dilatation of the pupil of the eye.
myelemia A form of leukemia in which there are many myelocytes (primitive white blood cells).
myelin The sheath surrounding certain nerves.
myelitis Inflammation of the spinal cord.
myelo- Referring to the bone marrow or spinal cord.

myeloblast A primitive cell in the bone marrow that eventually emerges as a white blood cell.

myelocyte A primitive cell that eventually develops into a mature white blood cell.

myelography X-ray of the spinal canal carried out after the injection of a dye that will show up on the x-ray film.

myeloma A malignant tumor of bone marrow.

myelomalacia Degeneration and softening of the spinal cord leading to paralysis.

myenteric Referring to the muscles in the wall of the intestines.

myesthesia Awareness of one's own muscle functionings.

myo- Referring to muscles.

myocarditis Inflammation of the heart muscles.

myocardium Heart muscle.

myoma A benign tumor of muscle.

myomalacia Degeneration of muscle.

myometrium The muscle of the wall of the uterus.

myopia Nearsightedness.

myosarcoma A malignant tumor of muscle.

myositis Muscle inflammation.

myotomy A surgical incision of muscle.

myotonia A spasm of muscle.

myringitis Inflammation of the eardrum.

myringotomy Surgical incision of the eardrum, performed to remove pus from the middle ear.

myxedema A metabolic disorder caused by insufficient function of the thyroid gland (hypothyroidism).

myxo- Referring to mucus, mucous glands, or mucous tissue.

myxoma A tumor of connective tissue.

myxosarcoma A malignant tumor of connective tissue.

N

nail The horny growths of tissue that protrude from the toes and fingertips.

nailbed The soft tissue beneath the nail.

nail, ingrown A condition in which the sharp edge of the nail, usually of the big toe, grows into the flesh alongside the nail.

nanism Dwarfism.

nape The back of the neck.

narcissism Love of oneself; sexual feelings for oneself.

narcolepsy A period of deep sleep, usually brought on by an epileptic attack.

narcosis A state of deep stupor produced by a drug.

narcotic A drug that produces sleep or stupor.

narcotism Narcotic addiction.

narcotize To produce an unconscious state.

nares The nostrils.

nasal Pertaining to the nose.

nasolabial Pertaining to the nose and lips.

nasolachrymal Referring to the nose and tear glands and ducts.

nasopharyngitis Inflammation of the nose and throat.

nasopharynx The nose and throat.

natality Birthrate.

natremia A condition in which there is too much sodium in the blood.

natural childbirth A method of childbirth in which as few artificial procedures as possible are carried out.

nausea The feeling that one may vomit.

navel The umbilicus; the site at which the child was attached to the mother by the umbilical cord.

navicular bone A boat-shaped bone of the wrist or ankle.

nearsightedness Myopia; a condition in which the eyeball is too long and the image falls short of the retina. Close objects are seen more clearly than distant objects.

neck That portion of the anatomy between the head and the chest.

necropsy Autopsy.

necrosis Death of tissue.

needle biopsy Removal of a small piece of tissue from a tumor with a specially devised needle.

negative result A method of indicating that a medical test is normal.

Neisserian infection Gonorrhea.

nematode Roundworm.

neonatal Newborn.

neonatal mortality. The death rate among newborns and infants during their first month of life.

neoplasm A tumor or growth.

nephrectomy Surgical removal of a kidney.

nephritis Inflammation of a kidney.

nephrolithiasis Stones in the kidney.

nephroma A malignant tumor of a kidney.

nephron The part of the kidney that secretes urine.

nephropexy An operation to replace a kidney into its normal position; carried out when a kidney has dropped out of position.

nephroptosis A "dropped" kidney.

nephrosis Degeneration of the kidney, a serious metabolic disease seen in infants and young children.

nerve The structure that transmits impulses and stimuli to and from the brain and spinal cord.

nerve, afferent A nerve that transmits impulses from the tissues to the brain and spinal cord.

nerve, autonomic A nerve of the involuntary system, which supplies the internal organs and other structures such as blood vessels.

nerve, cerebrospinal A nerve having its origin in the brain or spinal cord.

nerve, cranial A nerve that originates from the brain and exits through one of the openings in the skull.

nerve, efferent A nerve that transmits impulses from the brain and spinal cord to the tissues of the body.

nerve ending The point at which a nerve enters the structure it supplies.

nerve, motor A nerve that supplies muscles and causes them to contract.
nerve, parasympathetic A nerve of the involuntary system, such as those supplying the lungs and heart.
nerve, sensory A nerve that travels toward the spinal cord or brain and transmits sensations such as pain, heat, cold, and touch.
nerve, spinal A nerve having its origin in the spinal cord.
nerve, sympathetic A nerve of the sympathetic (involuntary) system, which causes blood vessels to contract and blood pressure to rise.
nerve tract The course of a nerve.
nervousness The condition of being overly excitable or sensitive.
neural Pertaining to nerves.
neuralgia Pain along a nerve.
neurasthenia Lack of energy; listlessness; fatigue.
neurectomy, presacral An operation wherein a small nerve in the lower abdomen is severed; undertaken to relieve excessive pain on menstruation.
neurilemma The covering or sheath of a nerve fiber.
neurilemmoma A tumor, usually benign, of the sheath of a nerve.
neuritis Inflammation of a nerve.
neurodermatitis A skin disease accompanied by an itching rash seen mainly on the neck, elbows, and knees of people who are nervous.
neurofibroma A nonmalignant tumor composed of nerves and fibrous tissue.
neurofibromatosis An inherited condition in which there are many tumors in the nerves to the skin and the tissues beneath the skin. Also called von Recklinghausen's disease.
neurogenic Arising from a nerve.
neurologist A physician who specializes in diseases of the nervous system.
neuroma A nerve tumor.
neuron A nerve.
neuropsychiatrist A physician who specializes in both nervous and mental diseases.
neurosis An emotional or psychological disorder. Not insanity.
neurosurgery Surgery of the brain, spinal cord, and nerves.
neurosyphilis Syphilis involving the brain or spinal cord.
neurotoxin A poison that affects a nerve or nerve tissue.
neutral Referring to a solution that is neither acid nor alkaline.
neutron An electrically neutral atomic particle.
neutropenia Decrease in the number of white blood cells in the circulation.
neutrophil A white blood cell.
nevus A mole.
newborn An infant up to the first three to five days of life.
new growth A tumor or neoplasm.
niacin Nicotinic acid; part of the vitamin-B complex.
nicotinic acid The vitamin that prevents the disease known as pellagra.
nictation Winking of the eyelids.
nidus A focus of infection.
Niemann-Pick disease A fatal disease affecting young children in which there is enlargement of the liver and spleen, anemia, and mental deterioration.
nightmare A horrible dream accompanied by agitation and fright.
night sweats Excessive perspiration during sleep.
nipple The outlet of the milk ducts in the breast.
nitremia An excess of nitrogen in the blood, as in uremia.
nitrogen (N) An element making up about 77 percent of the air one breathes.
nitrous oxide An anesthetic gas; "laughing gas."
noctambulation Sleepwalking.
nocturia Getting up at night to urinate.
nocturnal Occurring during the night.
node A small, round structure such as a lymph gland.
nodule A small node.
noma A severe, sometimes fatal ulcerating condition of the mouth.
nonallergenic Referring to a substance that will not cause an allergic reaction.
nonmalignant Not cancerous.
nonmotile Incapable of motion.
nonprotein nitrogen An important element of the blood.
nonpyogenic Referring to bacteria that do not produce pus.
nonspecific General.
nonsurgical Not requiring surgery.
nonunion Failure of broken fragments of bone to fuse.
nonviable Not able to live, as an embryo or fetus that has not yet reached the sixth month of development.
norm The normal; the average.
normal Conforming to a standard.
normoblast An immature red blood cell.
nose The organ of smell.
nostalgia Homesickness.
nostril One of the orifices of the nose.
notochord The structure in the embryo from which the spinal column develops.
Novocain A patented local anesthetic; procaine.
noxious Poisonous.
nuchal Referring to the back of the neck.
nuclear Referring to the nucleus or the center of the cell.
nucleolus A small, rounded spot within the nucleus of a cell.
nucleus The central living portion of a cell; that part containing the chromosomes and genes.
nulliparous Never having borne a child.
numbness Diminished sensation.
nurse A person who attends the sick.
nurse, dry A nurse who takes care of an infant but does not suckle him.
nurse, graduate A nurse holding a diploma from an approved school of nursing.

nurse, practical A nurse who is trained and licensed to care for patients but who has not received the R.N. degree.
nurse, registered A nurse who holds the R.N. degree from a school of nursing.
nurse, wet A nurse who suckles or breast-feeds an infant not her own.
nursling A nursing infant.
nutrient Nourishment.
nutrition The process of digestion and utilization of food substances.
nux vomica A stimulant drug containing strychnine.
nyctophobia Fear of the dark.
nystagmus A rapid, rhythmic, side-to-side movement of the eyeball seen in disorders of the brain.
nyxis Puncturing with a needle.

O

obesity Overweight.
obfuscation The process of becoming mentally disoriented or confused.
objective signs Conditions in an illness that can be seen or felt by the physician.
obliterate Surgically, to remove a part completely.
obsession A thought that continues in one's mind despite all attempts to forget it.
obstetrics The branch of medicine dealing with childbirth.
obstipation Absolute inability to move the bowels.
obstruction, intestinal A condition in which the passage of stool is obstructed.
obstruction, pyloric Obstruction of the outlet of the stomach seen in newborns. It is caused by an overgrowth of the muscles of the pylorus.
obstruction, ureteral Obstruction to the passage of urine along the ureter, usually due to a stone.
obtund To lessen or do away with, as anesthesia obtunds sensation.
obturator The opening in the pelvis located between the pubic and ischial bones.
occipital region The lower portion of the back of the head.
occiput The back of the head.
occlusion Shutting off, as of the blood flow to a part.
occult Not evident.
occupational disease A disease associated with the type of work or employment of a patient.
ocular Pertaining to the eye.
oculomotor Referring to the movement of the eye.
oculomotor nerve The third cranial nerve, which supplies muscles that move the eyeball.
odontoma A tumor originating from a tooth.
Oedipal Referring to the Oedipus complex, the psychoanalytic theory that in the development of the child there is a period in which love for the parent of the opposite sex and accompanying unconscious enmity for the parent of the same sex are extremely important.
ointment A salve.
olecranon The end of the ulna bone at the elbow.
olfactory Referring to the sense of smell.
olfactory nerve The first cranial nerve, which controls the sense of smell.
oligo- Scant; little.
oligomenorrhea Infrequent menstruation.
oligospermia A condition in which the number of sperm ejaculated is abnormally small.
oliguria The passage of a scant amount of urine.
-ology A suffix meaning "the science of."
-oma A suffix meaning "tumor."
omentum An apronlike, fatty membrane hanging down from the stomach and transverse colon in the abdominal cavity.
omphalectomy Surgical removal of the navel, often carried out in repairing a large hernia of the umbilicus.
omphalitis An inflammation of the navel.
omphalocele A birth deformity in which the umbilicus has failed to close and skin fails to grow over it.
onanism Masturbation.
onco- Relating to tumors.
oncology The science of tumors.
ontogeny The whole development of a single organism.
onychia Inflammation of the nailbed of a finger or toe.
onychophagy Nail biting.
oocyte An unfertilized egg cell.
oogenesis Development of an egg within the ovary before its expulsion.
oophorectomy Surgical removal of an ovary.
opacity Nontransparency.
opaque Nontransparent.
open reduction Setting a fracture by making a surgical incision and exposing the broken bones.
operable Able to be corrected or improved by surgery.
operation Any surgical procedure.
operative risk The chances of how well or how badly a patient will withstand surgery.
ophidism Poisoning due to snakebite.
ophthalmectomy Surgical removal of an eye.
ophthalmia Inflammation of the eye.
ophthalmia neonatorum Gonorrheal inflammation of the eyes of a newborn.
ophthalmologist A physician who specializes in diseases of the eye.
ophthalmoscope An instrument used to examine the interior of the eye.
opiate A medication containing opium or an opium derivative.
opisthotonos A spasm of the muscles of the back causing such arching that only the head and the feet touch the bed; seen in the convulsion of tetanus.
opium An extract of the poppy plant used as a medication to relieve pain and induce sleep.
opsonin A substance in the blood that acts on bacteria and makes them susceptible to destruction by white blood cells.

optical Pertaining to the sense of sight.
optician One who makes eyeglasses, lenses, or who refracts eyes to note the necessary type of eyeglass which should be worn.
optic nerve The second cranial nerve, which is the main nerve to the eye.
optic neuritis Inflammation and degeneration of the main nerve to the eye.
optimum The best condition.
optometer An instrument for determining errors in vision.
optometrist One who measures or refracts eyes to note the need for eyeglasses.
oral Referring to the mouth.
oral hypoglycemic drugs Drugs taken by mouth to lower blood sugar levels, now being prescribed in the treatment of certain cases of diabetes.
orbicular muscles Circular muscles that surround the eyes and the mouth.
orbit The bony socket in the skull in which the eye is set.
orchidectomy Surgical removal of a testicle.
orchidopexy An operation for undescended testicle.
orchitis Inflammation of a testicle.
organ A specialized body structure performing a specific function.
organic disease A disease associated with changes in structure rather than upset in function; the opposite of a functional disease.
organism Anything that lives.
orgasm The climax of a sexual act.
oriented Aware of one's surroundings.
orifice An opening in a body cavity, such as the nostrils or vagina.
oropharynx The mouth and throat.
ortho- Straight; normal.
orthodontist A dentist who specializes in straightening the teeth.
orthopedics The branch of medicine concerned with diseases and conditions of bones, muscles, tendons, etc.
orthopnea The need to sit up in order to breathe, usually associated with heart or lung disorders.
orthopsychiatry The branch of psychiatry that deals mainly with emotional or mental problems of children.
orthoptics Exercises to improve the function of the eye muscles.
orthostatic albuminuria Albumin in the urine in patients who stand in one position for long periods of time.
os A mouth; also, a bone.
os calcis The heelbone.
oscillation Vibration.
Osgood-Schlatter disease An inflammation of the tibia near the knee joint, seen mainly in adolescent boys.
osmology The study of the sense of smell.
osmosis The passage of a substance through a membrane from a dilute to a concentrated solution.
osseous Relating to bones.
ossicles The three small bones of hearing in the middle ear (malleus, incus, and stapes).
ossification The transformation of nonbony tissue into bony tissue.
osteitis Inflammation of bone.
osteitis deformans Inflammation of the bone, often accompanied by marked deformity.
osteitis fibrosa cystica Inflammation and deformation of bones secondary to excessive activity of the parathyroid glands.
osteo- Relating to bone.
osteoarthritis A form of arthritis associated with bone and cartilage degeneration; seen most often in aging people.
osteochondritis Inflammation of a bone and its cartilage.
osteochondroma A benign tumor of bone and cartilage.
osteochondrosis Degeneration of bone growth centers in the bones of rapidly growing children.
osteodystrophy Imperfect bone formation secondary to disease, as in rickets.
osteofibrosis Degeneration of the bone marrow.
osteogenesis imperfecta A birth deformity of unknown cause in which there is imperfect bone formation, brittleness of bones, and many fractures.
osteogenic sarcoma A highly malignant bone tumor.
osteoid osteoma A benign tumor occurring in the middle, softer portions of a bone.
osteoma A benign bone tumor.
osteomalacia Softening of bone.
osteomyelitis An infection of bone.
osteopath One who follows a branch of healing which states that functional and structural interdependence are essential for the maintenance of health. Osteopaths often treat disease by concentrating on the bones, muscles, and joints.
osteopetrosis Hardening of the bone. It is a rare inherited disease, also called marble bones.
osteoporosis A loss in bony substance producing softness of bones.
osteosarcoma A bone malignancy.
osteotomy A surgical incision into a bone.
otalgia An earache.
otic Relating to the ear.
otitis media Inflammation of the middle ear, often seen following upper-respiratory infections in children.
otolaryngology The study of the ear, nose, and throat.
otology The branch of medicine dealing with diseases of the ear.
-otomy A suffix meaning "surgical incision into."
otoplasty Plastic surgery on the ears.
otorrhea A discharge from the ears.
otosclerosis A form of deafness.
otoscope A lighted instrument for examining the ear canal and eardrum.
ovarian Referring to the ovaries.
ovarian follicle A sac or cavity within an ovary containing an egg.

ovariectomy Removal of an ovary.

ovary The female reproductive gland.

overbite A condition in which the teeth of the upper jaw overlap the teeth of the lower jaw markedly.

oviduct The Fallopian tube; the hollow tube, leading from the abdominal cavity to the uterine cavity, that transports the egg.

ovular Relating to an egg (ovum).

ovulation The process during which an egg is released from the ovary.

ovule The egg before it leaves the ovary.

ovum An egg.

oxidation The process of combining with oxygen.

oxygen An odorless gas necessary for life. Atmospheric air contains approximately 20 percent oxygen.

oxyhemoglobin A combination of oxygen and hemoglobin in red blood cells.

oxyuriasis An infestation of the intestine with pinworms, resulting in inflammation of the bowels and rectum.

oz. Ounce.

P

pacifier A rubber nipple given to an infant to satisfy his urge to suck.

pack A moist, wet dressing.

pad A gauze pad used as a dressing for a wound.

Paget's disease
1. Paget's disease of the bones is a disturbance in its metabolism associated with loss of calcium and eventually replacement in an irregular manner. This causes considerable thickening and bone deformity.
2. Paget's disease of the nipple is accompanied by thickening of the skin and scaling. It is due to underlying cancer of the breast.

pain Hurt.

palate The roof of the mouth.

palate, cleft A birth deformity in which the two sides of the palate fail to meet in the midline, thus leaving an opening between the nasal and mouth cavities.

palate, hard The part of the roof of the mouth that is covered by bone.

palate, soft The part of the roof of the mouth that is behind the hard palate and is composed of soft tissue.

palliation Relief of a condition without curing it.

palliative A medication given to relieve, not to cure.

pallor Paleness.

palm The inner surface of the hand.

palpable Able to be felt.

palpation The act of feeling.

palpebral Referring to the eyelids.

palpitation Feeling one's own heartbeat, usually associated with pounding, rapid heart action.

palsy Nerve paralysis; also, a tremor.

palsy, Bell's A paralysis of one side of the face, resulting in a drooping eyelid, inability to close the eyelid completely, and a twisting and drooping of the corner of the mouth.

palsy, birth Paralysis, usually of the shoulder and upper arm, caused by injury during childbirth.

palsy, bulbar A fatal disease in which there is degeneration of vital nerves in the brain.

palsy, cerebral Paralysis caused by a defect within the brain, often present from birth.

panarthritis Inflammation of many joints.

pancarditis Inflammation of all the structural components of the heart, seen in severe rheumatic fever.

pancreas An abdominal gland lying crosswise in the upper abdomen. It secretes enzymes into the intestine for the digestion of food, and it produces insulin, which is secreted into the bloodstream.

pancreatic cystic fibrosis An inherited disease of newborns that affects the pancreas and many other organs of the body. It is characterized by foul-smelling stools containing undigested fat. (Now called simply cystic fibrosis.)

pancreatitis Inflammation of the pancreas.

pandemic disease A disease occurring in epidemic proportions covering a very wide area of territory.

panniculus The layer of fat beneath the skin.

pansinusitis Inflammation of all the nasal sinuses.

panus An inflamed lymph node.

Papanicolaou test A cancer smear. The vagina and cervix of the uterus are swabbed with cotton and the cells so obtained are placed under the microscope to see if any of them are cancer cells.

papilla A small nipple-shaped prominence of tissue.

papilledema Swelling of the optic nerves in the back of the eye as seen through an ophthalmoscope.

papilloma A benign growth of surface-lining cells, such as mucous membrane or skin.

papule A pimple or pimplelike formation.

para- Next to; resembling.

para-aminosalicylic acid (PAS) A valuable drug in the treatment of tuberculosis.

paracentesis Tapping a body cavity with a needle in order to withdraw fluid.

paralysis Inability to use muscles because of disease and injury to the nerves that supply them.

paramecium A form of one-celled organism; a protozoan.

paramedial Located alongside the midline.

paranasal sinuses The sinuses near the nose.

paranoid state A state in which an individual has delusions of persecution.

paraphimosis Inflammation of the foreskin of the penis.

paraplegic An individual with both lower limbs paralyzed.

pararectal abscess An abscess alongside the rectum.

parasite An organism that lives at the expense of another.

parasitic disease A disease caused by an infestation with parasites, such as malaria, amebic dysentery, and worm diseases.

parasitology The study of parasitic organisms.

parasympathetic nerves The nerves of the autonomic or involuntary nervous system, which supply the eyes, glands, heart, and abdominal organs.

parathormone The hormone secreted by the parathyroid glands in the neck.

parathyroid glands Four small endocrine glands in the neck behind the thyroid. They secrete the hormone that controls calcium and phosphorus metabolism.

paratyphoid fever A disease resembling typhoid but caused by a different germ (salmonella).

paregoric A medication used to stop diarrhea and colic.

parenchymal tissue The part of an organ that is responsible for its main function.

parenteral medication Medicine given through a route other than the mouth.

paresis Incomplete or partial paralysis.

paresthesia A tingling, burning sensation.

parietal Referring to the wall of a cavity.

parietal bones Major bones of the skull lying behind the frontal bones. They make up the top of the head.

Parkinsonism A nervous disease involving a rhythmic tremor, masklike appearance to the face, rigidity of muscle action, and slowing of all body motion. Also called paralysis agitans or shaking palsy.

parodonitis Inflammation around a tooth.

paronychia Inflammation around a fingernail; a "run-around."

parotid gland A salivary gland located at the angle of the jaw.

parotitis Inflammation of the parotid gland.

parovarian Located next to the ovary.

paroxysm A convulsion; a severe spasm.

parrot fever A severe infection caused by a germ transmitted from parrots and other birds; psittacosis.

pars A part of an organ.

parthenogenesis Reproduction without fertilization.

parturition Childbirth.

PAS Para-aminosalicylic acid, an antituberculosis drug.

passage A channel through an organ or structure.

passive Caused without active effort.

pasteurization The process of destroying the harmful germs in milk by heating it for 40 minutes at 60° to 70°C.

patch test A skin test to discover sensitivity to irritants, performed by applying an irritant to the skin and covering it with an adhesive patch.

patella The kneecap.

patent Wide-open.

pathogenic Relating to the ability to cause disease.

pathognomonic Relating to special signs and symptoms that distinguish a particular disease from others.

pathologist A physician who specializes in the study of the nature of disease by studying tissues.

pathology The science dealing with the nature of disease on the basis of tissue examination.

patient One who is under the care of a physician.

patulous Open.

pectineal Referring to the region of the pubic bones.

pectoral muscles The chest muscles.

pectus A general term denoting the chest or breast.

pediatrician A physician who specializes in diseases of children.

pedicle graft A skin graft transferred from one part of the body to another by use of a stalk or pedicle.

pediculosis A skin condition caused by lice.

pediculosis capitis Lice on the scalp.

pediculosis corporis Lice on the body.

pediculosis palpebrarum Lice in the eyebrows.

pediculosis pubic Lice in the pubic hair.

pedology Pediatrics.

pedophilia Love of children; also, sexual feelings of an adult for a child.

pedunculated Attached by a narrow stalk.

pellagra A vitamin-deficiency disease caused by lack of nicotinic acid.

pelvimetry, X-ray X-rays taken before childbirth to determine the size of the walls of the pelvis and the child's head.

pelvis The bony ring formed by all the bones in the hip region, including the sacrum, coccyx, ilium, ischium, and pubic bones.

pelvis, renal The portion of the kidney where the ureter commences.

pemphigus A very serious skin disease associated with large blisters and areas of gangrene.

pendulous Hanging down.

penetrating Piercing, as a penetrating ulcer that is eating through the wall of an organ.

penicillin An antibiotic derived from the fungus *Penicillium notatum*.

penis The male sex organ.

penis envy In psychoanalysis, the envy of the female child for the organ she lacks.

Penrose drain A rubber drain used in surgical wounds.

Pentothal An intravenous general anesthetic.

pepsin An enzyme secreted by the intestinal tract that aids in the digestion of protein and other food substances.

peptic Referring to digestion.

peptic ulcer An ulcer of the stomach, duodenum, or lower end of the esophagus.

peptone A basic protein.

perception The ability to recognize and interpret stimuli.

percussion Tapping various parts of the body and noting the sound that is made.

percutaneous Through the skin.

perennial Lasting throughout the year; also, lasting for several years.

perforated Pierced; ruptured.

perfusion The pouring or injecting of a fluid into or through an organ or structure.
peri- Around; near.
perianal Located near the anus.
periarthritis Inflammation of the tissues surrounding a joint.
pericarditis Inflammation of the sheath surrounding the heart.
pericardium The sheath of tissue encasing the heart.
perichondritis Inflammation around the cartilage of a joint.
perinephric abscess An abscess located around the kidney.
perineum The tissue between the anus and scrotum in the male or between the anus and the vaginal opening in the female.
periosteum The thin tissue encasing bones.
periostitis Inflammation or infection of the periosteum.
peripheral Near the surface; distant; the opposite of proximal.
perisplenitis Inflammation of the covering of the spleen.
peristalsis Contractions of the intestines, occurring in waves, that propel the intestinal contents onward. A normal process.
perithelium Tissue surrounding small blood vessels and capillaries.
peritoneum The lining membrane of the abdominal cavity.
peritonitis Infection of the abdominal lining and cavity.
peritonitis, adhesive Inflammation of the abdominal lining resulting in the formation of adhesions.
peritonitis, aseptic Inflammation of the lining of the abdominal cavity caused by chemicals rather than bacteria.
peritonitis, diffuse Inflammation of the entire abdominal lining.
peritonitis, localized Inflammation of one area of the abdominal lining.
peritonitis, pelvic Inflammation of the abdominal lining associated with disease in the pelvic organs.
peritonitis, purulent Peritonitis associated with pus-forming bacteria.
peritonitis, septic Peritonitis associated with pus and a severe toxic reaction.
peritonsillar abscess Quinsy sore throat; an abscess of the tonsils that has spread to the tissues surrounding it.
perivascular Located around a blood vessel.
perlèche Cracking of the skin in the corners of the mouth, thought to be due to a vitamin-B deficiency.
permeable Allowing solutions and fine particles to pass through.
pernicious anemia Primary anemia; Addison's anemia; a specific type of anemia associated with lack of acid in the stomach.
pernio Chilblain.
peroneal Referring to the region on the outer side of the legs.
peroral Through the mouth.
per os By mouth.
peroxide A common name for hydrogen peroxide (H_2O_2).
per rectum Through the rectum.
perspire To sweat.
Perthes' disease A characteristic disease of the bone involving inflammation of the head and neck of the femur at the hip joint.
pertussis Whooping cough.
perversion A deviation from the usual.
pes Foot.
petechiae Small hemorrhages into the skin or mucous membranes.
petit mal A minor epileptic attack.
petrous bone Part of the temporal bone on the side of the skull.
Peyer's patches Patches of lymphlike tissue in the mucous membrane of the intestine.
phagocyte A cell that can eat or destroy foreign matter or bacteria.
phagocytosis The process whereby phagocytes destroy circulating viruses, foreign bodies, or bacteria.
phalanges The bones of the fingers or toes.
phallic Pertaining to the penis.
phallus The penis.
phantasy Fantasy; a mental impression based on imagination.
pharmacology The science dealing with the nature and action of drugs.
pharyngitis Sore throat; inflammation of the mucous membranes of the pharynx.
pharynx The area in the back of the nose and mouth; the throat.
phenobarbital One of the most popularly used barbiturate drugs, used to calm nerves and induce sleep.
phenomenon A sign or manifestation of a disease.
pheochromocytoma A tumor of the adrenal glands associated with marked increase in blood pressure.
phimosis A condition in which the foreskin cannot be withdrawn over the head of the penis.
phlebitis Inflammation of a vein.
phlebolith A calcified deposit in a vein.
phlebotomy Bloodletting.
phlegm Secretions of mucus from the lungs or bronchial tubes.
phlegmatic Slow; sluggish.
phobia An excessive fear.
phocomelia A birth deformity in which there is absence of an arm, forearm, thigh, or a leg, but the hand or the foot is present and attached directly to the body.
photophobia Inability to withstand bright light.
phrenetic Frantic.
phrenic Pertaining to the diaphragm.
phrenic nerves The nerves to the diaphragm.
phylogeny The complete development of a species.
physiatrics Physical medicine.
physic A laxative.
physical examination The inspection and examination of the body by a physician.
physiognomy Physical appearance.

physiology The science that studies the function of tissues and organs.
physiotherapy Treatment that utilizes physical agents.
phytobezoar A ball of foreign body found in the stomachs of people who have eaten large quantities of nondigestible materials such as hair.
phytosis A disease caused by a vegetable parasite, such as in athlete's foot.
pia mater The membrane covering the brain and spinal cord that contains the blood vessels.
Pick's disease Degeneration of the brain seen in infants.
pigeon breast A deformity of the breastbone causing it to resemble the breast of a pigeon.
pigeon-toe A foot deformity characterized by walking with the toes turned in.
pigmentation Discoloration of skin surfaces by pigment.
pile Hemorrhoid.
piliform Hairlike.
pilleus The membranes occasionally found covering the head of a newborn.
pilonidal cyst A sinus and cyst located at the base of the spine, usually containing an accumulation of hairs.
pilosis Excessive growth of hair.
pimple A small abscess.
pinch graft Skin grafting in which a small pinch of skin is placed over the raw area.
pineal gland A small gland in the base of the brain whose function is not clearly known. Tumors of this structure may occur in children and are accompanied by precocious sexual development.
pink-eye Conjunctivitis; inflammation of the eye due to a specific organism; also known as Koch-Weeks conjunctivitis.
pinna The outer ear.
pinworm A parasite that sometimes invades the intestinal tract, causing inflammation of the bowel and rectal itching.
pisiform A small bone in the wrist.
pituitary gland An important endocrine gland located at the base of the brain. Its hormones regulate growth and control the secretions of other endocrine glands, such as the thyroid, adrenals, ovaries, and testicles.
pityriasis rosea A skin disease sometimes accompanied by fever for a few weeks and characterized by pale-red patches over the body.
placebo A medicine having no active ingredients that is given for the purpose of pleasing or calming a patient.
placenta The structure by which the embryo is attached to the wall of the uterus; the afterbirth.
placenta, abruptio *See* abruptio placenta.
placenta previa A condition in which serious hemorrhage occurs during the latter part of pregnancy.
plague A highly contagious, often fatal epidemic disease with high fever, enlargement of the lymph glands, and mental confusion. It is transmitted to man by the bite of infected fleas from rats.
plane A natural dividing line between tissues.
plantar warts Warts on the sole of the foot.
plasma The fluid portion of the blood, minus the red and white blood cells.
Plasmodium The parasite that causes malaria.
plaster cast A hard appliance made of plaster of Paris to encase a limb that has been injured.
plastic surgery Surgery devoted to altering the shape of parts of the body or to the restoration of lost tissues.
platelets, blood Thrombocytes; the small colorless disks in circulating blood that aid in blood clotting.
platyhelminthes Flatworms; tapeworms.
platysma A thin sheet of muscle located beneath the skin of the chin and neck.
pledget A cotton ball.
pleomorphic Relating to malignant cells that have a common origin but widely different appearances.
plethoric Having an excess of blood.
pleura The membrane lining the chest cavity and covering the lungs.
pleurisy Inflammation of the lining of the chest cavity.
pleuritis Pleurisy.
pleurodynia A condition in which there is sudden severe pain in the side of the chest. It lasts a few days and disappears spontaneously.
plexus A network of nerves or blood vessels.
plicate In surgery, to fold tissue so it can form a double layer.
plug, mucous Secretion obstructing the bronchial tubes.
plumbism Lead poisoning.
pneumo- Air.
pneumococcus A germ causing pneumonia.
pneumoconioses Chronic inflammation of the lungs caused by the prolonged inhalation of certain types of dusts.
pneumoencephalography X-ray examination of the brain carried out after injecting air into the cerebrospinal space surrounding the brain.
pneumohemothorax Air and blood in the chest cavity surrounding the lungs.
pneumonectomy Removal of a lung surgically.
pneumonia Inflammation of the lungs, caused by the pneumonia germ, a virus, the influenza germ, or any other type of bacteria or virus.
pneumonitis Inflammation of the lungs.
pneumoperitoneum Air in the abdominal cavity.
pneumothorax Air in the chest cavity surrounding the lungs.
pockmark A scar left from a small pimple associated with chickenpox or smallpox.
podiatrist A specialist, not a physician, in conditions affecting the feet.
poikilocytes Irregularly shaped red blood cells.
poikilothermic Cold-blooded; unable to regulate body tem-

perature to counter the environment.

pointing Coming to a head (said of an abscess).

poisoning A toxic condition caused by bacteria, drugs, medications, spoiled foods, bites, and other agents.

poison ivy A vine that, on contact, can cause an allergic skin inflammation.

poison oak A plant that causes a skin inflammation similar to that caused by poison ivy.

poison sumac A shrub that causes a skin inflammation similar to that caused by poison ivy.

polio Poliomyelitis (infantile paralysis).

polioencephalitis Inflammation of the brain, especially the gray matter.

poliomyelitis A virus disease, often occurring in epidemics, affecting the central nervous system and musculature.

pollen The spores of flowering plants that are carried by the air. They may act as irritants to allergic people.

pollenosis Hay fever or asthma caused by sensitivity to pollen.

pollex The thumb.

poly- Many; excessive.

polyarthritis Inflammation of several joints.

polycystic kidneys A condition, present since birth, in which the kidneys have innumerable cysts. Eventually it may result in inadequate kidney function.

polycythemia A condition associated with too many red blood cells.

polydactyl Having more than the normal number of fingers or toes.

polydipsia Excessive thirst.

polyethylene A plastic material that can be molded into the shape of a tube. Such tubes are used for insertion into the stomach, for intravenous feedings, etc.

polymorphic Occurring in several forms.

polymorphonuclear leukocyte A type of white blood cell.

polyneuritis Inflammation of many nerves.

polyp A growth, usually nonmalignant, of mucous membranes.

polyphagia Excessive eating.

polyposis Having many polyps. Congenital polyposis is a birth deformity of the large bowel in which there are innumerable polyps on the mucous-membrane surface.

polysaccharide A carbohydrate.

polyserositis A condition noted in Pick's disease.

polyuria The passage of large quantities of urine.

polyvalent serum An antiserum containing several immunizing substances.

pons The base of the brain.

popliteal region The back of the knee.

pore The tiny opening of a sweat gland on the surface of the skin.

porosis A condition in which the solidity of bone is impaired.

porphyria An upset in metabolism resulting in the production of a chemical known as porphyrin. This may lead to abdominal colic, paralysis, mental disturbance, skin eruptions, and a characteristic finding of blackish urine.

portacaval shunt An operation, performed to relieve cirrhosis of the liver, in which the portal vein is stitched to the vena cava.

portal hypertension Obstruction to the flow of blood from the intestines through the liver.

portal system The veins leading from the intestines to the liver.

port-wine stain A reddish birthmark.

post- After.

posterior Located in the back, or toward the rear.

postmortem Autopsy.

postnasal drip A discharge of mucus or pus from the back of the nose into the throat.

postnatal The period immediately after birth.

postoperative After surgery.

postpartum After childbirth.

postprandial After eating.

post-traumatic After an injury.

potable Fit to drink.

potassemia Excess potassium in the blood.

potency Power; strength.

potentiation Improvement of the effects of one medication by adding another medication.

potion A liquid medication.

Pott's disease Tuberculosis of the spine.

Pott's fracture A common fracture occurring above the ankle and involving both the tibia and fibula.

pouch An anatomical area that forms a pocket or sac.

poultice A semisolid application to the skin for the purpose of bringing heat and added blood supply to the area.

Poupart's ligament The ligament in the groin extending from the pubic bone to the crest of the hipbone.

powder, Dover's A power containing ipecac, used to promote perspiration.

powder, dusting A powder applied to the skin to decrease irritation.

prandial Pertaining to a meal.

pre- Before; in front of.

preanesthetic medication That given to quiet the patient before anesthesia.

preauricular In front of the ear.

precancerous Tumor tissue that is benign but has the potential of becoming malignant.

precipitation A process by which a substance in solution is brought out of solution.

precocious Developing earlier than normal.

precordium The region overlying the heart.

predigested Treated for easier digestion.

predisposition A state of being particularly susceptible to a disease.

pre-eclampsia A toxic condition of pregnancy.

pregnancy The condition of having a developing baby inside the body.

pregnancy, abdominal A pregnancy in which the embryo is developing within the abdominal cavity rather than within the uterus.

pregnancy, ectopic A state in which the embryo is developing outside the uterus in the Fallopian tube.
pregnancy, ovarian That which takes place within the ovary.
pregnancy, tubal That which takes place in the Fallopian tube.
prehension The act of grabbing, as a newborn child will close his fingers around an object placed in his hand.
premalignant Precancerous.
premature Taking place before the proper time.
prematurity Delivery before 40 weeks of pregnancy have elapsed.
premenstrual Before menstruation.
premonition Foreknowledge.
prenatal care Care of the mother during pregnancy.
prenatal influence The theory that an unborn child can be influenced by events that happen to the mother.
prenatal period The period from the time of conception until the onset of labor.
preoperative procedures Measures carried out to prepare a patient for surgery.
prepatellar In front of the kneecap.
prepuce The foreskin of the penis.
prepyloric The region of the stomach just before the pylorus.
presbyopia Farsightedness.
prescription Written instructions concerning medications or drugs.
pressure Tension; pull.
pressure, abdominal Changes brought on by attempting to move the bowels or urinate, by coughing, by sneezing, etc.
pressure, blood The force exerted by the heart in pumping blood from its chambers.
pressure, intracranial The pressure of the brain and its blood supply on the bones of the skull.
pressure, intraocular The tension within the eyeball.
pressure, pulse The difference in blood pressure when the heart is contracting and when it is relaxing.
pressure, venous The pressure of blood in the veins.
presystolic The interval just before the heart contracts.
preventive medicine The branch of medicine that concerns itself with the prevention of disease.
priapism Erection of the male organ.
prickly heat A skin rash, seen particularly in children who are exposed to excessive heat and who perspire a great deal.
primary union Normal healing without infection.
primipara A woman who is having her first child.
p.r.n. A prescription abbreviation signifying "whenever necessary."
probe A slender metal instrument used to explore wounds or orifices.
procaine A local anesthetic agent.
process A prominence; bony overgrowth.
procreate To reproduce.
proctitis Inflammation of the anus and rectum.
proctoscope A hollow metal tube inserted into the anus and rectum for the purpose of examination and treatment.
prodromal symptoms Early manifestations of a disease before it has developed fully.
progenitor A parent or ancestor.
progeny Offspring.
prognathous Having a jaw that juts forward.
prognosis Prediction as to the duration, course, and outcome of a disease.
prolapse The falling down of an organ.
proliferation The growth of tissue, as a proliferation of skin over the raw edges of a wound.
promontory A projection.
pronate To turn into a face-down position. To pronate the arm is to turn the palm downward.
prone Lying face down.
propagate To reproduce.
prophylactic Preventive.
proprioceptive Referring to impulses from joints, tendons, and muscles.
proptosis Falling out of position.
prostate The male gland behind the outlet of the urinary bladder.
prosthesis An artificial part, such as an artificial limb.
prostrated Exhausted.
protean Having many appearances and forms.
protease An enzyme that digests proteins.
protein A basic food substance containing nitrogen, characteristic of all living matter.
Proteus A genus of bacteria.
prothrombin A body protein that goes to form thrombin, an essential substance in blood clotting.
protopathic Referring to a generalized sensation.
protoplasm The essential material making up living cells.
protozoa One-celled organisms. Some protozoa act as parasites and cause disease in humans.
protrusion A projection outward of a part of a body or organ.
proud flesh Overgrown tissue in a wound that has not yet healed. Also known as granulation tissue.
proximal Near the center of the body; opposite of peripheral or distal.
prurigo Chronic inflammation of the skin with severe itching.
pruritis Itching.
pruritis ani Itching of the anus.
pruritis vulvae Itching of the vulva surrounding the female genitals.
pseudo- False.
pseudohermaphrodite An individual born with internal genitals of one sex but external genitals that resemble those of the opposite sex.
pseudopolyposis Warty growths of the lining of the intestine seen in cases of ulcerative colitis.
psittacosis Parrot fever; a severe lung disease caused by a virus affecting parrots and other tropical birds.

psoas muscles Muscles arising from the abdominal aspects of the vertebra and running down along the posterior part of the abdomen to the pubic and thigh bones.

psoriasis A noncontagious, chronic skin disease that lasts throughout the patient's life.

psyche The mind.

psychiatric Referring to psychiatry.

psychiatrist A physician who specializes in disorders of the mind.

psychoanalysis A method of treating emotional disorders through analysis of the character, personality, and mind.

psychogenic disorder Illness of mental origin.

psychologist A specialist, not necessarily a physician, who studies the function of the mind.

psychology The study of the mind.

psychomotor Concerned with conscious, voluntary movements.

psychoneurosis A mental and emotional imbalance associated with anxiety states.

psychopathic Pertaining to severely disturbed behavior.

psychosis A mental disorder usually involving lack of insight; mental illness; insanity.

psychosomatic Pertaining to the mind and body.

psychotherapy Any treatment of mental or emotional disorders.

psychotic Insane; mentally ill.

pterygium A growth of mucous membrane extending over the inner portions of the eye.

ptomaine poisoning A food poisoning; a nonmedical term for gastroenteritis caused by eating spoiled foods.

ptosis The dropping or falling out of position of an organ, such as the drooping of an eyelid.

ptyalin The chemical in saliva that starts the process of starch digestion.

ptysis Spitting.

puberty That period of life when the sex organs begin to mature. It usually begins in females between 11 and 13 years of age and in males between 12 and 14 years of age.

pubescent Adolescent.

pubis The bones forming the front of the pelvis located at the bottom of the abdomen.

pudendum The external genitals, especially of the female.

puerile Childish.

puerperal fever An infection following childbirth.

puerperium Childbirth. Labor.

pulmonary Pertaining to the lungs.

pulmotor A machine to resuscitate those who have been asphyxiated.

pulsation A beating.

pulse The wave felt when the finger is placed over an artery. It results from the contractions and relaxations of the heart in rhythmic fashion.

pulvule A capsule of medicine.

pump, breast An apparatus to remove milk from a nursing breast.

pump, cardiac An apparatus used in heart surgery to circulate blood while the surgeon works on the heart.

pump, stomach An apparatus to empty the stomach.

punctate Marked with tiny dots.

puncture, lumbar A spinal tap.

puncture, sternal Entering the breastbone in order to get a sample of bone marrow.

puncture wound Any wound made with a pointed object.

pupil The place in the center of the eye through which light is admitted.

pupillary Pertaining to the pupil.

purgative Laxative.

purpura Hemorrhage into the skin, characterized by a bluish appearance to the skin.

purulent Containing pus.

pus The product of tissue broken down by the action of bacteria.

pustule A small abscess filled with pus.

putrefaction Decomposition of tissue.

pyelitis Infection of the outlet of the kidney.

pyelogram X-rays taken after specific dyes have been given to outline the kidneys and the kidney outlet.

pyelonephritis Inflammation involving the kidney and its outlet.

pyelophlebitis Inflammation of the portal vein.

pyemia A generalized condition associated with bacteria in the blood.

pyloric stenosis Constriction of the outlet of the stomach seen in newborns.

pylorospasm Severe spasm of sphincter muscles of the pylorus.

pylorus The far end of the stomach just before the duodenum.

pyoderma A pustular condition of the skin.

pyogenic Pus-forming.

pyorrhea Inflammation of the gums about the teeth.

pyretic Referring to elevated temperature; fever.

pyrexia Fever.

pyrogenic Causing fever.

pyuria Pus in the urine.

Q

Q fever An infection caused by one of the rickettsial bacteria, which are carried by ticks and lice. It is characterized by high fever, inflammation of the lungs, nausea, and vomiting.

q.h. A prescription symbol meaning "every hour."

q.i.d. A prescription symbol meaning "four times daily."

q.s. A prescription symbol meaning "as much as is sufficient."

qt. Quart.

quadrant A quarter of, such as a quadrant of the abdomen.

quadriceps The large muscles in the front of the thigh.

quadriplegia Paralysis of all four limbs.

quadruplet Any one of four children born at one birth.

quarantine The isolation and detaining of individuals who have been exposed to contagious diseases.

quartan Occurring every fourth day, as in certain types of malaria.
quick The fingernail bed.
quickening The first sensations a mother has of the movements of her unborn child.
Quick test A blood test to determine adequacy of liver function. Also, a test used to determine the ability of the blood to clot.
quinidine A medication used to stop irregularities of the heartbeat.
quinine A drug extracted from cinchona bark, formerly used in the treatment of malaria.
quinsy sore throat A severe infection of the tonsil associated with the formation of an abscess alongside it.
quintuplet Any one of five children born at one birth.
quotidian Occurring every day.
q.v. A prescription symbol meaning "as much as is desired."

R

rabid Having rabies.
rabies Hydrophobia; a fatal infectious disease of dogs, cats, and wild animals. It can be transmitted to man by the bite of an infected animal.
rachitic Having rickets.
rachitis Rickets.
radial Leading out from the center.
radiation The passage of energy through space. This energy may be transmitted by ultraviolet rays, gamma rays, cosmic rays, or x-rays.
radiation sickness Nausea, vomiting, and weakness as a reaction to large doses of x-rays or other radiation.
radiation therapy Treatment with x-rays or radium, cobalt, or other radioactive substances.
radicular Referring to the nerves originating in the spine.
radioactive Referring to any substance that emits radiant energy.
radiography The making of x-rays.
radioisotope A stable, non-radioactive element that is bombarded in a reactor with neutrons and other particles so as to make it radioactive.
radiologist A physician who specializes in the use of x-rays.
radiology The branch of medicine dealing with radioactive substances and their diagnostic and therapeutic use.
radio-opaque Not transparent to x-rays, such as barium and certain iodine preparations.
radioresistant Resisting the effects of radiation and therefore not destroyed by x-rays or other radioactivity.
radiosensitive Destroyable by radiation.
radiotherapy Radiation therapy.
radio-ulnar Pertaining to the bones of the forearm.
radium A radioactive metal made from pitchblende and used in the treatment of certain malignant diseases.
radius The outer bone of the forearm.
radon The radioactive element given off by radium.
ragweed The weed whose pollen causes hay fever in the United States.
rale A sound heard through a stethoscope placed over the chest when a patient is suffering from a lung condition such as pneumonia, bronchitis, or tuberculosis.
Ramstedt operation A surgical procedure in which the overgrown muscle surrounding the outlet of the stomach is slit.
ramus A branch, usually referring to the branch of a nerve.
ranula A cyst of the salivary gland beneath the tongue.
raphe A seam or ridge.
rarefaction of bone Loss of calcium in bone.
rat-bite fever A disease brought on by the bite of an infected rat. It may cause joint pain, swelling, and patches of redness in the skin.
rationalization A mental attempt to justify an unacceptable situation.
Raynaud's disease A disease, affecting women more than men, in which there is chronic constriction and spasm of the blood vessels in the fingers. It occasionally leads to gangrene of a finger tip.
RBC Red blood cells.
reaction Any response to stimulation.
reaction, anaphylactic An allergic response resulting from contact with a substance to which a person is sensitive.
reaction, coordinated Normal muscle responses.
reaction, immune A reaction to a test that shows that the individual is not susceptible.
reaction, local A reaction that occurs in the area where the stimulus has been applied.
reaction, manic-depressive Periods of great elation alternating with periods of grave depression.
reaction, paranoid A feeling of being persecuted.
reaction, schizophrenic A term used to describe a form of schizophrenia.
reaction time The period that elapses between a stimulus and the response to it.
reaction, transfusion The symptoms in the recipient caused by a transfusion of incompatible blood.
reagent Any substance used in chemical reactions.
recessive characteristic A characteristic that has a tendency not to be visible or active when inherited.
recovery room A room where patients recover from surgical procedures.
recrudescence A relapse in the course of a disease.
rectocele A hernia of the rectum resulting in its protrusion into the vagina.
rectum The lower terminal portion of the large bowel.
rectus abdominis The long straight muscles of the abdominal wall extending from the ribs down to the pubis.
recumbent Lying down; reclining.
recuperation Convalescence.
reduction Setting a fracture and bringing the broken fragments into realignment.
reduplication Doubling, such

as a birth deformity in which certain parts of the intestinal tract may be doubled.

reflex An involuntary response to a stimulus.

reflex, Achilles The ankle jerk.

reflex, Babinski An elevation, rather than bending, of the big toe when the sole of the foot is scratched; occurring in infants normally.

reflex, ciliary Changes in the size of the pupil of the eye.

reflex, conditioned An acquired reflex in which one responds automatically because of repetition (repeated association with the stimulus).

reflex, conjunctival Blinking of the eye when the surface of the eye is touched.

reflex, instinctive A natural reflex.

reflex, patellar Knee jerk.

reflex, protective An automatic reflex against something that threatens bodily harm.

reflex, skin Any skin reaction caused by irritation or stimulation.

reflex, sucking An instinctive reflex of a newborn when anything comes into contact with his lips.

reflex, vasomotor Contraction or dilatation of blood vessels in response to stimuli.

reflux Flowing in a backward direction.

refraction Testing the eyes for glasses.

refractory Referring to an illness that does not respond to treatment.

refrigeration Cooling.

regeneration The healing of tissues.

regimen A planned course of treatment.

region A part of the body. As the abdominal region.

regional ileitis An inflammatory disease involving the lower portion of the small intestine.

regurgitation A backward flow, often referring to milk or food that has been brought back up into the mouth after having been swallowed.

rehabilitation Treatment directed toward the restoration of someone who has had a prolonged illness.

reinfection Another infection with the same germ.

relapse The return of a condition after apparent recovery.

remedial Referring to something that attempts to cure.

remission A clearing up of a disease.

renal Pertaining to the kidneys.

renal colic An excruciating pain in the kidney region secondary to kidney stones.

rennin A substance found in the stomach juice that curdles milk.

reposition To place back in its normal place.

repression In psychology, a mental mechanism whereby the individual pushes out of his conscious mind ideas that are incompatible with his routine existence.

reproduction The process of producing one's own kind.

resectible Capable of being removed surgically.

resection Surgical removal.

reserve An ability or capacity for use on special occasions.

reserve, alkaline Chemicals in the blood that are able to neutralize acids.

reserve, cardiac The power of the heart to pump more blood than usual when it is necessary.

reserve, diminished The inability of an organ to respond when extraordinary effort is demanded of it.

resident physician A physician, in hospital training, learning a specialty of medicine or surgery. Resident training begins after completion of internship.

residual urine The urine remaining in the bladder after voiding.

resolution The clearing up of an infection.

resonance The vibrations that are heard over the chest when the lungs are clear and filled with air.

respiration Breathing.

respirator An iron lung; a machine that performs artificial respiration.

respiratory rate The number of breaths per minute.

respiratory system The nose, throat, larynx, trachea, bronchial tubes, and lungs.

resuscitation The revival of a patient who appears to be dead or almost dead.

resuture To stitch a wound again.

retching Attempting to vomit.

rete A network.

reticular Forming a structure resembling a network.

reticulocyte A young immature red blood cell.

reticuloendothelial system All of the phagocyte cells of the body, including cells located in the lymphatic channels, connective tissue, bone marrow, lungs, liver, and other structures.

reticulum-cell sarcoma A sarcoma derived from the cells of the reticuloendothelial system.

retina The innermost layer of the eye, the sensitive organ on which light rays are focused.

retinitis Inflammation of the retina of the eye.

retinoblastoma A malignant tumor of the retina of the eye.

retinoscope An instrument for determining errors in vision.

retractor An instrument devised for drawing back superficial tissues.

retro- In back of; behind.

retrobulbar Behind the eyeball.

retrocecal Behind the cecum.

retroflexed Bent backward.

retrograde Going in the opposite direction.

retrogression A deterioration of a tissue or structure.

retrolental fibroplasia Blindness in premature newborns, often associated with the breathing in of excessive quantities of oxygen.

retropharyngeal abscess Abscess behind the membranes in back of the throat.

retroverted Tipped backward.

reversion A biological term relating to a trait or characteristic inherited from a remote ancestor; a throwback.

revive To bring back to life.

rhabdomyoma A tumor of muscle.
Rh blood groups *See* Rh factor.
rheumatic fever An inflammatory disease of children associated with bouts of high fever, painful swelling of the joints, and inflammation of the heart.
rheumatic heart disease Inflammation of the heart secondary to rheumatic fever.
rheumatism A word used to describe many conditions associated with diseases of the tendons and joints.
rheumatoid arthritis Inflammation of joints associated with symptoms resembling rheumatism.
Rh factor A blood component. Its presence may be involved with the destruction of red blood cells in an unborn or newborn infant (erythroblastosis). It may also be involved in the causation of blood-transfusion reactions.
Rh-factor sensitization The process of becoming sensitized to Rh substances.
rhinitis Inflammation of the lining membrane of the nose.
rhinitis, acute The common cold.
rhinitis, allergic Hay fever.
rhinitis, vasomotor An allergic inflammation of the mucous membranes of the nose.
rhinoplasty Plastic surgery on the nose; nasoplasty.
rhinorrhea A running nose.
rhizotomy Surgery to cut the roots of spinal nerves, carried out to relieve incurable pain.
Rh-negative A term referring to people whose blood does not contain the Rh substance; 15 percent of people fall into this category.
rhonchus A loud wheezing sound heard when listening to the chest with a stethoscope.
Rh-positive A term referring to people whose blood contains the Rh substance; 85 percent of people are Rh-positive.
rhythm Regularity.
riboflavin Vitamin B_2. Lack of this vitamin causes dryness and cracking of the skin and inflammation of the eyes.
rickets A deficiency disease caused by lack of vitamin D.
rickettsial diseases A group of diseases caused by bacterialike organisms. These parasites are carried by ticks, lice, and other insects.
rigidity Stiffness of muscles.
ringworm A contagious disease caused by a fungus.
R.N. Registered nurse.
Rocky Mountain spotted fever A dangerous disease caused by the bite of an infected tick.
roentgen ray X-ray.
Rorschach test A test of personality, particularly effective in determining the presence of neurotic tendencies.
rose fever An allergic condition similar to hay fever.
roseola A contagious disease known as exanthem subitum.
roughage Food containing material that will not be absorbed from the intestinal tract.
roundworm A worm that sometimes inhabits the intestinal tract.
rubella German measles.
rubeola Measles.
Rubin test A test to note whether the Fallopian (uterine) tubes are open; carried out by injecting air into the cervix.
rubor Redness caused by inflammation.
rudimentary Merely partially formed; underdeveloped.
rugae Folds or ridges of tissue, as seen in the lining of the stomach.
rump The buttocks.
runaround A paronychial infection around the base of a nail.
rupture A hernia; tearing of a part.

S

Sabin vaccine A polio vaccine, given orally.
sac An anatomical term denoting a pouch.
sacrococcygeal region That area at the very bottom of the spine above the anal region.
sacroiliac Referring to the area where the sacrum and iliac bones form a joint.
sacrolumbar Referring to the region of the lower back and loins.
sacrum The shield-shaped bone composed of five fused vertebrae located toward the base of the vertebral column.
St. Vitus' dance Chorea, a disease characterized by jerky, involuntary movements of the muscles of the limbs, seen in some cases of rheumatic fever.
salicylate A drug that is often particularly useful in relieving pain and in bringing temperature down to normal. Aspirin is a salicylate.
saline solution Salt solution.
saliva The secretion of the salivary glands into the mouth.
salivary glands The glands that produce and secrete saliva. They are the parotid, the submaxillary, and the sublingual glands.
salivation The excretion of saliva.
Salk vaccine A polio vaccine, given by injection.
salmonella infection Paratyphoid fever; a disease with many of the symptoms of typhoid fever but much milder. It is caused by the *Salmonella* bacteria.
salpingitis Inflammation of the Fallopian tubes.
salpinx A tube.
salve An ointment.
sanity Mental balance.
saphenous veins The large system of veins in the legs and thighs that drains the superficial tissues of the lower limbs.
saprophytes Germs that live by eating dead tissue.
sarcoidosis A chronic disease of unknown origin affecting mostly young adults. It involves several organs but does not cause them to undergo degeneration.
sarcoma A malignant tumor made up of connective tissues.
sartorius muscle A lengthy muscle in the thigh that aids the act of crossing one leg over the other.
saturated Having as much of a solid or gas dissolved in a solution as the solution can take.
saturnism Lead poisoning.

satyr tip A pointed ear.
scabies A contagious skin condition caused by an insect that burrows under the superficial layers of skin. It causes great itching and is characterized by extensive scratch marks.
scalenus Muscles in the neck that arise near the spinal vertebrae and extend to the front portion of the first two ribs.
scalpel A surgical knife.
scapula The shoulder blade; wingbone.
scarlatina Scarlet fever.
scarlet fever A contagious disease of childhood caused by a streptococcus.
scatoma A hard lump of stool in the bowels.
scatophagy Eating feces.
Schick test A skin test to determine whether one is immune to diphtheria.
schistosomiasis A condition that is incurred by swimming in waters infested with a parasite of snails.
schizo- Split.
schizophrenia A form of mental illness in which there is a withdrawal from reality. It occurs mostly in adolescents and young adults.
Schultz-Charlton test A skin test to note if one is immune to scarlet fever.
sciatica A condition in which there is inflammation and severe pain in the lower back and coursing down the back of the legs, due to inflammation of the sciatic nerve.
sciatic nerve The large, long nerve originating in the spinal cord and supplying the muscles of the lower limbs.
scintiscanner A device for determining the presence of radioactive substances that have been given to the body.
scission The dividing or splitting of a cell; also, nuclear splitting.
sclera The white of the eye.
scleritis Inflammation of the white of the eye.
scleroderma A skin disease in which there are very hard patches with color changes.
sclerosis Hardening of tissues.
sclerotherapy The injection of a medication into a vein or other structure in order to produce a clot or hardening.
sclerotic Hardened.
scolex The head of a tapeworm.
scoliolordosis Curvature of the spine in which there is both side-to-side and front-to-back deformity.
scoliosis Abnormal curvature of the spine, often seen in adolescents.
scope Any device for examining an organ.
scopolamine "Truth serum." It produces a sleepy, relaxed state and is often given as a premedication before anesthesia.
scorbutic Pertaining to scurvy.
scotoma A blind spot on the retina of the eye.
scrofula An old term for tuberculosis of the lymph glands in the neck.
scrotum The pouch, located beneath the penis, that contains the testicles.
scrum-pox Impetigo.
scurvy A deficiency disease caused by lack of vitamin C. It is characterized by anemia, weakness, bleeding gums, and other bleeding tendencies.
sebaceous cysts Wens. Cysts in or just beneath the skin secondary to blockage of the ducts from the oil glands.
seborrheic dermatitis A skin disease caused by oversecretion of the sebaceous glands.
sebum The material secreted by sebaceous glands. It is an oily, waxy substance.
secrete To produce a special substance and to expel it.
section A slice of tissue.
secundines The afterbirth; the placenta and membranes.
sedative A drug given to calm the nerves.
sediment Any material that settles to the bottom of a liquid.
segment A portion of tissue.
segmentation Cleavage, as in the division of cells.
seizure A sudden attack, as a severe paroxysm of pain.
self-limited A term applied to a condition that lasts but a specific length of time and then disappears.
sella turcica The depression in the base of the skull that harbors the pituitary gland.
semen The fluid that carries the male sperm. It is stored in the seminal vesicles.
semi- Half.
semicircular canals The bony canals of the inner ear. They are important in maintaining the sense of balance.
semicomatose Partially unconscious.
semiconscious Partially conscious.
semilunar cartilages The cartilages lying on top of the tibial bone in the knee joint. These cartilages are often torn in athletic injuries.
seminal vesicles Small glands near the prostate where semen is stored before its discharge.
seminoma A tumor of the testicle, sometimes malignant.
semirecumbent Partially lying down.
senility Old age.
senna A mild laxative.
sensation A kind of feeling resulting from a particular type of stimulus.
sense The appreciation and realization of a sensation.
sense organ Special nerves equipped to receive and pass along specific stimuli.
sensitized Having developed a sensitivity to a stimulus. A person with hay fever is sensitized to the pollen of ragweed.
sensorium The part of the brain that receives and interprets sensations.
sensory Pertaining to sensation.
sepsis Bloodstream infection with bacteria.
septal defect An abnormal opening between the left and the right chambers of the heart.
septic Infected.
septicemia Living and growing bacteria in the bloodstream.
septum A partition.
sequelae Symptoms following the onset of a disease.
sequestration The passing out of the body of a dead piece of

tissue, such as sequestration of bone following osteomyelitis.

serology The branch of clinical medicine that studies the serum of the blood.

serosa The membranes that cover the heart, lungs, and intestines, as well as various body cavities.

serous fluid Material resembling the serum of the blood.

serum The part of the whole blood that remains after blood has clotted. It is yellowish in color.

serum, immune Serum containing antibodies against a specific disease. It is injected into patients to protect them from that disease.

serum sickness Illness following injection of a serum into a person who is allergic to something in the serum. Symptoms include pain in the joints, swelling at the site of the injection, hives, and fever.

sessile Having a broad base.

sex chromosomes The X and Y chromosomes, which determine one's sex. Half the sperm have a Y and half have an X chromosome; all ova contain an X chromosome.

shaking palsy A nervous disease involving a shaking, rhythmic tremor of the hands. Also called Parkinson's disease or paralysis agitans.

sheath A tissue covering.

shin The bony margin of the tibia on the front of the leg.

shingles Herpes zoster; a disease of the nerve endings in the skin, characterized by the formation of blisters and severe pain along the course of the involved nerve.

shock An upset caused by inadequate amounts of blood circulating in the bloodstream. It can be brought on by loss of blood, severe injury, or great anxiety. It is characterized by drop in blood pressure, rapid weak pulse, moist clammy skin, thirst, and great anxiety.

shock, anaphylactic Shock produced by injecting a medication to which the patient is sensitized.

shock, hematogenic Shock caused by great blood loss.

shock, insulin Shock caused by injecting too much insulin resulting in too little sugar in the circulating blood.

shock, irreversible Shock that has lasted so long that recovery is impossible.

shock, neurogenic Shock caused by excessive nerve stimulation.

shock, primary Shock occurring immediately after an injury.

shock, secondary Shock occurring several hours after an injury.

shock treatment Electric current administered to the brain, causing momentary unconsciousness and convulsions. Used to help mentally ill people.

shot A common expression meaning an injection or inoculation.

shoulder The region where the arm joins the body.

shunt A bypass; an alternate route.

sialodenitis Inflammation of a salivary gland.

sialorrhea Secretion or flow of saliva.

sibling A brother or sister.

sibling rivalry Rivalry between brothers, between sisters, or between sister and brother.

sickle-cell anemia A type of anemia characterized by a sickle shape to the red blood cells. It is seen mostly in Negroes and other dark-skinned peoples.

sicklemia Sickle-cell anemia.

sideropenia Iron deficiency in the blood.

sigmoid colon Part of the descending colon on the left side of the abdomen. It is the part of the large bowel just above the beginning of the rectum.

sigmoidoscope A long, hollow, lighted metal tube used to look into the rectum and sigmoid colon.

sign An objective evidence of a disease.

sign, Chvostek's In tetany, a spasm of the muscles of the face caused by tapping them.

sign, fontanel Bulging of the openings in the skulls of infants as seen in meningitis or in conditions in which pressure within the skull is increased.

sign, Kernig's In cases of meningitis, pain and resistance on attempts to straighten the knee completely when the thigh is flexed.

sign, Koplik's Spots in the mouth seen a day or two before the onset of measles.

sign, McBurney's In appendicitis, pain, tenderness, and muscle spasm over the appendix in the lower-right part of the abdomen.

sinew Tendon.

singultus Hiccoughs.

sinus A hollow body cavity; a channel.

sinusitis Inflammation of one of the sinuses around the nose.

sinusotomy An artificial opening drilled into a sinus for the purpose of allowing drainage of pus.

sinus rhythm Regular, normal heart rhythm.

Sister Kenny treatment A method of treating infantile paralysis that is directed toward the relief of muscle spasm by the application of moist compresses.

situs inversus A birth deformity in which the organs are on the opposite side from normal, such as a right-sided heart.

skeleton The bony support of the body.

skull The bony structure containing the brain.

sleeping sickness Inflammation of the brain; encephalitis.

sling A supporting bandage around a bodily part.

slough Dead tissue that separates from a wound.

smallpox A highly contagious disease tending to occur in epidemic form. It is characterized by skin eruptions, high fever, and severe toxemia.

smear Cells that have been spread onto a glass slide and prepared for microscopic examination.

smegma The material secreted by the sebaceous glands in the foreskin of the male penis or in the labia minora in the female.

sodium A metallic element found in large quantities in body fluids and cells.
sodium bicarbonate A mild alkali used extensively to neutralize excess stomach acid; ordinary baking soda.
sodium chloride Salt.
sodium citrate A solution added to transfusions to prevent them from clotting.
solar plexus A nerve center in the upper abdomen.
soleus muscle One of the two large muscles in the back of the leg.
soluble Capable of dissolving.
solution A mixture of a solid, liquid, or gas in a liquid.
solution, isotonic A solution corresponding in strength to a dissolved substance encountered in body tissues.
solution, Ringer's An artificially made solution containing many of the minerals found in body fluids.
solution, saturated A solution containing all the solids it can hold in a dissolved state.
somatic Pertaining to the body.
somatoplasm Body cells, as contrasted to cells found in the ovaries or testicles, which are called germ plasm.
somnambulism Sleepwalking.
somnolence Sleepiness.
soporific Causing deep sleep.
space An anatomical region.
space, dead The vacant space left behind after the removal of an organ or structure.
space, epidural The area just outside the spinal canal.
space, intercostal The space in between the ribs.
space, mediastinal The space in the chest in which the heart and great blood vessels are located.
space, palmar Compartments in the anterior portion of the hand.
space, peritoneal Areas in between the intestines and other abdominal organs.
space, perivascular Areas surrounding blood vessels.
space, popliteal The back of the knee.
space, retroperitoneal The area behind the abdomen in which the kidneys, adrenal glands, aorta, and vena cava are located.
space, retropharyngeal The area behind the throat.
space, subarachnoid The area surrounding the brain and spinal cord that contains cerebrospinal fluid.
space, subdural The space containing the blood vessels surrounding the brain.
space, subphrenic The space beneath the diaphragm.
spasm An abrupt and forceful contraction of a muscle.
spasm, clonic Muscle contractions and relaxations occurring intermittently.
spasm, tonic Muscle contractions that continue steadily.
spasmodic Pertaining to or characterized by spasms.
spastic Characterized by spasms.
spasticity Prolonged and continued contraction of a muscle.
specialist A physician who limits his practice to the study and treatment of one type or class of diseases. Also, one who confines his interest to specific organs or systems within the body.
specific gravity The weight of a volume of a substance compared to the weight of an equal volume of another substance (usually water) used as a standard.
speculum Any instrument inserted into a body opening so that the examining physician may look inside it.
sperm The male germ cell.
spermatic cord The tubular structure leading from the testicle to the seminal vesicle.
spermatocele A cyst of the testicle or epididymis.
spermatocyte The forerunner of the mature sperm cell.
spermatogenesis The process by which male sperm cells are formed.
sphenoid sinus The cavity in the skull behind and above the nose. It has an outlet that drains into the nasal cavity.
spherocytes Red blood cells that are round all over instead of having two concave sides. They are particularly fragile and are easily destroyed.
spherocytosis A disease in which the red blood cells are spherocytes and rupture easily. Also called hemolytic anemia or chronic familial jaundice.
sphincter A ringlike muscle that controls the opening and closing of a body orifice.
sphincter, anal The sphincter surrounding the anus.
sphincter, cardiac The sphincter surrounding the lower end of the esophagus at its entrance into the stomach.
sphincter of Oddi The sphincter surrounding the termination of the bile duct and pancreatic duct at the entrance to the duodenum.
sphincter, pyloric The sphincter surrounding the outlet of the stomach at its entrance into the duodenum.
sphincter, urethral The sphincter surrounding the urethra leading from the bladder to the outside.
sphincterotomy The surgical cutting of a sphincter.
sphygmomanometer A blood-pressure machine.
spicule A small, sharp piece of something hard, such as bone.
spike A sharp rise in temperature.
spina bifida A birth defect in which there is incomplete formation and fusion of the spinal canal. There is a hernia through which the spinal cord and nerves protrude.
spina bifida occulta A birth deformity in which there is incomplete formation of the spinal canal but no hernia or protrusion.
spinal accessory nerve The 11th cranial nerve, which supplies muscles in the neck.
spinal canal The area filled with spinal fluid immediately surrounding the spinal cord.
spinal cord The part of the central nervous system that is contained within the vertebral column.
spinal fusion An operation in which the spinal canal is fused and made more rigid. Often

done in scoliosis, where there is curvature of the spine.

spinalis muscles Muscles alongside the vertebrae, which help to straighten the head and spine.

spine The backbone or vertebral column.

spine, cervical The portion of the spine that is in the neck.

spine, dorsal The portion of the spine that is in the back of the chest; the thoracic spine.

spine, lumbar The portion of the spine that is in the lower back.

spine, sacrococcygeal The portion of the spine that forms the posterior wall of the pelvis.

spirochete A type of bacteria. The germ causing syphilis is a spirochete.

splanchnic nerves Nerves supplying the abdominal organs.

spleen An abdominal organ located in the upper-left portion of the abdomen. It is a hemolymph organ that, during the life of the embryo, produces blood cells. After birth, one of its functions is related to the disposal of worn-out red blood cells.

splenectomy Surgical removal of the spleen.

splenic artery The blood vessel supplying the spleen.

splenitis Inflammation of the spleen.

splenohepatomegaly Enlargement of both the spleen and liver.

splenomegaly Enlargement of the spleen.

splenorenal shunt Surgical connection of the large vein of the spleen to the large vein of the kidney in an attempt to relieve cirrhosis of the liver.

splint A support for an injured extremity or other part of the body.

splint, airplane A splint designed to keep the arm up and out from the side of the body.

splint, banjo A wire and rubberband splint to put traction on a broken finger.

splint, T A splint applied to the upper back in cases of fractured collarbones.

split-thickness graft A skin graft composed of all but the very deepest layers of the skin.

spondylolisthesis A deformity of the spinal column caused by the gliding forward of one vertebra over another.

spontaneous pneumothorax Air in the chest (pleural) cavity due to the rupture of a superficial blister on the surface of a lung.

sporadic Occurring once in a while.

spore The reproductive cell of certain lower organisms.

sprain A tear or rupture of a muscle, ligament, or joint.

spray A medicine that is applied by vaporizing it.

sprue A nutritional deficiency disease associated with anemia, large frothy stools, red tongue, loss of weight, and weakness.

sputum Mucous material spit out from the mouth that originates from the nose, throat, trachea, or lungs.

squamous Resembling in shape the scales of a fish.

squint Crossed eyes.

ss. A prescription symbol meaning "one-half."

stable Referring to a chemical or compound that resists destruction and maintains its normal composition.

stagnation A term applied to blood that is not flowing normally.

stain A dye used to color tissues that will be examined microscopically.

stalk An elongated portion of tissue, such as the stalk of a polyp.

stammer To speak haltingly; stutter.

stapes One of the three small bones of the middle ear.

stapes mobilization operation An operation to relieve deafness in which the small bones of hearing, such as the stapes bone, are freed of adhesions and manipulated so that they vibrate normally.

staphylococcus A type of bacteria found everywhere. It is one of the most common causes of pimples, boils, and other pus-forming infections.

stasis Stagnation.

static Quiescent, at rest, in equilibrium.

status A condition.

status asthmaticus Continuous unrelieved asthmatic attacks.

status epilepticus Repeated attacks of epilepsy.

status lymphaticus A state of suffocation and sudden death formerly thought to be caused by enlargement of the thymus gland. This theory is now outdated.

steapsin An enzyme originating in the pancreas that digests fats.

steatoma A sebaceous cyst.

steatorrhea Fatty feces.

stellate Star-shaped.

stenosis Constriction or narrowing of a passageway or opening.

stenosis, aortic Narrowing of the valve of the aorta.

stenosis, mitral Narrowing of the mitral valve of the heart.

stenosis, pyloric Narrowing of the outlet of the stomach.

stenosis, tricuspid Narrowing of the tricuspid valve of the heart.

Stensen's duct The tube leading from the parotid gland in the angle of the jaw to the inside of the cheek. It transports saliva to the mouth.

stercolith A hard piece of stool.

stereogram A three-dimensional x-ray picture.

sterile Germ-free.

sterilization Destruction of germs.

sternal puncture Inserting a specially devised needle into the marrow of the breastbone to obtain a sample of bone marrow.

sternoclavicular region Referring to both the collarbone and the breastbone.

sternocleidomastoid muscles The large muscles on either side of the neck extending from behind the ears to the junction of the breastbone and collarbone. Shortening of these muscles can lead to wry neck (torticollis).

sternotomy Cutting the sternum, an operative approach to the organs in the mediastinum.

sternum The breastbone.
steroids Drugs of hormone origin, especially those from the pituitary and adrenal glands. Cortisone and ACTH are steroid drugs.
stethoscope An instrument used by physicians to amplify sounds heard from the body, such as the heartbeat and breath.
stigma A sign signifying the existence of some special condition.
stillbirth The birth of a dead child.
Still's disease A chronic infectious arthritis in childhood.
stimulant Any drug whose action produces stimulation.
stimulation Causing an exciting reaction in the body.
stippling Small black dots seen in red blood cells in cases of lead poisoning.
stitch Suture.
stoma An opening.
stomach The part of the digestive tract located between the esophagus and the duodenum. It is dilated and saclike in shape, and its main function is to churn food and start the process of digestion.
stomachic A medication to stimulate the appetite.
stomatitis Inflammation of the mucous membranes of the mouth.
stomodeum The mouth of an embryo during early development.
stool Feces.
stool, fatty Feces containing large amounts of fat, seen in diseases of the pancreas.
stool, tarry Jet-black stools seen when there has been hemorrhage within the upper portion of the intestinal tract.
strabismus Crossed eyes.
strangulation Inability to breathe; also, death of a part because its circulation is cut off, as in strangulated hernia.
stratum A layer of tissues.
strawberry birthmark A birthmark caused by dilated blood vessels in the skin.
streptococcus A type of bacteria causing severe pus-forming infections.
streptomycin A powerful antibiotic drug.
stress reactions Abnormal conditions or disorders caused by undue strain or tension.
striated muscle Voluntary muscles, as in the arms and legs.
stricture An abnormal narrowing.
stridor Loud, harsh breathing caused by failure of the larynx to relax during respiration.
stripping The last of the milk to be gotten from a breast; also, an operative procedure for removing varicose veins.
stroke Apoplexy. The sudden rupture or clotting of a blood vessel to the brain. It may lead to unconsciousness, partial paralysis, and, in some instances, death.
stroma The connective tissue of an organ.
structure The arrangement of the elements that make up an organ or bodily part.
stunting Growth stoppage.
stupe A poultice; a compress often applied to the abdomen.
stupor Semiconsciousness.
stye An infection of an eyelid, usually resulting in abscess formation.
sub- Under; beneath.
subacromial Relating to the region just under the shoulder joint.
subacute Between acute and chronic.
subarachnoid hemorrhage Hemorrhage around the brain beneath the arachnoid membrane.
subarachnoid space The area beneath the arachnoid membrane, which covers the brain.
subclavian Beneath the clavicle (collarbone).
subclinical disease A condition whose signs and symptoms are so mild and slight that they go unnoticed.
subconscious The portion of the unconscious mind whose contents can be made conscious at will.
subcostal Beneath the ribs.
subcutaneous Underneath the skin.
subdiaphragmatic Underneath the diaphragm.
subdural Beneath the dural covering of the brain.
subdural hematoma A blood clot within the skull lying beneath the dura.
subjective Referring to symptoms that the patient states he is experiencing but that cannot be detected by the examining physician.
sublethal Less than fatal.
sublingual Located beneath the tongue.
subluxation A slight dislocation of a joint or bone.
submandibular Underneath the lower jaw.
submaxillary Lying underneath the lower jaw.
submental Beneath the chin.
submucosa Connective tissue lying beneath a mucous membrane.
submucous resection An operation on the nose to correct a deviated septum.
subnormal Below normal.
suboccipital Under the back of the head.
subscapular Beneath the shoulderblades.
subserous Beneath the outer covering (serosa) of an organ.
subsidence The disappearance or subsiding of symptoms.
substernal Beneath the breastbone.
subtotal Less than complete.
subungual Beneath the fingernail.
succus entericus Intestinal juices that contain the enzymes that digest food.
suckle To nurse from a breast.
sudation Sweating.
sudorific A medication to bring about perspiration.
suffocate To be unable to draw air into the lungs.
suffusion The pouring out of body fluids into the tissues.
sulcus A groove or lined depression.
sulfa drugs A group of chemical drugs that have excellent powers in inhibiting the growth of infectious bacteria.
sulfonamides The sulfa drugs.
sunstroke Being overcome by excessive heat.
super- Upon; above; too much.

superego A term referring to one of the three basic divisions of the personality; the conscience.
superfecundation One pregnancy taking place while another is in progress.
superfetation The implantation and growth of a fertilized egg in a uterus that is already pregnant.
superficial Near the surface.
superinfection A second infection by a different germ occurring as a complication of the first infection.
superior Referring to an organ that is located above another organ.
supernumerary Referring to an extra organ or part, as a sixth finger or toe.
supersaturated Containing more solid dissolved in solution than the solution can ordinarily hold.
supersonic Referring to sound waves of such high frequency that they cannot be heard.
supinate To turn the palm of the hand upward. Opposite of pronate.
supine Lying with the face up.
supplementary vitamins Vitamins given by pill or injection to patients who lack a sufficient amount of vitamins in their bodies.
suppository, rectal A medication prepared for insertion into the rectum.
suppository, vaginal A medication prepared for insertion into the vagina.
suppression The stoppage of a secretion or excretion.
suppurate To form pus.
suppurative wound A wound from which pus is discharged.
supraclavicular Just above the collarbone.
supraorbital Above the eye.
suprapubic Above the pubic bones; the lowermost portion of the abdomen.
suprarenal Just above the kidneys.
suprascapular Located just above the shoulderblade.
suprasternal notch The depression just above the breastbone at the base of the neck.
surface tension The tension on the top of a liquid.
surgery The branch of medicine dealing with operative treatment for disease.
susceptibility The tendency to develop a disease when exposed to it. The opposite of immunity.
suspension A liquid in which tiny solid particles float.
suture To stitch tissue surgically.
sweat test Examination of sweat for its chemical composition. Performed on infants in cases of suspected cystic fibrosis.
sycosis Inflammation of the hair roots.
Sydenham's chorea Purposeless, involuntary movements of the muscles of the face, arms, and legs.
symbiosis The living together of organisms of different species for their mutual benefit.
symbol An abbreviation for a chemical element; also, a sign.
symmetry Similarity between the two sides of the body.
sympathetic nervous system The involuntary nervous system, including nerves that control blood-vessel contractions, heart rate, perspiration, etc.
sympathetic ophthalmia Severe inflammation of an eye, often leading to blindness, caused by an injury or disease of the other eye.
symphysis The joining together or meeting of two bones, as the symphysis pubis where the two pubic bones meet each other below the abdomen.
symptom An evidence of a disease.
symptomatic treatment Treatment directed toward relieving the patient's complaints rather than eliminating the basic cause of the illness.
symptomatology All of the symptoms that constitute a particular illness.
symptom complex All the symptoms of a disease.
synapse The area where one nerve ends and another begins.
synchondrosis A junction of two bones in which cartilage lies in between, as the joining of the bones in the sacroiliac joint.
syncope Fainting.
syndactyly Webbed fingers or toes.
syndrome A group of symptoms and signs that, when they appear simultaneously, form a definite pattern of a specific disease or abnormality.
synergy Cooperative action, as of two or more chemicals or organs.
synostosis The union of two or more bones that originally were separate.
synovial fluid The clear amber fluid usually present in small quantities in a joint.
synovioma A malignant tumor originating in the membrane or covering sheaths (synovial membranes) of joints or tendons.
synovitis Inflammation of a joint lining.
synthesis Formation of complex substances out of simple substances.
syphilis A communicable venereal disease.
syphilis, acquired Syphilis caught from another.
syphilis, congenital Syphilis present at birth and acquired during development in the uterus.
syringe The glass, plastic, or metal container and the plunger that, when attached to a needle, are used to inject substances into the body.
syringomyelia A disease of the spinal cord in which there are many and extensive partial paralyses of various structures in the body.
system A set of body organs performing one main function.
systemic Referring to a condition or disease involving the entire body.
systole The phase of heartbeat during which the heart contracts.
systolic blood pressure The force with which blood is pumped when the heart is contracting.

T

tachycardia Rapid heartbeat.
tactile Referring to the sense of touch.
taenia Tapeworms.
taenia coli The long bands of fibrous tissue that extend along the outside of the large bowel.
taint An inherited tendency toward the development of a disease.
talipes Deformity of the foot, such as clubfoot.
tampon A cotton sponge often used to plug a cavity.
tamponade Stoppage of discharge or flow of blood by inserting a cotton sponge.
tantrum Fit of uncontrollable rage.
tapeworm A long, narrow, flat worm that lives in the intestinal tract of humans.
tapping The insertion of a needle into a body cavity.
tarsalgia Pain in the foot.
tarsus The ankle.
TAT Tetanus antitoxin; also, Thematic Apperception Test, a psychological test.
Tay-Sach's disease Amaurotic familial idiocy. A progressive fatal disease occurring in infants.
TB Tuberculosis.
technique A method used in performing surgery.
telangiectasis Small, reddish areas on the skin caused by enlargement and dilatation of blood capillaries.
temperature Body heat. Normal is 98.6°F.
temporal Referring to the region of the temple on the skull; the side of the head in front of and slightly above the ear.
temperomandibular joint The junction of the lower jawbone and the temporal bone at the side of the head in front of the ear.
tenderness Pain on touching a part.
tendinoplasty A plastic operation on a tendon, often performed in cases of paralysis or where there is a contracture of the tendon.
tendon The fibrous portion of muscles that extends to their attachment to bone.
tenesmus Pain and spasms when attempting to pass urine or evacuate the bowels.
tenoplasty Plastic surgery or repair of a tendon.
tenosynovitis Inflammation or infection of a tendon and its sheath.
tenotomy Cutting a tendon, sometimes performed to lengthen the structure.
tension Stretching or straining.
tension, intraocular The tension of the fluid within the eyeball.
tentorium The fibrous tissue shelf separating the two main portions of the brain, the cerebrum and the cerebellum.
tepid Lukewarm.
teratoma A tumor composed of tissue that usually does not grow in the region where the tumor is located. Thus, a teratoma in the ovary may contain hair, teeth, stomach tissue, etc. Teratomas are formed of embryonic tissue.
term The end of the ninth month of pregnancy, when delivery is expected.
terminal The end.
terminology A method for naming and classifying terms.
tertian Occurring every other day.
test A procedure to aid in making a diagnosis.
test, agglutination A test to demonstrate the presence of antibodies in the blood.
test, albumin The presence of albumin in the urine may indicate kidney disease.
test, alkaline phosphatase A blood test indicating obstruction to the flow of bile into the intestine.
test, allergy Any test used to demonstrate the presence of an allergy.
test, amylase A blood test that may indicate inflammation of the pancreas.
test, amyloid A test that, when elevated, indicates the presence of degeneration in certain organs of the body.
test, aptitude A psychological test to determine the potential ability of an individual in a special field of endeavor.
test, auditory A test of the ability to hear with an audiometer.
test, Benedict's A urine test for the presence of sugar.
test, benzidine A test for the presence of blood.
test, bilirubin A blood test for the presence of bile pigments.
test, Binet-Simon An I.Q. test.
test, biopsy The surgical removal of tissue in order to examine it microscopically and make a diagnosis.
test, bleeding-time Puncturing the finger and noting how long it takes for bleeding to stop.
test, Cattell infant's A test for the intelligence of infants under two years of age.
test, circulation-time A test to determine how rapidly blood circulates throughout the body.
test, clearance A test of the efficiency of the kidney in clearing certain substances from the circulating blood.
test, cold-agglutination A test for blood antibodies.
test, color-vision The viewing of multicolored cards to determine if one is color-blind.
test, concentration-dilution A test of the adequacy of kidney function.
test, conjunctival An allergic test in which the substance suspected of being the cause of the allergy is dropped into the eye.
test, Coombs A blood test to determine Rh antibodies.
test, cross-matching A test to determine whether the donor's and recipient's blood will mix without clotting.
test, Davidsohn differential A test to determine the presence of infectious mononucleosis.
test, Dick A skin test to determine susceptibility to scarlet fever.
test, ferric chloride A urine test to determine the presence of acidosis.

test, fragility A test to note the strength of red blood cells.
test, galactose-tolerance A test of liver function to see if it can utilize milk sugar.
test, Gesell A psychological test of the mental development of children under five years of age.
test, glucose-tolerance A blood test to determine the presence of diabetes or a tendency toward its development. It is also used to determine the presence of hypoglycemia.
test, guaiac A test for the presence of blood in the stool or urine.
test, heterophile A test to detect the presence of infectious mononucleosis.
test, histamine The injection of histamine normally causes secretion of hydrochloric acid in the stomach.
test, icterus-index A test for the presence of bile pigments in the blood.
test, indigo carmine A blood test to detect the adequacy of kidney function.
test, intelligence Any one of many psychological tests to determine the degree of intelligence.
test, Kahn A blood test for the presence of syphilis.
test, Kline A blood test for syphilis.
test, L.E. A blood test for the presence of lupus erythematosus.
test, Mantoux A skin-sensitivity test for tuberculosis.
test, Mazzini A test for syphilis.
test, patch An allergy test in which the substance suspected of causing the allergy is applied to the skin and held in place for a day or two with an adhesive patch.
test, paternity A test attempting to prove that a particular man might be the father of a child. Such tests can prove conclusively that a particular man is *not* the father of the child.
test, penicillin-sensitivity A test to discover an individual's sensitivity to penicillin.
test, potassium-tolerance A potassium salt is swallowed. If the patient has inadequate adrenal-gland function, the potassium blood quantity is markedly increased.
test, prothrombin-time A blood test to determine the adequacy of the blood-clotting mechanism.
test, Rh A blood test for the presence of the Rh factor. It is now performed on all pregnant women.
test, Rorschach A psychological test for the presence of neurotic tendencies.
test, Schick A skin test to determine susceptibility to diphtheria.
test, scratch An allergy test in which the skin is scratched and the substance suspected of causing the allergy is applied to the scratched area.
test, sedimentation The time it takes blood cells in a glass tube to settle out and separate from the serum.
test, Stanford-Binet An I.Q. test.
test, thymol-turbidity A liver-function test.
test, tourniquet A test to note capillary resistance.
test, tuberculin A skin test to determine the presence of the germ causing tuberculosis in the system.
test, vital-capacity A test to determine the adequacy of lung function.
test, von Pirquet A skin test for the presence of the tuberculosis germ in the body.
test, Wassermann A blood test for the presence of syphilis.
test, Widal A test for the presence of typhoid fever.
testicle A male organ that produces sperm, located in the scrotum.
testicle, undescended A testicle that has not descended into the scrotal sac but remains in the abdomen or groin.
testis The testicle.
testosterone The male sex hormone.
tetanus Lockjaw; an often fatal infectious disease caused by the tetanus germ.
tetany A disease caused by insufficient calcium in the blood. It is characterized by muscle spasms and convulsions. In infants, tetany may be caused by lack of vitamin D in the diet.
tetralogy of Fallot A birth deformity of the heart involving defects in the blood vessels and walls of the heart chambers. In certain cases, this condition can be corrected through surgery.
thalassemia Cooley's anemia; Mediterranean anemia; a hereditary disease characterized by enlargement of the spleen, underdevelopment of the body, and marked anemia.
theca The covering or sheath of a tendon.
thecitis Tendon-sheath inflammation.
thelasis Suckling at the breast.
thelitis Inflammation of a nipple.
thelium The nipple.
thenar region The palm of the hand, especially that region located adjacent to the base of the thumb.
theory A credible, scientific idea.
therapeusis The science of treatment of disease.
therapy Treatment.
therapy, chemo- Treatment of disease by chemicals, as with the sulfa drugs.
therapy, electroshock Causing convulsions and unconsciousness; a form of treatment sometimes used on mentally ill patients.
therapy, endocrine Treatment of disease through the giving of hormones.
therapy, group The psychiatric treatment of several patients at the same time.
therapy, occupational Treatment of a disease by getting the patient to keep himself busy.
therapy, oxygen Applying an oxygen mask or tent.
therapy, physical Treatment of disease utilizing physical aids such as heat, light, water, and electricity.
therapy, radiation Treatment

with x-rays, radium, or other radioactive substances.

therapy, replacement The use of hormones to replace those the body has stopped producing.

thermal Relating to heat.

thermolabile Referring to a substance that is readily destroyed by heat.

thermometer An instrument for measuring temperature.

thermostable Referring to a substance that is not easily destroyed by heat.

thermotherapy Treatment of a condition by utilizing heat.

thiamin Vitamin B_1.

thigh The part of the leg extending from the groin to the knee.

Thomsen's disease A lack of muscle function and coordination due to a defect present from birth; a hereditary condition.

thoracentesis Tapping the chest cavity with a needle to withdraw accumulated fluids.

thoracic Referring to the chest.

thoracic duct The main lymph channel in the chest. It collects lymph from organs in the abdomen and chest and empties into the large subclavian vein in the neck.

thoraco- Relating to the chest.

thoraco-acromial Referring to the tip of the shoulder and the chest.

thoracolumbar spine The part of the spine that extends from the chest down to the sacrum.

thoracoplasty An operation upon the chest wall in which several ribs are removed; sometimes performed in cases of tuberculosis in order to collapse the lung and keep it at rest.

thoracotomy A surgical incision into the chest cavity.

thorax The chest.

threshold The level of stimulation that will produce a response.

thrill A vibration felt by the physician's examining hand when placed on a heart in which there is a murmur.

throat The pharynx.

thrombin A chemical enzyme that becomes active when blood leaves its natural place within the blood vessels. Thrombin is necessary for blood clotting.

thromboangiitis obliterans Buerger's disease. A chronic inflammatory disease of the arteries and veins; sometimes leading to gangrene of portions of the lower limbs.

thrombocyte A blood platelet.

thrombocytopenic purpura A generalized disease associated with hemorrhage under the skin, improper blood clotting, and a deficiency of blood platelets. Most cases can be cured by surgical removal of the spleen.

thrombocytosis An excess number of blood platelets.

thromboendarteriectomy An operation upon a sclerotic (hardened) artery in which the vessel is opened and the inner layer is reamed out. This may lead to improved flow of blood through it.

thrombokinase A chemical found in the blood that is essential to the formation of thrombin.

thrombolysis Dissolution of a blood clot.

thrombopenia Decrease in the number of blood platelets.

thrombophlebitis Inflammation of a vein with blood-clot formation.

thrombose To clot.

thrombosis Formation of a clot.

thrombus A clot of blood.

throwback The appearance of a type that resembles a primitive ancestor.

thrush A fungus infection (monilia) of the mouth often seen in children.

thymectomy Surgical removal of the thymus gland in the chest.

thymic Referring to the thymus gland.

thymoma A tumor of the thymus gland.

thymus gland A lymph gland located beneath the breastbone in newborns. Its main function is carried out during development of the embryo, and it normally undergoes degeneration during the first two years of life.

thyroglossal cyst A cyst in the front of the neck composed of cells originating from the tongue and thyroid gland. It usually occurs in children and young adults.

thyrohyoid Referring to the thyroid cartilage, which makes up a portion of the voicebox and the hyoid bone under the chin.

thyroidectomy Surgical removal of the thyroid gland or a portion of it.

thyroid gland The endocrine gland located in the front of the neck. It regulates body metabolism and secretes a hormone known as thyroxin.

thyroxin The hormone manufactured by the thyroid gland.

tibia The larger of the two legbones, located on the inner side of the leg.

tibialis muscles Two long muscles of the leg responsible for flexing and extending the foot.

tibiofibular Pertaining to the tibia and fibula, the bones of the legs.

tic Twitching; a habit spasm.

ticks Insects or bugs that live on plants or animals. Their bite often transmits disease to man.

t.i.d. A prescription symbol meaning "three times daily."

timothy A grass growing in the United States. Its pollen causes hay fever during June and July.

tincture A ten-percent alcoholic solution of a medication.

tinea Ringworm.

tinnitus Ringing in the ears.

tissue An aggregation of cells that are similar in type.

tocopherol Vitamin E; wheatgerm oil.

tolerance The ability to endure the influence of a medication or drug.

tomogram An x-ray taken to get a clear picture mainly of one plane of the body.

tongue The muscle of speech arising from the floor of the mouth and back of the throat.

tongue, bifid A birth deformity in which the front portion of the tongue is split in two.

tongue, coated A whitish coat on the tongue.
tongue, furred Same as above.
tongue, geographic A birth deformity in which there are thickened areas and deep furrows in the surface of the tongue.
tongue, hairy A tongue that is brownish in color and has long wavy projections on its surface.
tongue, strawberry The reddened tongue seen in scarlet fever.
tongue-tie A tongue that has an abnormally short frenum.
tonic A medication given to stimulate; also, referring to a continuous muscle contraction or spasm.
tonicity The state of relaxation or contraction of a muscle or other organ.
tonsillectomy Removal of the tonsils.
tonsillitis Inflammation or infection of the tonsils.
tonsils Lymph glands located in the mouth near the back of the tongue.
tonus The normal degree of contraction present in most muscles.
tooth, bicuspid A premolar tooth.
tooth, canine One of two sharp, pointed teeth on each side of the front four incisors.
tooth, deciduous Baby tooth.
tooth, impacted One lying obliquely.
tooth, incisor One of the front four teeth in the upper and lower jaws.
tooth, molar A back tooth.
tooth, premolar A tooth before the molars.
tooth, wisdom The last molar, usually not erupting until adulthood is reached.
torpid Sluggish.
torsion A twisting.
torsion of the testicle An acute condition in which the cord leading to the testicle becomes twisted. Immediate surgery is necessary to save the testicle.
torso The trunk of the body.
torticollis Wryneck; a spasm or contraction of the muscles on one side of the neck.
tourniquet An apparatus for controlling hemorrhage.
toxemia A condition characterized by poisonous products (toxins) in the blood.
toxic Poisonous.
toxin The poison manufactured by a bacterium or other form of animal or vegetable life.
toxoid A toxin that has been inactivated but that retains its ability to stimulate the formation of antibodies within the body.
trachea The windpipe.
tracheitis Inflammation of the trachea.
tracheobronchitis Inflammation of the trachea and bronchial tubes.
tracheotomy A surgical incision into the trachea, performed to relieve suffocation.
trachoma A virus disease of the eyelids, seen most often in Asian and African countries.
tract A pathway.
traction Pulling or exerting force to stretch a part.
tragus The small cartilage pointing backward over the opening of the external ear.
trance A hypnotic state.
tranquilizer A drug given to calm the nerves.
trans- Through; across.
transection A cutting across.
transference A feeling of affection and love, or hostility and hate, that a patient displays toward his psychiatrist.
transfusion The giving of blood from a donor to a recipient.
transfusion reaction One caused by giving incompatible blood.
transillumination The lighting up of an organ or part of the body as an aid to diagnosis.
transmigration The passage of cells from their usual habitat out into the tissues.
transmissible A condition that can be given to another.
transmutation The method by which one species of animal life develops into another; evolution.
transpiration Exhaled air.
transplant Tissue taken from one part of the body and put into another; a graft.
transverse Across; at right angles to the longitudinal axis of the body.
transverse colon The part of the large bowel that lies across the upper abdomen.
trapezius muscles Large muscles arising from the back of the head and vertebrae in the neck and chest and extending to the collarbone and wingbones.
trauma Injury.
trembling Muscle quivering.
tremor A shaking of a hand, arm, leg, or head due to muscle quivering.
trench mouth Vincent's infection; ulceration of the gums and mucous membrane of the throat, caused by a specific germ, *Fusobacterium*.
Trendelenburg position Lying supine with the feet elevated.
trepanning An operation in which a hole is bored into the skull.
trephining An operation in which a coin-shaped hole is bored into the skull.
trepidation Anxiety; fear.
triad A combination of three symptoms or signs that makes the diagnosis of a disease.
triceps The muscles of the back of the upper arm that extend to the elbow.
trichiasis A disease of the eyelashes that irritates the eyeball; also, an anal condition caused by irritation from hairs about the anus.
trichinosis A parasitic disease affecting muscles and causing nausea, vomiting, dizziness, and diarrhea. Caused by eating infested ham or pork.
trichobezoar A ball of hair in the stomach or intestine. Due to eating one's own hair.
trichomonas vaginitis Inflammation of the vagina caused by an infection with the *Trichomonas vaginalis* organism.
trichophagy Eating hair.
trichophytosis Fungus infection of hair, often occurring in the scalps of children.
trichuriasis Infestation with roundworms.
tricuspid Having three cusps,

as the tricuspid valve of the heart.

trifacial nerve The trigeminal nerve.

trigeminal nerve The fifth cranial nerve, which supplies the face and jaws.

trigeminal neuralgia Neuritis of the trigeminal (fifth cranial) nerve, characterized by severe pain in the face occurring in sudden paroxysms. Tic doloureux.

trigone The triangular area at the base of the urinary bladder.

trimester Three-month period.

triplet One of three infants born at the same time.

trismus Lockjaw.

troche A lozenge soothing to an inflamed throat.

trochlear nerve The fourth cranial nerve, which supplies the muscles going to the upper outer portion of the eyeball.

trophic Pertaining to nutrition.

truncated Shortened.

truss A support, worn to keep in a hernia.

Trypanosoma A parasite causing Chagas' disease. It is transmitted by insect bites.

trypsin An intestinal enzyme that digests proteins.

tsetse fly The African fly that sometimes carries the agent causing African sleeping sickness.

tsp. Teaspoonful.

tubal pregnancy Ectopic pregnancy. Pregnancy taking place in the Fallopian (uterine) tubes.

tube, eustachian The auditory tube.

tubercle Inflammatory reaction caused by the tuberculosis germ.

tubercle, Darwin's A small projection of cartilage in the upper portion of the outer ear.

tuberculin test A skin test to determine the presence of the tuberculosis germ.

tuberculosis Any infection caused by the tuberculosis germ. It may involve the lungs or any other organ of the body.

tuberculosis, active That which is causing symptoms.

tuberculosis, arrested That which was once active but has been brought under control.

tuberculosis, avian That type found in birds.

tuberculosis, bovine That type found in cattle.

tuberculosis, disseminated That which has spread throughout the body.

tuberculosis, extrapulmonary That which occurs outside the lungs.

tuberculosis, inactive That which has healed and causes no symptoms.

tuberculosis, primary The first infection, almost always in childhood.

tuberculosis, pulmonary Lung tuberculosis.

tubule A small tube.

tularemia A severe infectious disease caused by handling infected rabbits and rodents.

tumefaction A swelling.

tumor A swelling; a growth.

tunica vaginalis The covering membranes of the testicle.

turbid Cloudy.

turgid Swollen as a result of having excess blood in an organ or part.

tympanic membrane The eardrum.

tympanic nerve The nerve supplying the middle ear.

tympanitic Sounding like a drum.

typhoid fever A disease caused by the typhoid bacillus.

typhus fever A disease caused by rickettsia. (It has no relation to typhoid fever.)

typical Following the usual pattern.

typing Determining the blood group of an individual before giving him a transfusion.

U

ulcer An absence of the normal lining of a body or mucous-membrane surface.

ulcer, peptic Ulcer occurring in the esophagus, stomach, or duodenum.

ulcer, trophic Ulcer caused by lack of blood supply to a part.

ulcerative colitis A specific form of colitis, chronic in nature, associated with bloody diarrhea, anemia, and ulcerations in the large bowel.

ulna The long bone on the inside of the forearm.

umbilectomy Surgical removal of the navel.

umbilical cord The cord going from the embryo's navel to the placenta.

umbilicus The navel.

unconscious Asleep; under anesthesia; in coma.

unction An ointment.

undescended testicle A testicle that has not come down into the scrotal sac.

undulant fever Mediterranean fever; Malta fever; brucellosis.

unguentum An ointment.

unilateral On one side of the body.

unilocular Referring to one pocket, as an abscess having but one cavity.

union The healing of tissues; fractured bones that have knit.

urachal cyst A cystic remnant of the urachus.

urachus A structure seen in the embryo extending from the bladder to the navel. Normally, it undergoes fibrosis and disappears by the time of birth.

urea A carbon compound found normally in the blood and urine.

uremia A disease caused by inability of the kidneys to eliminate waste products.

ureter A tube leading from a kidney to the bladder.

urethra A tube leading from the bladder to the outside.

urethritis Inflammation of the urethra.

urethroplasty A plastic operation upon the urethra, as in hypospadias or epispadias.

urgency Frequent desire to urinate.

uric acid A normal chemical constituent of the blood.

urinalysis Physical and chemical examination of the urine.

urine The liquid excreted by the kidneys.

urobilin Bile pigments excreted in the urine.

urogenital Referring to the urinary and genital organs (kidney, ureter, bladder, prostate, penis, urethra, etc.).

urography X-ray visualization of the urinary tract.

urologist A physician who specializes in diseases of the urogenital system.

urticaria Hives; an allergic condition of the skin characterized by the formation of large blotches or welts, which itch.

uterine Pertaining to the womb (uterus).

uterus The womb; the female organ in which the embryo develops.

uvea The part of the eye that contains the iris and blood vessels.

uvula The cone-shaped piece of tissue that hangs down from the soft palate in the back of the mouth.

uvulectomy Surgical removal of an elongated uvula.

uvulitis Inflammation of the uvula.

V

vaccinate To immunize against a disease.

vaccine Killed or markedly weakened bacteria or viruses in solution.

vaccine, autogenous A vaccine prepared from the patient's own bacteria.

vaccine, BCG A vaccine to protect against tuberculosis.

vaccine, cholera A vaccine to protect against cholera.

vaccine, cowpox A vaccine given to prevent smallpox.

vaccine, multivalent A vaccine containing several different types of bacteria in order to protect simultaneously against several different conditions.

vaccine, pertussis Whooping-cough vaccine.

vaccine, poliomyelitis Vaccine to protect against infantile paralysis.

vaccine, polyvalent A vaccine made from several different groups of the same bacteria.

vaccine, rabies The vaccine given in many doses over a period of two to three weeks to protect against rabies.

vaccine, Rocky Mountain spotted fever A vaccine prepared from the infected bodies of the ticks that cause the disease.

vaccine, Sabin An oral vaccine for the prevention of infantile paralysis.

vaccine, Salk A vaccine to protect against infantile paralysis; given by injection.

vaccine, smallpox A vaccine that prevents smallpox. It is prepared from cows infected with cowpox.

vaccine, staphylococcus That prepared from killed staphylococcal germs.

vaccine, T.A.B. Also called triple vaccine. It protects against typhoid fever, paratyphoid-A fever, and paratyphoid-B fever.

vaccine, typhus Vaccination against typhus fever.

vaccinia A virus disease of cattle that, when used to inoculate man, induces immunity to smallpox.

vagal Referring to the vagus nerve, the largest in the body.

vagina The female mucous-membrane canal leading from the vulva to the cervix of the uterus.

vaginitis Inflammation of the vagina.

vagotomy Cutting of the vagus nerve. An operation sometimes performed to relieve the symptoms of an ulcer and decrease the amount of acid secreted by the stomach.

vagus nerve The tenth cranial nerve, which supplies the heart, lungs, and the abdominal organs.

valgus The turning out of the foot.

valley fever Coccidioidomycosis. Also called San Joaquin Valley fever.

valve An anatomical fold in an organ or blood vessel that keeps the contents flowing in just one direction.

valve, aortic One situated in the left ventricle of the heart.

valve, bicuspid Mitral valve between the left atrium and ventricle.

valve, Houston's Folds in the mucous membrane in the rectum.

valve, ileocecal The valve between the end of the small intestine and the beginning of the large intestine.

valve, mitral The bicuspid valve between the left atrium and left ventricle.

valve, pulmonary The heart valve located at the exit of the right ventricle.

valve, pyloric The fold of mucous membrane between the end of the stomach and the beginning of the duodenum (small intestine).

valve, tricuspid The heart valve located between the right atrium and right ventricle.

valvulotomy The surgical cutting of a heart valve to relieve constriction.

vaporize To heat a substance so that it turns into steam.

varicella Chickenpox.

varices Varicose veins.

varicocele Varicose veins along spermatic cord and scrotum.

varicose veins Enlarged, dilated veins whose valves are damaged.

variola Smallpox.

varix A varicose vein.

varus A turned-in foot deformity.

vas deferens The tube carrying sperm from the testicles to the seminal vesicles.

vascular system Blood-vessel system.

vasoconstriction The narrowing and contraction of blood vessels.

vasodepressor A medication that lowers blood pressure.

vasodilatation Dilatation or enlargement of blood vessels.

vasomotor mechanism Mechanism regulating the contraction or dilatation of blood vessels.

vasopressor An agent that causes constriction of blood vessels and a rise in blood pressure.

vasospasm Narrowing or constriction of a blood vessel due to spasm.

VD Venereal disease.
vector An insect or other form of animal life that acts as a "go-between" in the transmission of germs to humans.
vegetative nervous system Autonomic nervous system.
vehicle A substance, usually a liquid, used as a mixer for an active drug.
veins The blood vessels that transport blood from the tissues back to the heart.
vena cava, inferior The large vein in the abdomen that transports blood back to the heart from structures and organs located below the diaphragm.
vena cava, superior The large vein above the heart that transports blood from the head, neck, and upper extremities to the heart.
venereal disease Disease acquired through sexual intercourse, such as syphilis and gonorrhea.
venesection Removing blood from a vein (bloodletting).
venipuncture Placement of a needle into a vein.
venogram X-ray of a vein.
venostasis Stoppage of the flow of blood through a vein.
ventilate To supply oxygen to the lungs.
ventral Referring to the front of the body.
ventricle A cavity or pouch, as the ventricle of the heart.
ventricular fibrillation A heart irregularity originating in a ventricle.
ventricular septal defect The birth deformity in which there is an abnormal opening between the left and right ventricles of the heart.
ventriculography A method of demonstrating the ventricles of the brain by x-ray.
venule A small vein.
vermifuge A medication used to kill worms in the intestinal tract.
vermin Lice.
verucca Warts.
version Altering the position of the fetus in the uterus before delivery.
vertebra One of the bones forming the spinal column.
vertex The top of the skull.
vertex presentation The most common position of the unborn child during labor, in which the back of the head presents to the vaginal outlet.
vertigo Dizziness.
vesical Relating to the urinary bladder.
vesication Blister formation.
vesicle A small blister; also, a small saclike container, such as the seminal vesicle, which holds the semen.
vestige An anatomical part that represents a primitive structure.
viable Able to live.
vibrion septique A germ causing gas gangrene, a most dangerous type of infection.
vibrissae The hairs in the nose.
villus A stalklike growth of tissue originating from a mucous membrane.
Vincent's angina Ulcerations of the mouth and throat associated with high fever and toxicity.
viosterol Vitamin D.
viremia Infection of the bloodstream with a virus.
virgin A female who has never experienced sexual relations.
virile Masculine-appearing.
virilism Applicable to a pseudohermaphrodite who is, in actuality, a female, but who has external genitals having many of the characteristics of the male.
virology The study of diseases caused by viruses.
virulent Able to cause disease; a powerful germ.
virus An organism, smaller than bacteria, capable of causing various infectious or contagious diseases.
viscera Organs, such as those in the chest or abdomen.
viscid Sticky; thick.
viscosity The quality of being thick and sticky.
viscus Any internal organ.
vital Relating to life; alive.
vitamin An organic compound or chemical, found in various foodstuffs, that is essential for the maintenance of normal life.
vitamin-A deficiency In the young, it leads to inadequate growth. In all people, it interferes with accuracy of vision and causes inflammation of the surface of the eyeball (xerophthalmia).
vitamin-B_1 deficiency Thiamine deficiency resulting in beriberi.
vitamin-B_2 deficiency Results in cracking of the skin at the corners of the mouth, chapped and dry hands, and scaling of the skin.
vitamin-B_6 deficiency Clinically, this deficiency occurs almost exclusively in infants. It may cause convulsions, stunted growth, and severe anemia.
vitamin-B_{12} deficiency This may cause severe anemia and associated nerve symptoms.
vitamin-C deficiency Causes scurvy.
vitamin-D deficiency Deficiency of this vitamin causes rickets with bone deformities.
vitamin-K deficiency Lack of this vitamin results in failure of the blood-clotting mechanisms and may cause brain hemorrhage in newborns.
vitelline duct The primitive portion of the developing embryo that eventually goes to form the umbilical cord.
vitiligo A skin condition characterized by patchy loss of pigment.
vitreous humor The jellylike transparent substance filling the inside of the eyeball.
vocal cords Two bands of tissue in the larynx that make speech possible by their expansion and contraction.
voicebox The larynx.
void To pass urine.
volar Pertaining to the palm or sole surfaces.
volatile A substance that is easily converted into a vapor.
volvulus A twist of the bowel, sometimes leading to gangrene.
vomer bones The bones separating the two sides of the nose.
vomit To throw up the contents of the stomach.
von Recklinghausen's disease A hereditary disease characterized by the formation of small

tumors along the course of nerves beneath the skin.

vulva The external female sex organs, including the major and minor lips, the clitoris, and the opening of the vagina.

vulvovaginitis Inflammation of both the vulva and the vagina.

W

walking iron A metal attachment to a leg cast that permits the patient to walk while still in the plaster.

walleye A condition in which one or both eyes are off-center and point in an outward direction.

wart An overgrowth of skin localized in a rounded area; a veruccus.

Wassermann test A test for syphilis.

water balance The mechanism whereby there is a balance between the amount of fluid that is taken into the body and the amount that is excreted.

WBC White blood cell.

wean To discontinue breast or bottle feeding.

webbed fingers or toes Birth deformities in which there is a thin membrane connecting two or more fingers or toes.

Weil's disease Jaundice caused by infection with a spirochete germ.

wens Sebaceous cysts located just beneath the skin.

wet nurse A woman who breast feeds another woman's infant.

Wharton's duct The tube leading from the submaxillary gland to the mouth. It transports saliva.

wheal The individual hive seen on the body surface in some allergic conditions.

whiplash injury A sprain of the muscles and tendons of the back of the neck, caused by a sudden blow from the rear such as when the rear of one's automobile is smashed into.

white matter Nerve fibers in the tissues of the brain.

whitlow An infection of the fingertip.

whooping cough Pertussis. A contagious disease lasting several weeks, characterized by paroxysms of severe coughing and a whooping sound on deep inspiration.

Wilm's tumor A malignant tumor of the kidney, seen in infants.

Wirsung's duct The tube leading from the pancreas to the intestines.

Wolffian duct The primitive duct of the kidney in the embryo that goes to form the ureter.

womb The uterus.

wryneck *See* torticollis.

X

xanthelasma A benign, yellowish, flat growth on the eyelids.

xanthochromia Yellowish discoloration of the spinal fluid caused by brain hemorrhage.

xanthoma A yellow, benign skin tumor.

xanthomatosis A deposit of yellow xanthoma cells throughout the tissues and organs of the body. Also called Hand-Schüller-Christian disease.

xanthosis Yellow color of the skin due to eating carrots, squash, etc.

X chromosome The sex chromosome, or the 23d chromosome. When a male sperm contains the X chromosome and fertilizes an egg, the offspring will be a girl.

xenology The study of parasites.

xenophobia Fear of strangers.

xeroderma An excessively dry skin.

xerophthalmia Thickening of the conjunctiva of the eye secondary to vitamin-A deficiency.

xerosis Dryness of the skin.

xerostomia Dry mouth.

xiphisternum The downward projection of bone at the end of the breastbone.

xiphoid The lowermost extent of the breastbone.

X-rays Light rays of short length that are passed by an electrical generator through a glass vacuum tube. Such rays are able to penetrate body tissues. Also called roentgen rays.

Y

yaws A tropical infection caused by a germ resembling the germ of syphilis. It is not, however, a venereal disease.

Y chromosome The sex chromosome found in approximately half the male sperm. When a sperm containing a Y sex chromosome fertilizes an egg, the offspring will be a boy.

yellow fever An acute infectious disease caused by a virus that gets into the body through the bite of an infected mosquito. It is characterized by chills, fever, aches and pains, jaundice, vomiting, and hemorrhage from mucous membranes. Uremia and death often occur.

yellow jack Yellow fever.

yellow jaundice Same as jaundice.

yolk sac A primitive sac in embryos, lasting only during the early stages of development. Early blood cells are formed in the yolk sac.

Z

zinc oxide A medication, usually used in ointment form, that relieves many skin irritations.

Z-plasty An operative procedure to repair skin scars and to remove skin contractures.

zygoma The cheekbone.

zygote A term referring to the fertilized egg before it starts to divide and multiply.

Index

Acknowledgments to Sources of Illustrations

The editor wishes to express his appreciation to the Jewish Hospital of Brooklyn, the Adelphi Hospital, and their personnel for the kind permission and cooperation which was granted in taking photographs of certain of their facilities. Thanks are also here expressed to the following individuals and organizations for photographs and illustrations reproduced in this encyclopedia: The American Cancer Society, Inc., New York; The American Museum of Natural History, New York; Clinitest, Ames Co., Inc., Elkhart, Indiana; Clay-Adams, Inc., New York; Doho Chemical Corp., New York; Department of Rheumatoid Diseases, Bellevue Hospital, New York; Deputy Commissioner of Community Relations, Police Department, City of New York; L. W. Frohlich and Company, New York; Dr. Otto Kestler; Dr. I. Newton Kugelmass; E. S. Livingston, Ltd., London; The Maico Co.; March of Dimes, New York; New York University Medical Center, New York; Parke, Davis & Co.; Dr. George H. Percival; Chas. Pfizer & Co., Inc., New York; Dr. Franklin H. Top.